Mosby's Atlas and Text of

Clinical Imaging

Mosby's Atlas and Text of

Clinical Imaging

Jamie Weir MBBS DMRD FRCP(Ed) FRCR
Clinical Professor of Radiology
Aberdeen Teaching Hospitals
Aberdeen, UK

Alison D Murray MB ChB MRCP FRCR
Senior Lecturer, University of Aberdeen and
Honorary Consultant Radiologist to
Aberdeen Royal Hospitals NHS Trust
Aberdeen, UK

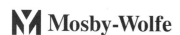 **Mosby-Wolfe**

London Chicago Philadelphia St Louis Sydney Tokyo

4.99

Project Manager	Sarah Gray
Development Editor	Simon Pritchard
Designer	Paul Phillips
Layout Artist	Gisli Thor
Cover Design	Paul Phillips
Illustration	Mike Saiz
Production	Siobhán Egan
Index	Laurence Errington
Copyeditor	Sue Lowry
Publisher	Geoff Greenwood

Copyright © 1998 Mosby International Ltd.

Published in 1998 by Mosby–Wolfe, an imprint of Mosby International Ltd.

Printed by Grafos SA, Arte sobre papel, Barcelona, Spain.

ISBN 0 7234 2555 8

For full details of all Mosby titles, please write to Mosby International, Lynton House, 7–12 Tavistock Square, London WC1H 9LB, UK.

A CIP catalogue record for this book is available from the British Library.

Library of Congress Cataloging-in-Publication Data applied for

Contents

Foreword

A century after the discovery of X-rays by Wilhelm Röntgen, clinical imaging holds out a more exciting prospect than ever before. Modern medical practice requires that we investigate and treat patients in an ever more efficient and effective manner. Central to this strategy is an awareness of the presence, nature, and extent of disease, much of which is obtainable through radiological imaging. Thus radiology lies at the heart of modern medicine.

This atlas and text represents an innovative initial approach to radiology, providing a succinct summary of the main radiological features of each clinical disease process. The consistent organization of the contents will make it particularly useful to the medical student addressing a clinical case study.

The Royal College of Radiologists exists to raise the standards of practice in our specialty through training and education. This book aims to educate the medical student and engender an appreciation of the ways in which current imaging techniques are used to assist in diagnosing disease and managing patients. I commend it to the reader.

Michael Brindle MD MRAD FRCR
President, Royal College of Radiologists
September 1997

Preface

The techniques and technology of 'Imaging' are crucial to the understanding and treatment of a wide range of medical conditions. This atlas and text is intended to portray the characteristics of disease in a way appropriate to current medical undergraduate curricula. There has been a move away from pure didactic teaching of fact to be learnt by rote, to a more logical problem-solving educational environment. This is reflected in our text by integration of the radiological appearances of disease in a structured form. For ease of use, the outline for each of the 10 system-based chapters is aetiological, with analysis of common symptoms and signs and points of importance being noted where appropriate.

Technical considerations, patient consent and preparation, contrast media, contraindications, and hazards are summarized in the appendix at the end of the text, so avoiding repetition in each chapter. All doctors should be aware of the role of imaging in the diagnostic process and also of its limitations and potential risks, in order that they may discuss imaging investigations with patients in an informed manner. One of the purposes of this text is to enable that process to be carried out. Imaging often provides a fascinating insight into disease processes, and it is our intention that this text will stimulate the reader to explore further the possibilities that modern imaging provides, both in diagnostic and in therapeutic fields.

Jamie Weir
Alison Murray
September 1997

Acknowledgements

We wish to thank June Gibb and Diane Honeyman for their typing of the manuscript; Drs Gillian Needham and Karen Duncan for their help in the sections on the Breast, and Obstetrics and Gynaecology, respectively; Geoff Greenwood and Simon Pritchard of Mosby for their patience and forbearance during the production of this manuscript; and lastly, our long-suffering families who helped, cajoled, and encouraged us to get the project finished!

Sincere thanks also to the many colleagues who contributed images: Mr HR Atta, Dr AP Bayliss, Dr Philip Booth, Dr John Brunton, Mr Iain Cadle, Dr Heather Deans, Professor Fiona J Gilbert, Dr Lesley Gomersall, Dr Suzanne McClelland, Dr Fergus McKiddie, Dr Nigel McMillan, Dr Olive J Robb, Dr Elizabeth JN Stockdale, Dr Francis W Smith, Dr Peter Thorpe.

Abbreviations

CT	Computed tomography	IVDSA	Intravenous digital subtraction angiography
DSA	Digital subtraction angiography	IVU	Intravenous urogram
ERCP	Endoscopic retrograde cholangiopancreatography	MR	Magnetic resonance
HRCT	High-resolution computed tomography	PET	Positron emission tomography
IADSA	Intra-arterial digital subtraction angiography	SPECT	Single photon emission computed tomography

Dedicated to

Ewan, Holly, and Mhairi,

Jenny, Katie, Stephanie, and Nikki

chapter 1

Thorax

Part 1. Respiratory system

CONGENITAL ABNORMALITIES

TRACHEO-OESOPHAGEAL FISTULA

Tracheo-oesophageal fistula associated with oesophageal atresia is the most common form of this anomaly and presents in the neonatal period. The 'H' fistula, with patent trachea and oesophagus but with a communication between the two, is easily recognized but rare (it represents only approximately 5% of the cases), and often presents later. Other associated congenital anomalies are common; the systems involved may be remembered by the acronym VACTEL: *Vertebral Anal Cardiac Tracheo Esophageal Limb*.

SEQUESTRATION

Lung tissue that fails to connect to the bronchial tree and is associated with an anomalous systemic arterial blood supply from the aorta, either above or below the diaphragm, is described as sequestrated. There are two main forms of sequestration, termed intralobar and extralobar, depending on the relative position of the pleura. The intralobar form of the anomaly is the most common; the extralobar types are rare. Symptoms are usually caused by the abnormal lung tissue becoming infected, leading to recurrent pneumonia, often in the teenage years. The most common location of the anomaly is at the left lower lobe (**Fig. 1.1**); it is less common on the right, and extremely rare in the upper lobes.

LUNG AGENESIS

Lung agenesis is a rare condition that may be asymptomatic, but is often associated with other congenital anomalies, particularly tracheo-oesophageal fistula.

CONGENITAL LOBAR EMPHYSEMA

Congenital abnormal bronchial wall development may lead to narrowing of a bronchus, with intermittent obstruction. The resulting ball-valve effect, whereby air enters the bronchus but cannot get out because of the bronchial wall collapse, produces lobar emphysema. The upper lobes of the lung are affected most commonly and the increased size of the affected lobe may cause it to compress surrounding structures.

PULMONARY HYPOPLASIA

Bilateral pulmonary hypoplasia develops *in utero* as a result of reduced fetal breathing caused by such diverse conditions as neurological disease, reduced amniotic fluid volume, or diaphragmatic anomalies. Potter's syndrome comprises oligohydramnios, renal agenesis, abnormal skin and facies, and pulmonary hypoplasia.

Unilateral pulmonary hypoplasia (Macleod's syndrome) often affects the right lung; hypoplastic or absent pulmonary artery and bronchial circulation result in impaired perfusion (**Fig. 1.2**). Ventilation will also be reduced.

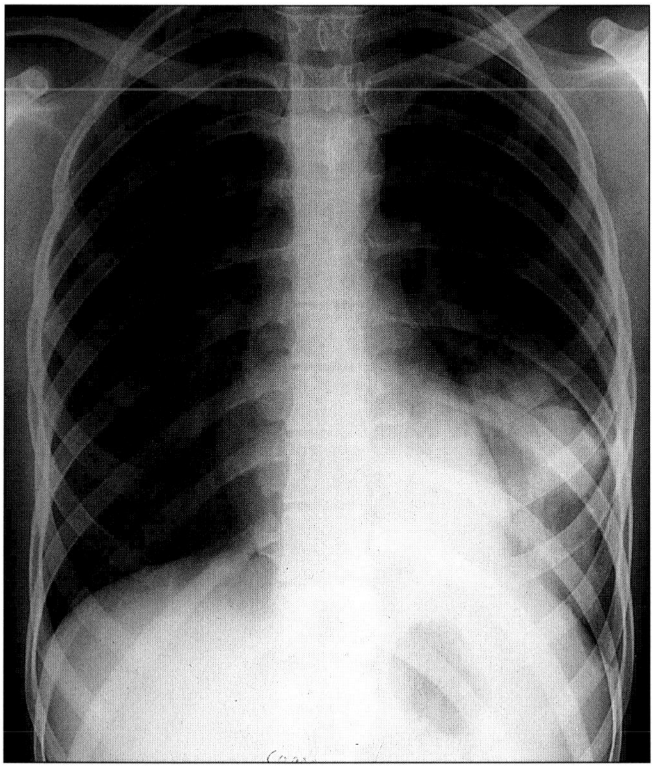

Fig. 1.1 Sequestrated segment in an 18-year-old girl presenting with recurrent left lower lobe pneumonia. Consolidation is present in the posterior basal segment of the left lower lobe; arteriography demonstrated anomalous vessels from the aorta supplying the sequestration.

ADENOMATOID MALFORMATION

Cystic adenomatoid malformation of the lung is rare, but potentially fatal. It is caused by expansile hamartomatous tissue with cystic spaces occupying part of a lobe or lung. It is the expansile nature of the lesion, producing compression of surrounding structures, that causes the problems. On a chest radiograph the lesion shows as a solid mass, occasionally with cystic air spaces, causing displacement of the mediastinum; it must be differentiated from diaphragmatic herniae (*see* page 4).

BRONCHOGENIC CYST

Bronchogenic cyst is an uncommon condition presenting from infancy right through to adult life. It consists of a duplication of part of the tracheobronchial tree, having a lining of respiratory epithelium and containing (often viscous) mucoid material. Most bronchogenic cysts occur in the mediastinium or hilar area and produce symptoms by compression of surrounding structures (**Fig. 1.3**). They may become infected, resulting in production of purulent sputum, fever, and dyspnoea. The chest radiograph reveals a mediastinal or hilar mass

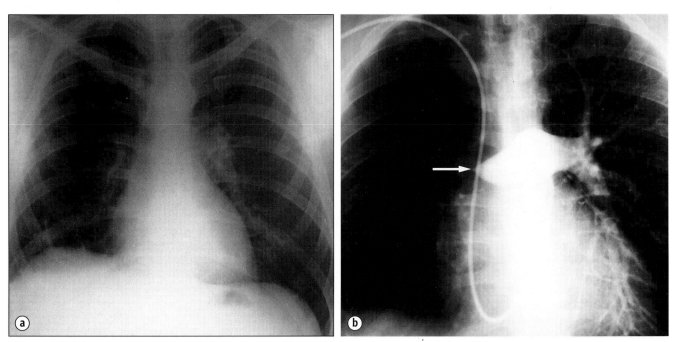

Fig. 1.2 (a) *Right pulmonary artery hypoplasia in a 20-year-old man, demonstrating a small right lung with an abnormal vasculature.* ***(b)*** *The pulmonary angiogram confirmed lack of development of the right pulmonary artery (arrow).*

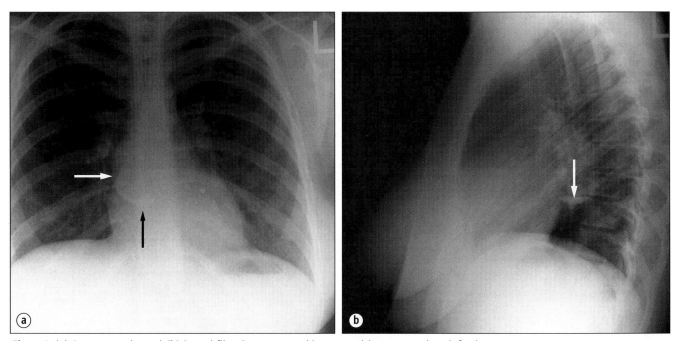

Fig. 1.3 (a) *Posteroanterior and* ***(b)*** *lateral films in a 24-year-old woman with recurrent chest infections. There is a mass in the middle mediastinum (arrows) projected over the right hilum that, on the lateral film, is seen to show a high-density fluid level indicating calcium within the bronchogenic cyst (arrow).*

that is round, well defined, and sometimes shows an air–fluid level if infection has occurred.

TRACHEOMEGALY AND ASSOCIATED SYNDROMES

Dilatation of the major airways (tracheomegaly) is seen in the Mounier-Kuhn syndrome, in which there is recurrent infection, leading to weakness in the tracheobronchial tree and bronchiectasis (**Fig. 1.4**).

Patients with the ciliary dyskinesia syndrome also have dilated airways, with bronchiectasis and immotile sperm. Kartagener's syndrome (dextrocardia, bronchiectasis, and sinusitis) is a form of the same disease (**Fig. 1.5**). In Young's syndrome, patients have infertility and azoospermia in addition to dilated airways, but ciliary function is normal.

Dilatation of the trachea and major bronchi are more common than was previously recognized, occurring in approximately 10% of patients with classical bronchiectasis.

CYSTIC FIBROSIS

Cystic fibrosis is an autosomal recessive condition affecting approximately 1 in 1500 children. The exocrine function of organs such the pancreas is severely impaired, resulting in the production of thick, tenacious mucous. The most severely affected systems are the respiratory, hepatobiliary, and reproductive tracts. Pulmonary manifestations progress from infancy and are often the cause of death in childhood, although many of the patients now reach adult life. Abnormal mucous plugging of the bronchi leads to obstruction, bronchial dilatation (bronchiectasis), and infection, often with *Staphylococcus aureus* or *Pseudomonas aeruginosa* (**Fig. 1.6**). Infection may result in the formation of cavities. Respiratory failure is often the terminal event. Lung and heart–lung transplants are among the available treatments, but results are variable and lack of donors is an unresolved problem.

ARTERIOVENOUS FISTULAE

Arteriovenous malformations are in most cases (90%) associated with the Rendu–Osler–Weber syndrome (hereditary haemorrhagic telangectasia, HHT) and are usually multiple. The lesions allow blood to bypass the normal lung capillary bed, giving right-to-left shunting and cyanosis in addition to removing the normal filtration function of the lung, which in turn allows bacteria to pass directly into the

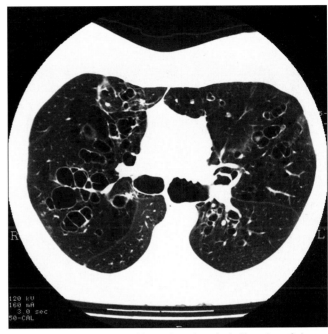

Fig. 1.4 *Severe cystic bronchiectasis and marked dilatation of the major bronchi with irregular walls, in a 46-year-old woman. The diagnosis is Mounier-Kuhn syndrome with tracheobronchomegaly and bronchiectasis.*

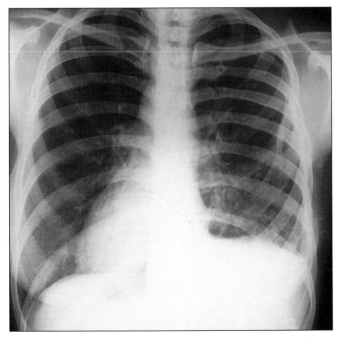

Fig. 1.5 *Dextrocardia in Kartagener's syndrome. The patient had undergone previous left thoracotomy for bronchiectasis.*

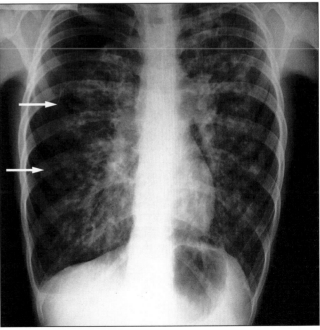

Fig. 1.6 *Cystic fibrosis in a 15-year-old, with pseudomonas infection, bronchiectasis, and a right pneumothorax (arrows).*

arterial circulation and form septic emboli. A brain abscess is a common site for an infected right-to-left embolus. On a chest radiograph, the fistula margins show lobules of variable size with, importantly, prominent serpiginous arterial feeding and venous drainage vessels extending towards the hilum of the lung (**Fig. 1.7**). Other clinical features of the autosomal dominant HHT include telangectatic lesions on the lips, nasal passages, and upper gastrointestinal tracts, together with cirrhosis of the liver, hepatomas, and splenomegaly.

CONGENITAL DIAPHRAGMATIC HERNIA

A congenital defect in the posterior part of the diaphragm may result in a large amount of abdominal contents entering the chest, causing severe respiratory difficulty and, in the neonatal period, presenting as a surgical emergency (**Fig. 1.8**). This type of diaphragmatic hernia is usually left-sided, often containing stomach and small bowel, but right-sided lesions may occur, having the liver and omentum as the hernial contents.

A Bochdalek hernia is a remnant of the pleuroperitoneal canal. The name is often given to the large neonatal herniae described above; however, smaller, more localized posterior herniae may present incidentally at any age, and contain perinephric fat, a high kidney or, rarely, gut (**Fig. 1.9**).

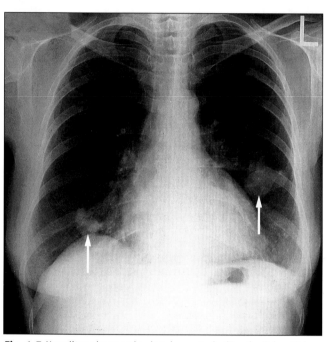

Fig. 1.7 *Hereditary haemorrhagic telangectasia (Rendu–Osler–Weber syndrome), demonstrating multiple bilateral arteriovenous malformations (arrows).*

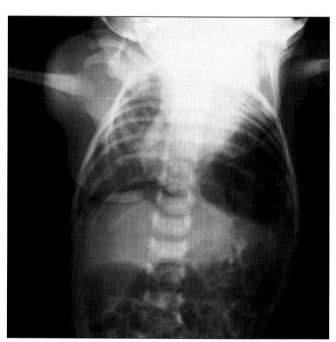

Fig. 1.8 *Congenital diaphragmatic hernia, with bowel throughout the left hemithorax.*

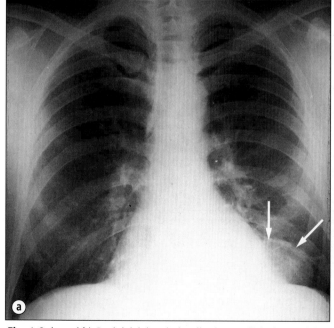

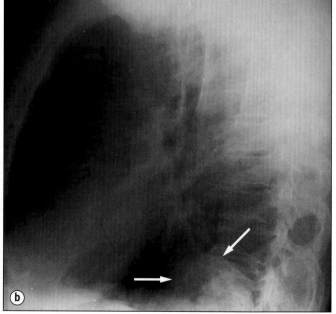

Fig. 1.9 *(**a** and **b**) Bochdalek hernia localized posteriorly (arrows) in a 65-year-old man.*

The anterior hernia of Morgagni protrudes through a space between the diaphragm and its anterior attachment to the sternum and costal margin. This hernia may contain omental fat, transverse colon, or liver; it presents at any age and is usually asymptomatic (**Fig. 1.10**). Strangulation of a loop of transverse colon has been reported as a complication of this hernia.

RESPIRATORY DISTRESS IN THE NEWBORN
The most important of the respiratory distress syndromes of the newborn is Infantile Respiratory Distress Syndrome (IRDS), which occurs primarily in premature babies and in babies born to diabetic mothers.

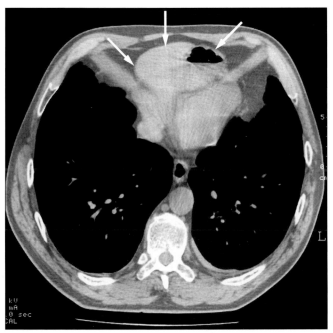

Fig. 1.10 *CT scan of a 61-year-old man, demonstrating an anterior hernia of Morgagni containing transverse colon (arrows).*

There is a lack of lung surfactant, resulting in atelectasis (revealed on radiographs by an air bronchogram) associated with ground-glass opacification, which is attributable to collapsed distal air spaces (**Fig. 1.11**). The lungs may become stiff and, in these patients, complications of ventilation such as pneumothorax, pneumomediastinum, and pulmonary interstitial emphysema may ensue, often with fatal consequences.

A further complication of IRDS is the opening up of the ductus arteriosus, with subsequent shunting leading to heart failure and pulmonary plethora. If high concentrations of oxygen are given at high pressure over a considerable period of time, bronchopulmonary dysplasia may occur and result in severe, long-term lung damage.

Other causes of respiratory distress in the newborn include masses in the neck or chest, intrinsic tracheal wall abnormalities, parenchymal pulmonary abnormalities, chest deformity, aspiration, and any cause of upper airway obstruction.

TRAUMA

SKELETAL TRAUMA
Rib fractures are common after trauma, the majority being simple and uncomplicated. Fractures involving the first three ribs result from considerable force that may also be associated with venous and arterial damage. Similarly, fractures of the lower ribs may also indicate damage to the upper abdominal organs, the liver, spleen, or kidneys. Depending on the force and type of trauma, rib fractures may cause penetrating lung damage, resulting in a pneumothorax, or bleeding into either the pleural space or the lung itself. Flail segments are caused by multiple rib fractures; they result in indrawing of the chest on inspiration and consequent respiratory compromise, which may be severe (**Fig. 1.12**).

PNEUMOTHORAX
Pneumothorax caused by trauma is less common than the spontaneous variety, which has a wide aetiology. The most common form of primary spontaneous pneumothorax results from a small

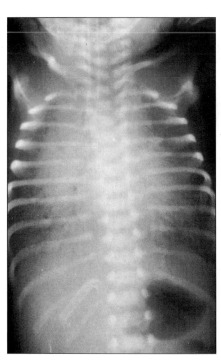

Fig. 1.11 *Infantile respiratory distress syndrome in a 3-day-old neonate, demonstrating widespread opacification of the lung fields extending from the hilar areas.*

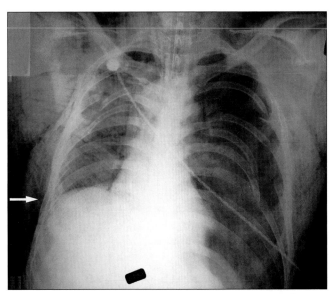

Fig. 1.12 *Severe bilateral chest injuries caused by a road traffic accident: multiple bilateral rib fractures, a left-sided pneumothorax, widespread surgical emphysema (arrow), and pulmonary contusion most marked on the right.*

subpleural bleb, bulla, or cyst (**Fig. 1.13**). The majority resolve spontaneously, by aspiration of the air through a needle, or by the insertion of a chest drain with suction. There is a significant recurrence rate and contralateral air leaks may also occur.

A tension pneumothorax may be traumatic or spontaneous, and presents as a clinical emergency. On inspiration, air leaks into the pleural space by means of a ball-valve-like mechanism that closes on expiration. The result is a collection of air under high pressure in the pleural space. As the air space grows, it displaces surrounding structures such as the mediastinum, heart, and diaphragm, and can be fatal if not treated immediately by the percutaneous insertion of a chest drain (**Fig. 1.14**).

DIAPHRAGMATIC RUPTURE

Blunt or penetrating trauma to the lower chest or upper abdomen may result in a ruptured hemidiaphragm.

Injuries to the left hemidiaphragm are more common than those to the right, because of the protective nature of the liver. Both may be difficult to diagnose clinically and by imaging. Herniation of the gut, which may also strangulate, occurs on the left side, either immediately after the injury or many years later. Ultrasound has been shown to provide specific first-line diagnosis of this condition, it should be combined with a chest radiograph, although the latter reveals only 50% of such ruptures (**Fig. 1.15**).

FAT EMBOLISM

Fat embolism is an indirect effect of multiple skeletal trauma involving fractures of the long bones. Damage to the bone marrow results in fat particles entering the venous system and passing through the right heart to lodge in the pulmonary capillary bed. The fat blocks the distal blood supply, causing an inflammatory reaction and acute lung damage. The development of hypoxia, respiratory distress, cyanosis, and acute cor pulmonale in a patient with recent (within the past 72 hours) multiple long bone or pelvic fractures determines a diagnosis of fat embolism syndrome. This sequence of events proves fatal in a significant proportion of patients (**Fig. 1.16**).

INFECTION

DEFINITIONS

'Consolidation' and 'collapse' of the lung often occur together, but have very different methods of causation.

Consolidation is said to occur when alveolar air is replaced by another material, so rendering the area radiographically opaque.

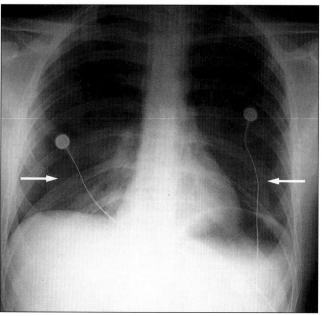

Fig. 1.13 *Bilateral spontaneous pneumothoraces in a young adult with no history of trauma. The edges of the lungs are outlined (arrows).*

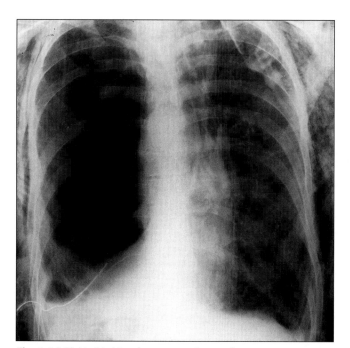

Fig. 1.14 *Right-sided tension pneumothorax after pneumonectomy, with bronchopleural fistula, severe surgical emphysema, and a right basal intercostal drainage tube that is blocked.*

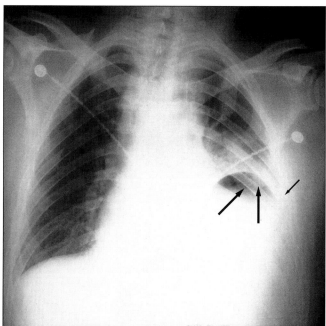

Fig. 1.15 *Rupture of the left hemidiaphragm as a result of trauma, demonstrating gas in the stomach fundus high in the left chest (large arrows), with a small pleural effusion (small arrow) and some consolidation in the left middle and lower zones.*

'Material' here may comprise fluid (both transudate and exudate), pus, blood, neoplastic tissue, lymph, parasites, fungus and, rarely, other agents (e.g. alveolar proteinosis).

Collapse of the lung implies loss of volume of part or all of a lobe or lung, often associated with movement of adjacent structures. It usually occurs when a bronchus is blocked and the lung distal to the block becomes unaerated, with subsequent reduction in size.

Several clinical points should be borne in mind when a patient has an infection of the lungs:

- Does the patient have a pre-existing lung or systemic condition?
- Does the patient have altered immunity?
- Does the patient come from an area of the world associated with particular kinds of infection?
- Has the patient recently travelled to known areas of infection?

Answers to these questions are crucial to interpretation of the chest radiograph, as many kinds of infection affect the lungs, but the majority show no specific radiological features.

Consolidation is the major abnormality of the vast majority of primary lung infections. The infection may be bacterial, viral, rickettsial, fungal, protozoal, or helminthic. Depending on the infecting agent, the manifestations on a chest radiograph may be protean and entirely non-specific or, as with infections such as secondary tuberculosis, characteristic signs may be apparent.

BACTERIAL INFECTIONS

Bacterial infections are common and may be acquired in the community or in hospital.

Streptococcal pneumonia often affects the lower lobes of the lung, rarely cavitates, and usually clears within 2 weeks; it occurs in adults and children. In contrast, staphylococcal pneumonia is often bilateral, may cavitate, takes longer to clear, and is associated with patients already unwell from systemic, immunological or other debilitating conditions such as cancer (**Fig. 1.17**).

Haemophilus influenzae often infects patients with pre-existing lung disease, whereas patients with cystic fibrosis commonly are infected with *Pseudomonas aeruginosa* (*see* Fig. 1.6).

Anaerobic lung infection is usually acquired by aspiration, but may be blood-borne; it persists for a considerable period of time (months), often cavitates, and may produce a lung abscess (**Fig. 1.18**).

Klebsiella pneumonia is a severe infection and is characterized by expansion of a lobe or lung; it is one of the rare pneumonias to cause this sign.

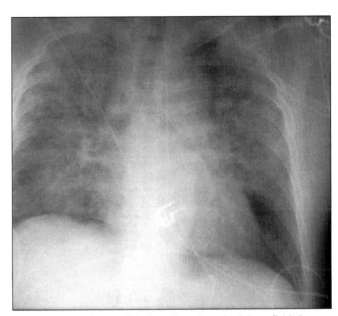

Fig. 1.16 *Multiple consolidations throughout both lung fields in an intensive-care patient, with fat emboli resulting from multiple pelvic and femoral fractures.*

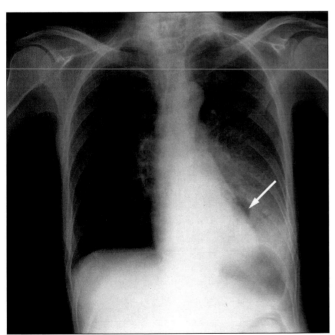

Fig. 1.17 *Left lower lobe staphylococcal pneumonia with cavitation (arrow), in an elderly patient with carcinomatosis.*

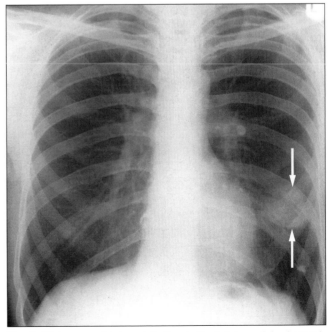

Fig. 1.18 *An anaerobic lung infection in the left lower lobe (arrows) which was present for approximately 2 years. The diagnosis was made by fine-needle lung biopsy.*

Tuberculosis

Primary

The initial infection in tuberculosis (TB) causes the classic Ghon focus, an area of consolidation that heals by fibrosis and calcification, and which may be present in any part of the lung. This lesion is associated with hilar and mediastinal lymphadenopathy, features not associated with the secondary or chronic form of TB (**Fig. 1.19**). An isolated pleural effusion may also be seen in primary TB infection.

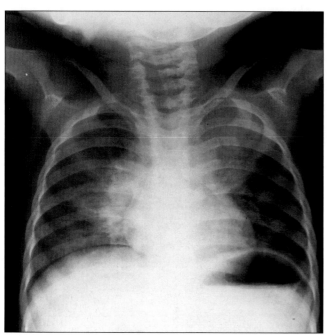

Fig. 1.19 *Primary tuberculosis in a child, demonstrating consolidation in the left upper lobe and mediastinal and hilar lymphadenopathy.*

Secondary (chronic, relapsing)

The classical postprimary infection develops in the apices of the lungs—usually the upper lobes or occasionally the lower lobes—where lung perfusion is at its worst and growing conditions for the infective organism are thus at their best. The consolidated areas cavitate, progressively lose volume, and lead to extensive broncho-pneumonia if not treated. Healing is by caseation, fibrosis, and calcification, leaving small areas of scarred lung (**Fig. 1.20**).

Miliary tuberculosis

Miliary TB is caused by haematogenous spread of the tubercle that, in the lung, manifests as multiple small nodules about 1 mm in size throughout the lung fields. With appropriate treatment, the nodules clear, leaving unaffected lung (**Fig. 1.21**).

Tuberculoma

Tuberculomas are solid lesions, often calcified, that may be the residue of primary or secondary infection and may harbour, deep within the lesion, active tubercle bacilli that can remain dormant for many years, only to reactivate later.

Atypical mycobacteria

Chest radiographic appearances differ little from that of *Mycobacterium tuberculosis*; all produce areas of consolidation and cavitation. Their importance lies in their associations; for example, patients with AIDS are susceptible to *M. avium intercellulare*. These atypical mycobacteria are resistant to first-, second- and even third-line drugs.

RICKETTSIAE, CHLAMYDIAE AND MYCOPLASMA
Rickettsiae

Q fever, caused by *Coxiella burnetii*, may lead to pneumonia, but there are no specific associated features.

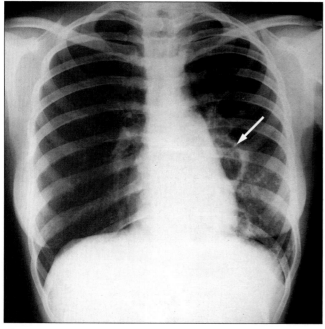

Fig. 1.20 *Cavitating tuberculous infection (arrow) in the left lower lobe, with surrounding consolidation.*

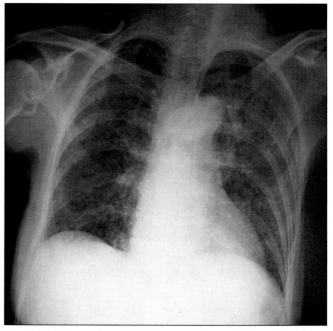

Fig. 1.21 *Miliary tuberculosis, demonstrating multiple small nodules throughout both lung fields.*

Chlamydiae

Chlamydia trachomatis infection may occur in infants, to whom it is spread from the mother, or in immunocompromised patients with or without AIDS. There are no specific radiographic features associated with this infection.

Infection with *Chlamydia psittaci* (psittacosis) is acquired from infected parrots or parakeets. It is characterized by nodular consolidation with hilar lymphadenopathy, and leads to a steadily worsening progression of disease if the cause is not removed.

Mycoplasma pneumonia

Mycoplasma pneumoniae causes a common community-acquired pneumonia characterized by consolidation, hilar lymphadenopathy, and interstitial infiltrates.

VIRAL PNEUMONIAS

The majority of viral pneumonias present a non-specific pattern of bronchopneumonia, often severe, that is associated with little or no sputum production and a poor response to antibiotics. Two main groups of causative viruses are recognized, depending on form of their nucleic acid: RNA-based or DNA-based.

Measles, respiratory syncytial virus, and influenza are the main lung infections in the RNA-based group.

Cytomegalovirus (CMV), chicken pox (herpes varicellae), herpes simplex and adenoviruses are the most common causative organisms in the DNA-based group. Most of them cause widespread nodular shadowing that may coalesce and progress to destructive lung disease (**Figs 1.22** and **1.23**).

ACTINOMYCOSIS AND NOCARDIOSIS

The organisms causing actinomycosis and nocardiosis are classified separately, but have features similar to those of fungi. The infections present on chest radiographs as solid peripheral lesions crossing tissue boundaries. The conditions are often progressive, and healing of the lesions is accompanied by marked fibrosis.

FUNGAL PNEUMONIAS
Aspergillosis

Aspergillosis exists in three main forms in the lung.

Allergic bronchopulmonary aspergillosis

Allergic bronchopulmonary aspergillosis produces a hypersensitivity reaction involving asthma, eosinophilia, and mucoid impaction of the airways. Airway casts are produced that are filled with fungus and eosinophils. Bronchiectasis is a common feature resulting from the chronic damage to the airways (**Fig. 1.24**).

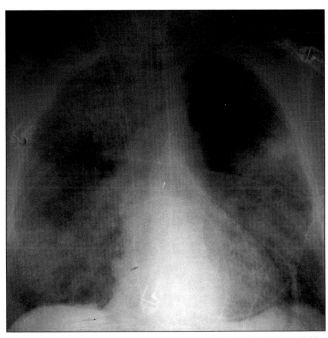

Fig. 1.22 *Widespread patchy consolidation throughout both lung fields in acute CMV pneumonia. The patient was in an intensive-care unit.*

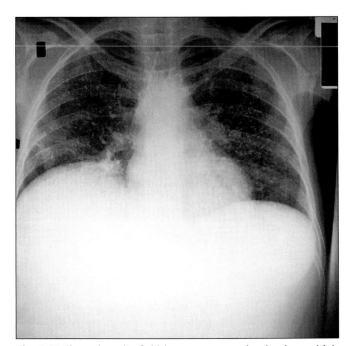

Fig. 1.23 *The end result of chicken pox pneumonia, showing multiple small calcific densities throughout both lung fields.*

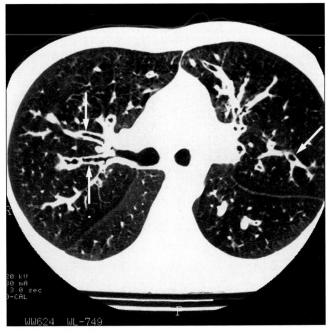

Fig. 1.24 *Allergic bronchopulmonary aspergillosis in a 30-year-old man, showing bronchiectasis with dilatation and bronchial wall thickening of all bronchi in the upper lobes (arrows).*

Mycetoma

Fungal invasion of the wall of a cavity within the lung, often following TB, results in the formation of a mycetoma or 'fungus ball' (**Fig. 1.25**). Persistent, heavy bleeding is one of the main clinical features of this lesion.

Invasive aspergillosis

Patients who are immunocompromised by AIDS or after treatment for cancer are susceptible to the *Aspergillus* fungus. This organism can directly invade the lung parenchyma, causing dense, often cavitated areas of consolidation. The resulting aspergillosis has a fatal outcome unless diagnosed early.

Histoplasmosis

Most cases of histoplasmosis occur in North America. They present incidentally as multiple calcified nodules on a chest radiograph that resembles that of chicken pox pneumonia. The acute form of the disease may be asymptomatic and show radiographically as areas of pneumonia, lymphadenopathy, and calcification.

Other fungal infections

Mucormycosis, candidiasis and cryptococcosis are almost always associated with severely ill, immunocompromised patients. They show as non-specific areas of consolidation that may cavitate, often with rapidly fatal consequences (**Fig. 1.26**).

PROTOZOAN INFECTIONS
Pneumocystis carinii pneumonia

Significant infection with *Pneumocystis carinii* pneumonia occurs only when the host has severe immunodeficiency, for example in patients with AIDS, in whom it is a common opportunistic infection and may occur in isolation or in combination with *M. tuberculosis* or the atypical forms of TB. On the chest radiograph, appearances vary from normal, through ground-glass opacification, to cystic bullous formation (**Figs 1.27** and **1.28**).

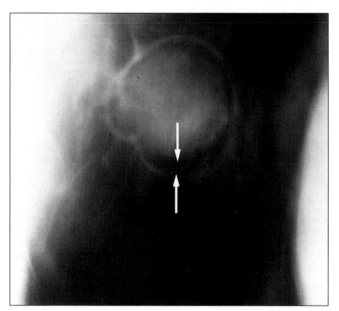

Fig. 1.25 *Tomogram of a mycetoma within a pre-existing lung cavity, demonstrating air between the fungus ball and the wall of the cavity (arrows).*

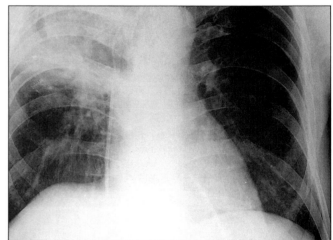

Fig. 1.26 *Mucormycosis. Cavitating fungus pneumonia in the right upper lobe in a patient with acute leukaemia.*

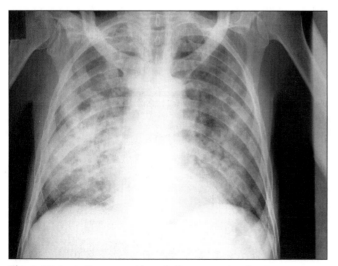

Fig. 1.27 *Acute* Pneumocystis carinii *pneumonia, showing widespread patchy consolidation throughout both lung fields, extending from the hilar areas.*

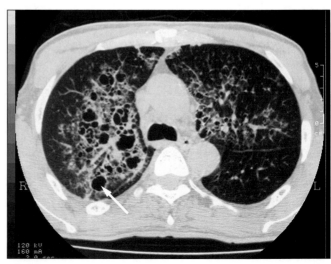

Fig. 1.28 *CT scan of a patient with* Pneumocystis carinii *pneumonia (PCP) and AIDS. There is consolidation in both lung fields, with cystic cavity formation (arrow) resulting from previous PCP infections.*

Amoebiasis

Amoeba is a common infective agent world wide, but amoebiasis rarely involves the lung, only doing so when a liver abscess penetrates the diaphragm, causing pleural and pulmonary spread of the disease.

HELMINTHIC INFESTATIONS
Hydatid disease

The liver is the organ most commonly infected by the *Echinococcus*; the lung takes second place. The hydatid cyst that forms in the lung has an oval or round appearance. If there are several present, multiple infestations are implicated. Anaphylactic shock is a potential hazard of attempts to take biopsy samples of these cysts (**Fig. 1.29**).

Worms

There are many worm infestations that can affect the lungs, often causing relatively non-specific clinical and radiological features, some of which are associated with eosinophilia. The organisms involved include *Wuchereria bancrofti*, *Schistosoma mansoni*, *Sch. haematobium*, and the lung fluke, *Paragonimus westermani*.

INFLAMMATORY CONDITIONS

CHRONIC BRONCHITIS

Among patients presenting with chronic bronchitis, 50% have a normal chest radiograph. The remainder have a mixture of patchy focal areas of consolidation, excessive clarity of bronchovascular markings as a result of surrounding destructive lung disease, and thickened bronchial walls (although the last feature is not visible on a chest radiograph until the thickening is considerable).

EMPHYSEMA

Although emphysema is not strictly inflammatory, its inclusion here forms a logical progression from the foregoing description of chronic bronchitis, as the two conditions commonly co-exist. Emphysema is a pathological condition, with enlargement of the air spaces distal to the terminal bronchus and destruction of alveolar spaces resulting in 'cavity' formation. Types of emphysema include periacinar (bullous lung disease), panacinar (widespread, severe and associated with α_1-antitrypsin deficiency), centriacinar (upper lobe disease), and irregular types (various forms and mixtures of disease types). Examples of radiographs from patients with emphysema are presented in **Figures 1.30–1.32**.

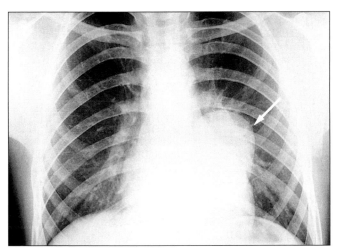

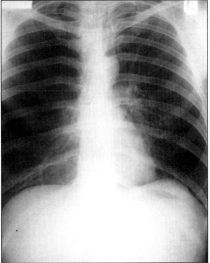

Fig. 1.30 Bullous emphysema of the right upper lobe, with compression of the right lower lobe.

Fig. 1.29 A rounded opacity (arrow) in the left lower lobe in a 15-year-old boy exposed to hydatid disease.

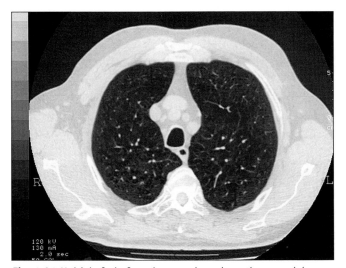

Fig. 1.31 Multiple foci of emphysema throughout the upper lobes.

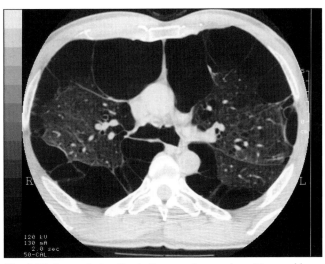

Fig. 1.32 Severe destructive bullous emphysema in a 48-year-old man who subsequently underwent lung transplantation.

Clinically, the severity of emphysema depends on the amount of disease present, which may or may not be visible on a chest radiograph. High-resolution CT (HRCT) gives better definition of the extent of lung destruction and shows the characteristic tissue patterns, together with the classic sign of overexpansion of the lung, which is irreversible.

ASTHMA

Asthma may be intrinsic or extrinsic. It produces hyperinflated lung fields on a chest radiograph but, unlike emphysema, the distribution of bronchovascular markings is normal and there are no areas of abnormal lung parenchyma. In an acute asthmatic attack, mediastinal emphysema (**Fig. 1.33**) may occur as a result of air being forced into the interstitium of the lung and passing through the lung hilum and into the mediastinum. A pneumothorax may also occur, but this complication is rare.

Extrinsic forms of asthma often have the same radiographic appearances, but occasionally other changes such as fleeting areas of consolidation may be seen, for example in Loeffler's pneumonitis.

BRONCHIECTASIS

Bronchiectasis is an inflammatory condition of the airways that is characterized by irreversible, dilated bronchi, often with increased wall thickness. The disease may be localized or generalized, with the pathology being essentially obstructive or non-obstructive. The wide

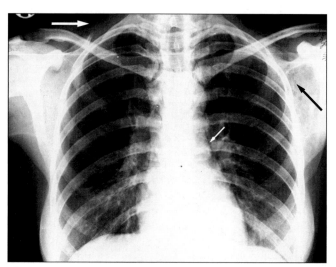

Fig. 1.33 *Acute asthma, with mediastinal (small arrow) and surgical emphysema around the neck and axillae (large arrows).*

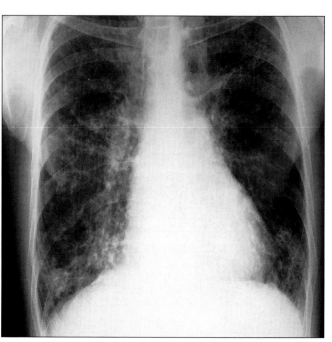

Fig. 1.34 *Severe bilateral bronchiectasis, with widespread air-space infection.*

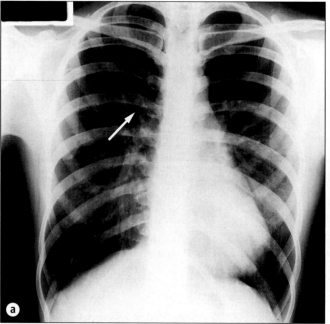

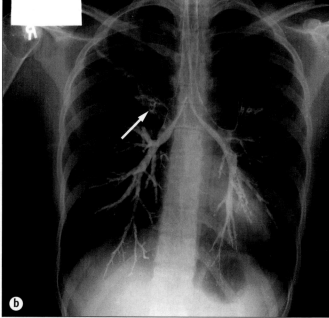

Fig. 1.35 (a) *Chest radiograph of a 23-year-old woman with previous tuberculosis in the right upper lobe and evidence of loss of volume of that lobe, with ring shadows (arrow).* **(b)** *Bronchogram of the same patient, demonstrating post-tuberculous bronchiectasis of the right upper lobe (arrow).*

aetiology varies from congenital to postinfective, obstructive, immunological, allergic, and many miscellaneous conditions.

Clinically, patients with bronchiectasis complain of recurrent chest infections and the production of copious purulent sputum. Bronchial wall thickening may be visible on the chest radiograph (Figs 1.34 and 1.35), dilated bronchi appearing as cylindrical, saccular or irregular lesions. Often, patchy inflammatory shadowing can be seen surrounding the bronchi, indicative of concurrent parenchymal infection. Previously, diagnosis was made by bronchography, but since the advent of HRCT (1–2 mm axial sections), this technique has been superseded, much to the relief of patients! (Figs 1.36 and 1.37).

EXTRINSIC ALLERGIC ALVEOLITIS

Extrinsic allergic alveolitis is an increasingly common problem world wide, perhaps partly because of increased recognition of the condition, but also because of the substantial number of organic compounds that are implicated as 'sensitizing' the lung. Classic conditions such as 'farmer's lung' and 'bird fancier's lung'—caused, respectively, by thermophilic actinomycetes and avian protein—have been joined by more esoteric examples such as 'prawn blower's lung' (caused by proteinaceous air-borne particles released during the preparation of prawns) and 'black fat tobacco smoker's lung'.

Radiologically and clinically, the disease may be acute, subacute, or chronic. Acute or subacute exposure produces multiple small nodules that are about 2 mm in diameter, bilateral, and widespread, giving a ground-glass appearance in some cases. HRCT reveals a typical distribution of alveolar shadowing (Fig. 1.38). The nodules may clear or persist. The chronic form of the disease manifests itself by fibrosis with loss of volume, usually affecting the upper lobes of the lung, and often accompanied by reticulo-nodular shadowing and bronchiectasis.

SARCOIDOSIS

Sarcoidosis is a multisystem disease of non-caseating granulomas of unknown aetiology, although it is probably immunologically based. Lymphadenopathy, usually comprising bilateral bronchopulmonary nodes combined with some enlargement of the mediastinal nodes, is the most common radiological manifestation (Fig. 1.39). This lymphadenopathy can either disappear rapidly or last months, years or decades; having resolved, it may recur. About 50% of patients with sarcoidosis develop parenchymal pulmonary nodules, often mid-zone in distribution, which can also be very variable in size, distribution, and duration (Fig. 1.40).

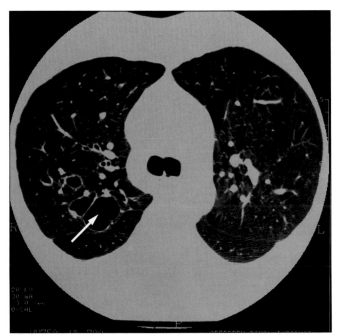

Fig. 1.36 Localized cystic bronchiectasis in a 45-year-old man, affecting the posterior segment of the right upper lobe (arrow).

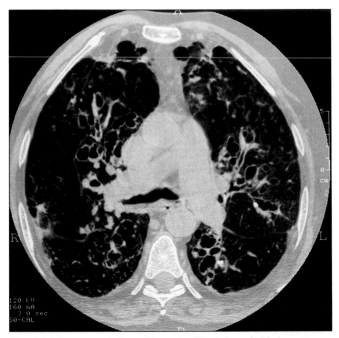

Fig. 1.37 Severe cystic bronchiectasis of both lung fields in a 72-year-old man.

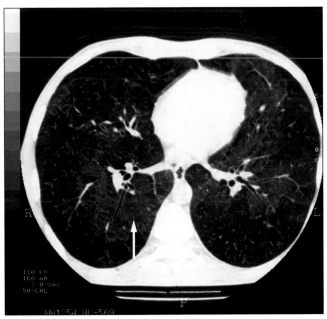

Fig. 1.38 Extrinsic allergic alveolitis. CT scan through the lung bases in a 39-year-old, demonstrating ground-glass consolidation (arrow) and increased lung density because of the alveolitis. There are normal lung fields more peripherally.

Sarcoid granulomas may heal by fibrosis, but only a small number of patients develop significant fibrosis, honeycombing, and endstage lung disease. The diagnosis of sarcoidosis is either clinical or histological by lymph node biopsy, often via mediastinoscopy.

IDIOPATHIC PULMONARY FIBROSIS

The cause of idiopathic pulmonary fibrosis (IPF) is unknown. It is characterized by progressive change from early inflammatory lesions in the alveolar septa to fibrosis, collagen deposition, and capillary destruction. A rapidly progressing form of the disease was known as Hamman Rich syndrome, but its true relationship with IPF is now in question.

Radiologically, reticulo-nodular shadowing, often basal, is the early predominant feature of IPF, visible on chest radiographs (**Figs 1.41 and 1.42**) but revealed more clearly on HRCT (**Figs 1.43 and 1.44**). The disease is usually bilateral, but variable in its degree of severity between sides. Volume loss and linear basal shadows caused by the development of fibrosis are later features, with subsequent progression to endstage honeycomb lung.

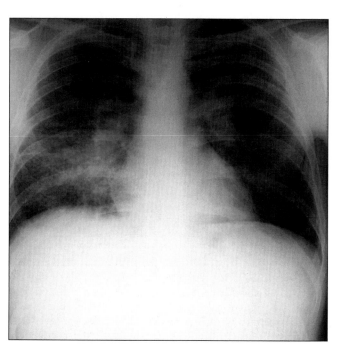

Fig. 1.39 Sarcoidosis. Bilateral hilar lymphadenopathy, with nodular shadowing in the right base and left upper lobe.

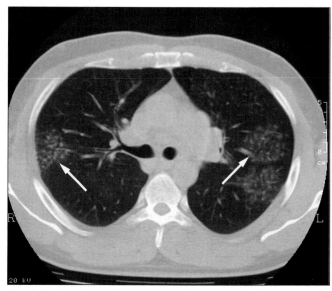

Fig. 1.40 Sarcoidosis. There are multiple enlarged nodes in the mediastinum and left hilum; multiple pulmonary nodules (arrows) in both middle zones.

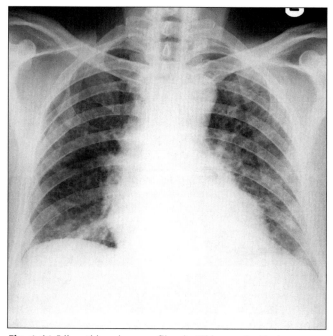

Fig. 1.41 Idiopathic pulmonary fibrosis. Widespread reticular shadowing throughout both lung fields, with loss of volume.

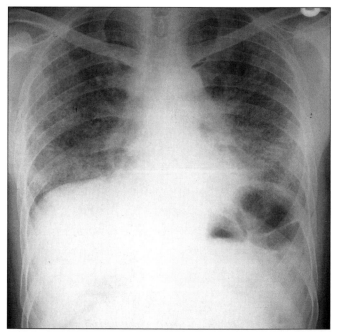

Fig. 1.42 Idiopathic pulmonary fibrosis. There is reticulo-nodular shadowing throughout both lung fields, with marked loss of volume of both lungs.

RHEUMATOID ARTHRITIS

Involvement of the thorax in rheumatoid arthritis is relatively common; pleural effusions are the most frequent abnormality. Lung manifestations include basal fibrosing alveolitis, and rheumatoid nodules (**Fig. 1.45**).

Caplan's syndrome is the name given to a condition seen in coal miners with rheumatoid disease that is characterized by the presence of large pulmonary nodules.

SYSTEMIC LUPUS ERYTHEMATOSUS

Systemic lupus erythematosus (SLE) is a multisystem vascular disorder that includes signs of pericardial and pleural effusions. Lung involvement can occur in either an acute or a chronic form, showing mainly non-specific areas of consolidation. There is also a high incidence of pneumonia, both bacterial and non-bacterial, in these immunocompromised patients.

SCLERODERMA

Scleroderma produces a fine reticular fibrotic pattern at the lung bases, with loss of volume. Pleural thickening and effusion are common.

SJÖGREN'S SYNDROME

Dry eyes and a dry mouth in middle-aged women are the classic features of the autoimmune disease known as Sjögren's syndrome. In

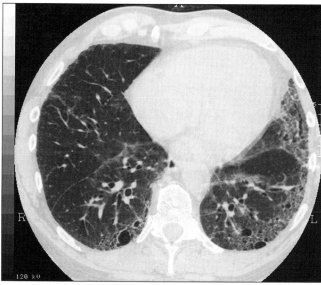

Fig. 1.43 *Idiopathic pulmonary fibrosis. CT scan through the lung bases, demonstrating cystic lesions in both lung bases, more marked on the left, and with relatively normal central areas.*

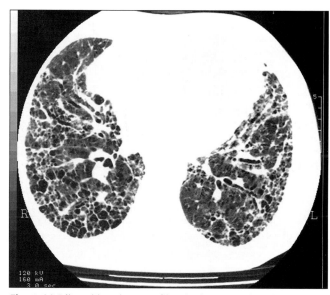

Fig. 1.44 *Idiopathic pulmonary fibrosis, demonstrating thick-walled cystic structures throughout both lower lobes, with evidence of increased alveolar opacification indicative of active disease superimposed on chronic disease.*

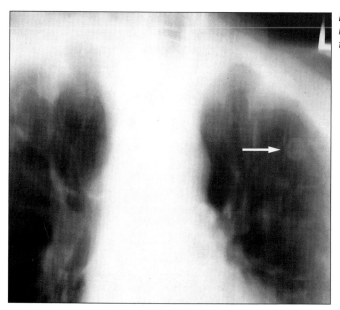

Fig. 1.45 *Rheumatoid nodules. Tomogram demonstrating multiple nodules in both lung fields. In the left upper lobe, one of the nodules is cavitating (arrows).*

about 33% of the patients, chest signs occur, including pneumonia and interstitial lung disease.

RELAPSING POLYCHRONDRITIS

Relapsing polychrondritis is a rare condition with progressive destruction of the cartilages in the ear, nose, larynx, and tracheo-bronchial tree (Fig. 1.46).

WEGENER'S GRANULOMATOSIS

An immunological response to as yet unidentified antigens is the probable cause of Wegener's granulomatosis, a midline disease with necrotizing granulomatous destruction of the upper and lower respiratory tracts. The majority of patients test positive for cyto-plasmic antineutrophil cytoplasmic antibodies (cANCA), and have lung involvement in their disease, as revealed by bronchial wall thickening, focal nodules, and consolidated areas of lung parenchyma. Diagnosis is by biopsy.

CHURG–STRAUSS SYNDROME

Necrotizing vasculitis, asthma, and eosinophilia characterize the fairly rare condition known as Churg–Strauss syndrome. Changes in the lung include transient focal areas of consolidation, diffuse pulmonary haemorrhage, and pleural effusions in 30% of cases.

BEHÇET'S SYNDROME

Behçet's syndrome is a rare, vasculitic syndrome comprising ulceration of the mouth and genitalia, specific skin and eye lesions, and arthritis. Lung involvement does occur, but is uncommon.

GOODPASTURE'S SYNDROME

Goodpasture's syndrome is the name given to glomerulonephritis combined with pulmonary haemorrhage caused by the antibody to basement membrane. It usually occurs in young males, whose chest radiographs show bilateral central air-space shadowing, as a result of haemorrhage and pulmonary oedema.

VASCULAR DISORDERS

PULMONARY HYPERTENSION

Pulmonary hypertension is best thought of as two separate conditions, pulmonary venous hypertension (PVHT) and pulmonary arterial hypertension (PAHT), which may co-exist, but have different aetiologies and radiological appearances.

PULMONARY VENOUS HYPERTENSION

Any obstruction to the venous drainage of the lungs results in increased pulmonary venous pressure. Thus, if the anatomical pathway is followed, the obstruction may be anywhere from the left atrium, through the left ventricle, to the aorta. The obstruction may be structural (e.g. mitral valve stenosis) or functional (e.g. the increased left ventricular end-diastolic pressure that occurs in left heart failure).

The consequence of the obstruction is that venous pressure is increased, which in turn leads to upper lobe blood diversion and the formation of pulmonary oedema, both alveolar and interstitial. If the condition is chronic, changes occur in the lung parenchyma, with formation of nodules and ossification (Fig. 1.47).

PULMONARY ARTERIAL HYPERTENSION

Increased pressure in the pulmonary arterial circulation results from three main types of disease.

The most common cause of PAHT is PVHT. Any increase in pulmonary venous pressure is transmitted across the capillary bed and thus causes an increase in pulmonary arterial pressure.

Conditions such as emphysema, primary pulmonary hypertension, and thromboembolic disease result in destruction of the pulmonary capillary bed, increasing the pulmonary vascular resistance and hence the pulmonary arterial pressure.

Ventricular septal defect, atrial septal defect, and patent ductus arteriosus are common causes of left-to-right shunts with an increased flow that leads, at some stage, to increased pulmonary arterial pressure.

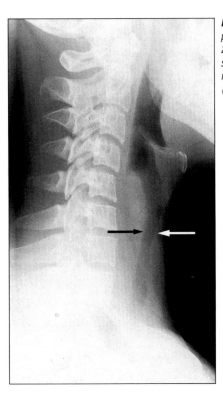

Fig. 1.46 Relapsing polychondritis in a 22-year-old woman, showing markedly narrowed trachea (arrows).

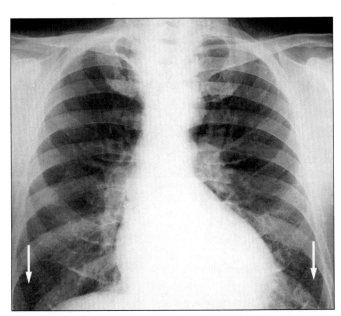

Fig. 1.47 Upper lobe venous blood diversion, with pulmonary venous hypertension and evidence of cardiac failure at the lung bases (septal lines – arrows), in a patient with left heart failure.

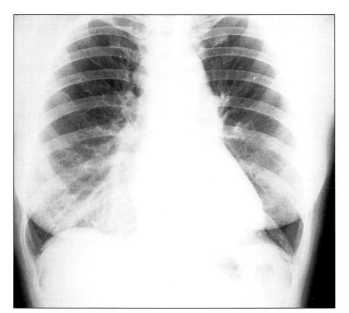

Fig. 1.48 *Pulmonary embolism. The chest radiograph shows some minor reduction in blood flow to the left lung, in a patient with clinically suspected left pulmonary embolism.*

THROMBOEMBOLIC DISEASE; PULMONARY INFARCTION

Pulmonary emboli are common, resulting in considerable morbidity and mortality in hospital patients. The majority of emboli arise in the veins of the lower limb and pelvis. Pulmonary emboli may be small or large, single or multiple, acute or chronic, and all may or may not cause pulmonary infarction. In view of the wide range of the disease, it is not surprising that the clinical symptoms and signs are protean and often non-specific.

Radiological features include, importantly, a normal chest radiograph, but also areas of consolidation, a pleural effusion, pulmonary oligaemia and, rarely, the typical triangular subpleural area of consolidation. The chest radiograph is therefore of limited value in diagnosing a pulmonary embolus, but should always be performed before a ventilation– perfusion lung scan, so that results of the two investigations can be viewed together (**Fig. 1.48**).

The imaging investigation practised most widely for diagnosing a pulmonary embolus is simultaneous ventilation and perfusion radionuclide scanning. The value of this technique lies in its ability to reveal areas of ventilation–perfusion mismatch—that is, areas in which ventilation is normal despite reduced or absent perfusion as a result of blockage of the appropriate pulmonary artery and its branches by the embolus (**Fig. 1.49**). If the radionuclide scans are indeterminate and clinical suspicion of a pulmonary embolus remains high, the gold-standard test is a pulmonary angiogram (**Figs 1.50–1.52**). The rise in intravenous drug abuse has lead to an increasing incidence of septic pulmonary emboli, which on imaging may be multiple and cavitating.

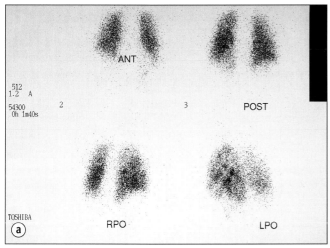

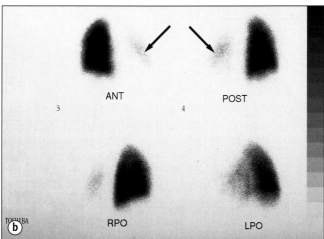

Fig. 1.49 *Same patient as in Figure 1.48.* **(a)** *Ventilation scan shows normal appearances.* **(b)** *Perfusion scan demonstrates marked reduction in blood flow to the left lung (arrows), consistent with pulmonary embolism.*

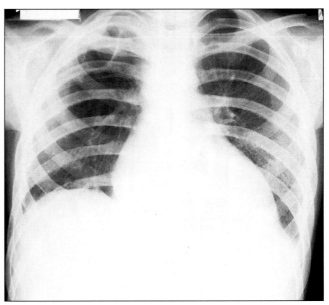

Fig. 1.50 *Chronic pulmonary emboli with marked reduction in vascularity to the right lung.*

17

COR PULMONALE

Cor pulmonale is the name of the clinical condition applied to patients who have right heart disease caused by acute or chronic lung disease. When the pulmonary artery pressure increases, the main pulmonary arteries dilate, the peripheral vessels shut down, the vascular resistance increases, the pressure increases further—and so the spiral continues. The right ventricle becomes hypertrophied and, when heart failure intervenes, it dilates, resulting in systemic venous distension.

An important point to remember when looking at an isolated chest radiograph is that there is no correlation between main pulmonary artery size and the pressure within. An atrial septal defect with a large shunt will have large central pulmonary arteries, yet the pulmonary artery pressure may be normal. Conversely, a patient with severe (systemic) pulmonary arterial hypertension, as occurs for example in some forms of ventricular septal defect, may have normal-sized main pulmonary arteries.

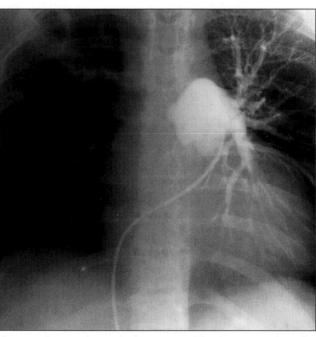

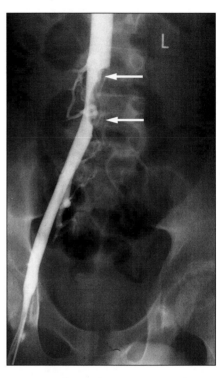

Fig. 1.52 *In the same patient as in the preceding two figures, venography demonstrates a large lobular filling defect of the lower inferior vena cava arising from the left common iliac vein (arrows), indicating the site of embolus.*

Fig. 1.51 *Same patient as in Figure 1.49, with pulmonary angiography demonstrating failure of any circulation to the right lung.*

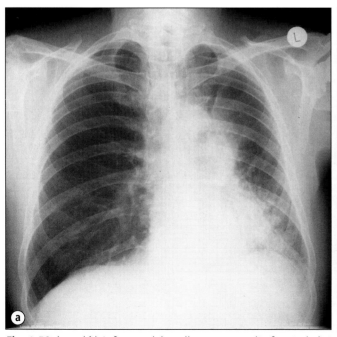

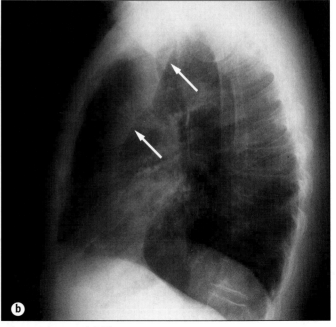

Fig. 1.53 *(a and b) Left upper lobe collapse as a result of central obstructing carcinoma. (a) The posteroanterior chest film demonstrates mediastinal shift to the left and loss of the normal left heart border as a result of the upper lobe collapse. (b) The lateral film demonstrates anterior displacement of the oblique fissure (arrows), with a consolidated upper lobe anteriorly.*

NEOPLASTIC DISEASE

PRIMARY LUNG TUMOURS

Primary lung carcinomas are of two main types radiologically. A central lesion causes obstructive symptoms and signs, tends to present early, and carries a worse prognosis because of its position. A peripheral lesion presents late, does not cause obstruction but may involve the chest wall, yet is potentially curable by surgery (**Figs 1.53** and **1.54**).

The pathological diagnosis of carcinoma of the lung is usually made on bronchoscopic biopsy. Peripheral lesions located beyond the reach of the bronchoscope may be amenable to fine-needle lung aspiration biopsy for cytological examination. The two major complications of percutaneous biopsy are pneumothorax and haemorrhage, both potentially serious but remediable. The technique should not be undertaken if the patient's lung function is too poor to sustain a pneumothorax as a complication, or if the patient either is taking anticoagulants or has a bleeding disorder.

Staging

The 'TNM' classification is used for staging carcinoma of the bronchus: T for tumour, N for nodal disease, and M for metastases. An abbreviated TNM staging classification is shown in **Figure 1.55**. Patients with stages 1–3A carcinoma are considered suitable for surgery; those with stages 3B and 4 have disease that is too advanced for surgical resection and cure.

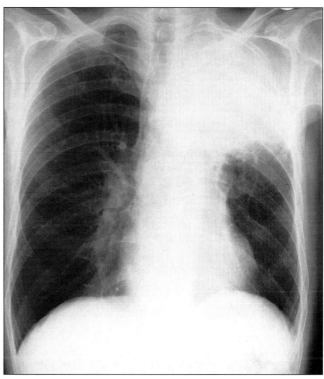

Fig. 1.54 *A large left apical mass, with displacement of the trachea to the right and indentation of the left main bronchus. The diagnosis is left upper lobe carcinoma.*

Fig. 1.55 *Lung carcinoma staging.*

Lung carcinoma staging			
T1	less than 3 cm		
T2	more than 3 cm/extends to hilar region/invades visceral pleura/partial atelectasis		
T3	Chest wall, diaphragm, pericardium, mediastinal pleura, total atelectasis		
T4	Mediastinum, heart, great vessels, trachea, oesophagus, malignant effusion		
N1	Peribronchial, ipsilateral hilar		
N2	Ipsilateral mediastinal		
N3	Contralateral mediastinal, scalene or supraclavicular		
M0	No distant metastasis		
M1	Distant metastasis		
T1N0M0 T2N0M0	Stage 1	Resectable	Surgery
T1N1M0 T1N1M0	Stage 2	Resectable	Surgery
T1N2M0 T2N2M0 T3 (N0,N1,N2) M0	Stage 3A	Potentially resectable	Surgery
Any T N3M0 T4 Any N M0	Stage 3B	Unresectable Not curable	Medical treatment
Any T Any N M1	Stage 4	Unresectable Not curable	Medical treatment

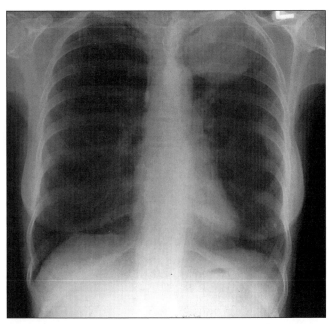

Fig. 1.56 *Pancoast tumour at the left apex, destroying the posterior aspects of the left 3rd and 4th ribs.*

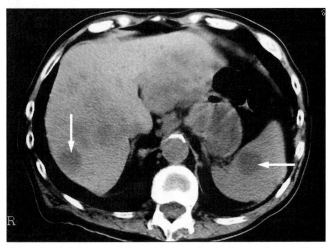

Fig. 1.57 *Multiple low-attenuation areas in the liver and spleen in a 78-year-old man with metastatic bronchial carcinoma.*

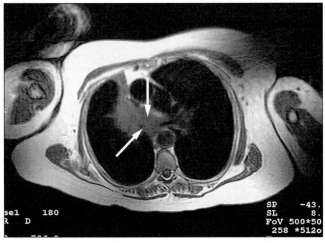

Fig. 1.58 *MRI axial scan demonstrating a soft-tissue mass surrounding the right main bronchus (arrows) extending into the fat of the mediastinum. Inoperable bronchogenic carcinoma.*

Bronchial carcinoma spreads essentially by local, lymphatic and haematogenous means. The importance of local spread depends on the site of the primary tumour. If the tumour is situated in the apex of the upper lobe, spread can occur through the upper ribs and invade the brachial plexus; arm pain and Horner's syndrome are two of the clinical symptoms of this type of lesion, known as a Pancoast tumour (**Fig. 1.56**).

Lymphatic spread is through the bronchopulmonary nodes, with subsequent spread into the mediastinal nodal groups eventually leading to extrathoracic nodal spread. The further the spread, the worse the prognosis, which is always poor in this condition: 50% survival for typical stage 1 patients, deteriorating to less than 5% 5 years' overall survival for all types and stages.

Haematogenous spread is common to liver (**Fig. 1.57**), bone marrow, brain and adrenals in addition to the ipsilateral or contralateral lung, or both. Radiological evaluation of staging therefore involves CT for chest and adrenals, ultrasound for the liver, radionuclide scanning for the bones and, in some centres, CT for the brain. MR imaging shows better definition of mediastinal involvement by central tumours (**Fig. 1.58**). All these procedures may be undertaken before surgery to assess the stage of the disease and avoid surgery in those patients whose disease is too advanced for it to be of benefit.

Occasionally, a lung tumour may present with a condition known as hypertrophic pulmonary osteoarthropathy (HPOA). The patient may experience bone pain, often in the distal arm or leg, and there are fairly characteristic appearances of a periosteal reaction on the radiograph.

SECONDARY MALIGNANCY

The pulmonary capillary bed acts as a filter for all the venous blood and it is therefore not surprising that many tumours that spread by tumour emboli lodge in the lungs and grow (**Figs 1.59** and **1.60**). Indeed, the tumours found most commonly in the lungs are secondaries. Although most secondary deposits in the lung fields give no indication of their origin, those that cavitate may be squamous, and others that ossify usually result from bone-producing tumours such as osteogenic sarcoma.

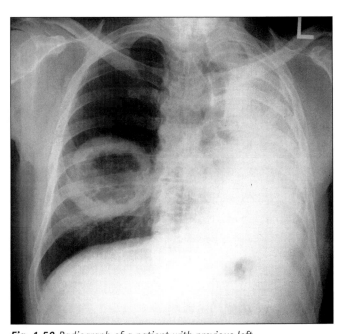

Fig. 1.59 *Radiograph of a patient with previous left pneumonectomy. There is a large cavitating squamous deposit in the right lung.*

Lymphangitis carcinomatosa

When malignant cells invade the lymphatic channels in the lung parenchyma and cause obstruction, the result is lymphangitis carcinomatosa. The reticulo-nodular shadowing, which may be localized or generalized and with or without lymphadenopathy, is best visualized on HRCT (Fig. 1.61). Common tumours involved in this type of metastatic spread are those of the bronchus, breast, prostate, colon, and pancreas.

BENIGN LUNG TUMOURS
Hamartoma

A hamartoma is a benign tumour containing cartilage, blood vessels, fat, and epithelium. Such tumours grow slowly, often contain calcifications, and never become malignant (Fig. 1.62).

Carcinoid tumour

Carcinoid tumours are neuroendocrine in origin and, in the majority of cases, remain benign, although aggressive malignant types do occur, and they may metastasize. Radiologically, the tumour may be small, occluding a bronchus (Fig. 1.63), or discovered incidentally as a peripheral coin lesion that may contain calcification.

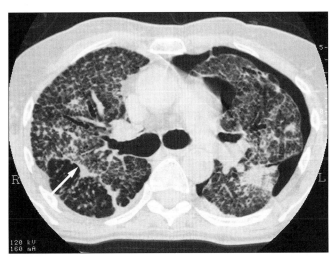

Fig. 1.61 Lymphangitis carcinomatosa. High-resolution CT scan demonstrating marked thickening of the interstitium of the lung fields (arrow). There is a left pneumothorax caused by lung biopsy.

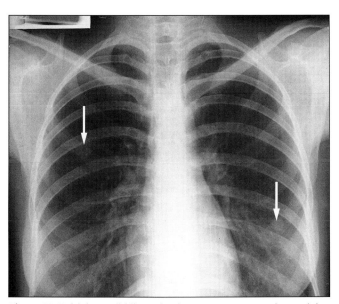

Fig. 1.60 Multiple small bilateral pulmonary metastases (arrows) in a young female patient with no known primary tumour.

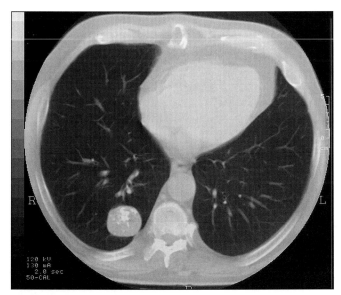

Fig. 1.62 Well-circumscribed 4 cm mass containing popcorn calcification situated in the posterior basal segment of the right lower lobe in a 73-year-old asymptomatic man. Typical hamartomatous appearance, confirmed on percutaneous lung biopsy.

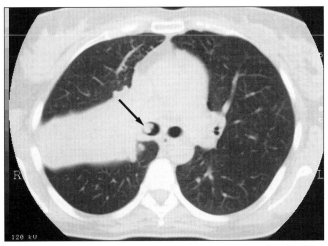

Fig. 1.63 Carcinoid tumour (bronchial adenoma): a small polypoid lesion projecting from the origin of the right upper lobe bronchus (arrow) into the right main bronchus. There is distal consolidation of the posterior aspect of the right upper lobe.

LYMPHOPROLIFERATIVE DISORDERS
Lymphoma

Hodgkin's disease

In Hodgkin's disease, in contrast to the common finding of enlarged bronchopulmonary and mediastinal nodes, primary involvement of the lung is relatively rare, and does not occur unless there is obvious accompanying nodal disease (**Figs 1.64–1.66**) (*see* page 29).

Non-Hodgkin's disease

Non-Hodgkin's disease rarely involves the lung as a primary focus of the disease, but may do so without nodal disease, unlike Hodgkin's disease.

MISCELLANEOUS MALIGNANCIES
Kaposi's sarcoma

Primary lung involvement of Kaposi's sarcoma is becoming recognized more commonly as the number of AIDS patients increases. Appearances on the chest radiograph are non-specific and include focal areas of infiltration and nodules (**Fig. 1.67**). The diagnosis is often complicated by the co-existence of opportunistic lung infections.

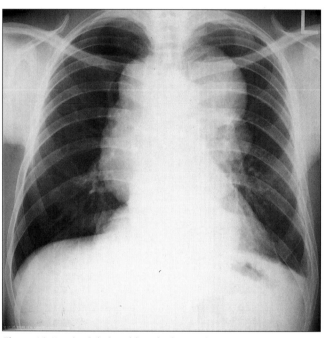

Fig. 1.64 *Massive lobulated lymphadenopathy in a young adolescent man. The diagnosis is Hodgkin's disease.*

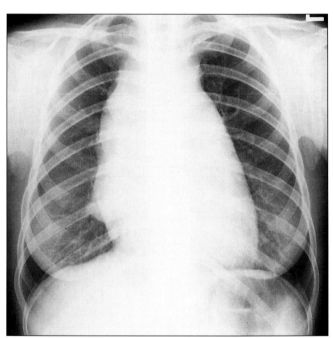

Fig. 1.65 *Widespread mediastinal involvement in Hodgkin's disease, in a 20-year-old woman.*

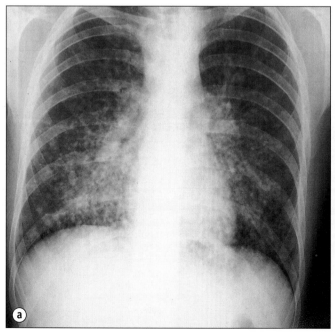

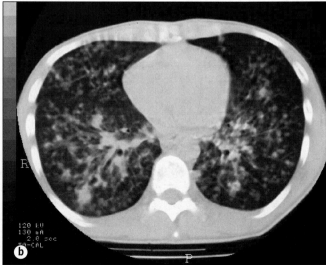

Fig. 1.66 (**a** *and* **b**) *Multiple nodules throughout the lung fields in a 21-year-old man with acute Hodgkin's lymphoma of the lungs. CT demonstrates the nodules of primary Hodgkin's tumour.*

DRUG-RELATED AND INDUSTRIAL LUNG DISEASES

DRUGS

Numerous drugs are known to cause pulmonary damage. Their classification is based largely on what adverse effect the drug causes: hypersensitivity reactions, pulmonary oedema, a diffuse alveolitis, SLE reactions, or a pulmonary vasculitis.

Types 1 and 3 are the most common of the hypersensitivity reactions, and are seen with drugs such as methotrexate and bleomycin (**Fig. 1.68**). Pulmonary oedema results from chemical or hormonal reactions, and is seen, for example, with cyclophosphamide. Diffuse alveolar damage is associated with nitrofurantoin and amiodarone (**Fig. 1.69**). SLE-like syndromes occur with anticonvulsants and antibacterial agents. Pulmonary vasculitis is associated typically with busulphan.

INDUSTRIAL LUNG DISEASES

This group of diseases can be subdivided into those having organic or non-organic causes. Those, such as farmer's lung, with organic causes have been considered above; this section will concern the inorganic dusts.

Coal miner's pneumoconiosis

The presence of nodules on the chest radiograph is the most characteristic radiological finding in all forms of inorganic dust disease, with the exception of diseases caused by exposure to asbestos. The fine, soft-tissue nodules found in the lungs of coal miners result from the inhalation of coal dust, which in itself is relatively inactive (**Fig. 1.70**), and are in sharp contrast to the fibrosis and massive shadows that typify disease occurring when the coal dust is mixed with silica. Exposure to beryllium causes chest radiographic appearances similar to those of sarcoidosis.

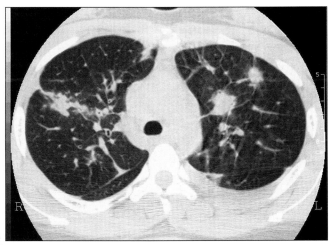

Fig. 1.67 Kaposi's sarcoma in a patient with AIDS. CT demonstrates multiple, ill-defined solid nodules in both lung fields, in biopsy-proven Kaposi's sarcoma.

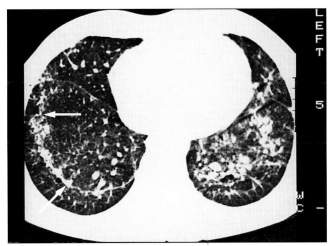

Fig. 1.68 Bleomycin toxicity, showing crescentic fibrotic shadows (arrows) in the periphery of both lung fields.

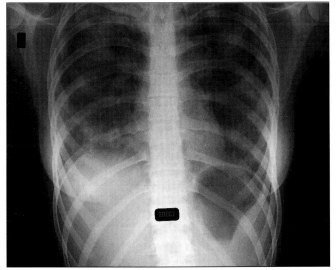

Fig. 1.69 A drug-induced hypersensitivity reaction, with widespread opacification of both lung fields.

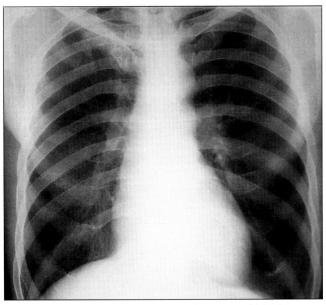

Fig. 1.70 Coal miner's pneumoconiosis. There are multiple, low-density nodules throughout both lung fields.

Silicosis

Silicosis is caused by the active response of the lung to silica particles. The radiograph commonly shows dense bands of fibrosis with intervening emphysema, and eggshell calcification of the hilar lymph nodes (**Fig.1.71**). There is an increased incidence of lung carcinoma in these patients.

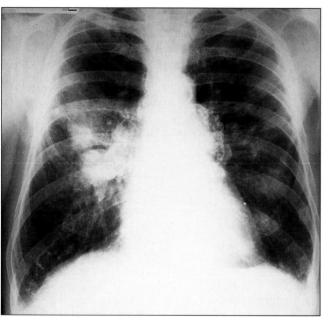

Fig. 1.71 *Silicosis. Nodules with pulmonary fibrosis and eggshell calcification of hilar glands.*

Stannosis

Stannosis results from exposure to tin and is characterized by nodules that are highly radiodense because of the high atomic number of tin.

Exposure to asbestos

Exposure to asbestos particles may predate the disease induced by many decades, thus it is important to take a full history in patients suspected of having this condition or its complications. Asbestos-related disease relates primarily to the benign pleural disease of thickening, calcification, and effusion. The term 'asbestosis' is reserved for pulmonary fibrosis and visceral pleural fibrosis (**Figs 1.72 and 1.73**), and is associated with an increased incidence of meso-thelioma (*see* page 28).

Other inhaled agents

Accidental inhalation of smoke in fires is common. The chest radiograph often remains normal, but acute pulmonary oedema, progressing to adult respiratory distress syndrome and areas of collapse, may develop. Drowning, with fresh or sea water entering the lungs, causes acute pulmonary oedema as a result of the difference in fluid osmolalities. Pulmonary oedema is also the main finding in patients who aspirate gastric contents.

MISCELLANEOUS CONDITIONS

INTENSIVE CARE

Chest radiographs obtained in patients in intensive care units or high dependency units, and in others requiring mobile radiography, appear very different from standard posteroanterior view chest radiographs obtained from erect patients. Radiographs in the former patients are anteroposterior in view and, in consequence, magnification of the mediastinal structures renders measurement of heart size invalid.

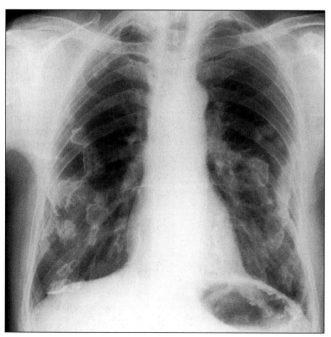

Fig. 1.72 *Result of exposure to asbestos, showing bilateral calcified pleural plaques.*

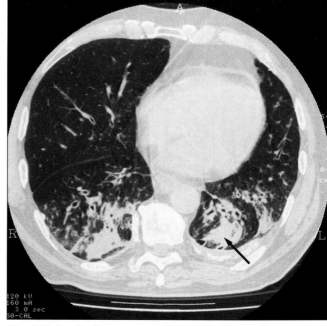

Fig. 1.73 *Result of exposure to asbestos. The CT scan demonstrates pleural thickening and calcification posteriorly, particularly at the left base, with areas of rounded atelectasis in the lung fields (arrow).*

Patients who are unconscious also undergo radiography in the supine position, which is associated with a different distribution of pulmonary blood flow and higher diaphragmatic shadows. **Figures 1.74a** and **1.74b** offer a comparison of chest radiographs obtained in the same patient from the standard and the anteroposterior, supine views; both radiographs were taken within 2 hours and both are normal!

CYSTIC LUNG DISEASE

There are several conditions that cause reticulo-nodular cystic lung disease, particularly well shown on HRCT. Langerhans' cell histiocytosis (histiocytosis X) is a systemic disorder in which the lungs show widespread thin-walled air spaces, with alveolar destruction and nodulation (**Figs 1.75** and **1.76**).

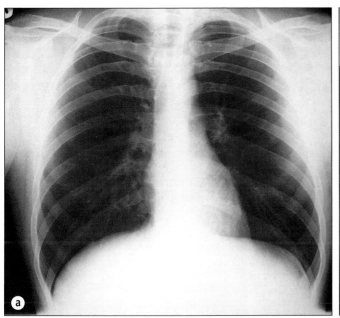
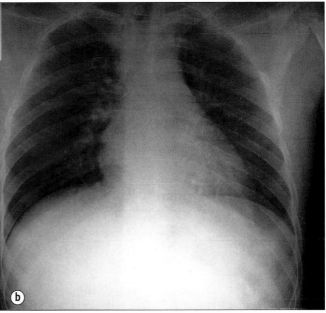

Fig. 1.74 (a) Normal posteroanterior chest radiograph, taken with the patient erect. *(b)* The same patient 2 hours later. Radiograph from the anteroposterior projection, with the patient in the supine position. Note the change in the blood flow pattern to a more even distribution to the upper lobes, and the apparent increase in heart size as a result of the magnification effect of an anteroposterior film.

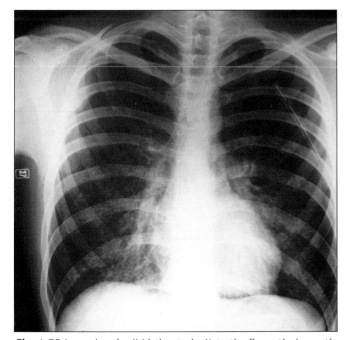
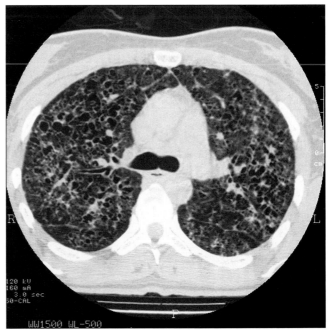

Fig. 1.75 Langerhans' cell histiocytosis. Note the fine reticular cystic pattern throughout both lung fields, with a left-sided pneumothorax and drainage tube.

Fig. 1.76 High-resolution CT scan of histiocytosis, demonstrating multiple thick-walled cystic spaces throughout both lung fields in a 32-year-old woman.

Neurofibromatosis (type 1) also causes a cystic lung disease similar to fibrosing alveolitis. Extremely rarely, similar appearances are found in a small percentage of patients with tuberous sclerosis (**Fig. 1.77**).

Lymphangioleiomyomatosis is the last of these conditions causing widespread cystic air-space shadowing. It occurs only in women, usually aged between 20 and 40 years.

INTERVENTIONAL AND THERAPEUTIC PROCEDURES

Percutaneous lung biopsy has been mentioned (*see* page 19).

Embolization of arteriovenous fistulae in the Rendu–Osler–Weber syndrome can be accomplished by catheterization of the appropriate pulmonary artery and the release of metal coils that lodge in the fistulae, causing thrombosis and hence closure of the shunt.

Other interventional techniques include the injection of appropriate drugs into mycetoma cavities and video-assisted thoracoscopic techniques.

Patients with stridor due to large airway narrowing, often caused by malignancy, can have metallic stents placed in the airway, thereby opening the narrowed site, relieving the stridor, and greatly improving the quality of their lives (**Fig. 1.78**).

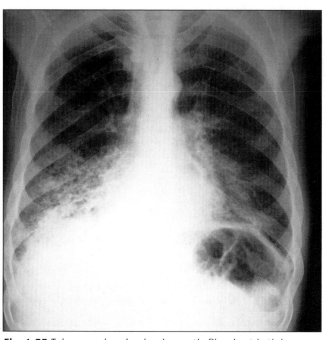

Fig. 1.77 *Tuberous sclerosis, showing cystic fibrosis at both lung bases.*

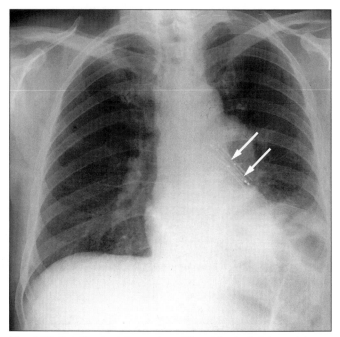

Fig. 1.78 *Metallic stent (arrows) positioned in the left lower lobe bronchus in a patient with left lower lobe carcinoma.*

Part 2. Pleura

CONGENITAL ABNORMALITIES

Common anomalies of the pleura include an azygos lobe, the fissure comprising four layers of pleura and accessory fissures, usually in the lower lobes. The condition is only of consequence to thoracic surgeons at the time of thoracotomy.

PLEURAL DISORDERS

PLEURAL EFFUSION

Pleural fluid may be a transudate or an exudate, contain blood, pus, chyle or other substances, and be caused by several conditions. It tends to accumulate in the most dependent parts of the pleural cavity; when the patient is in the erect position, these are the posterior costophrenic recesses. The best radiological view to observe fluid is thus a lateral one, as significant amounts (e.g. 500 ml) of fluid may not be obvious on a standard posteroanterior view (**Fig. 1.79**). All fluid looks the same on imaging, and it is often not possible to differentiate types of fluid or their aetiology. Fluid may become loculated, particularly if infective, and pleural thickening may occur quite rapidly (**Figs 1.80a** and **b**). Aspiration of the fluid should usually be accompanied by a pleural biopsy, as this additional procedure aids diagnosis substantially.

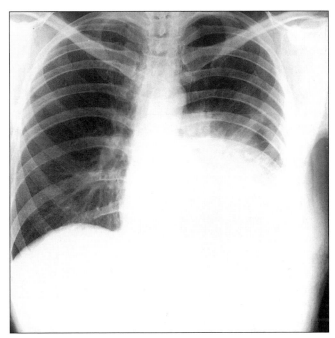

Fig. 1.79 Left pleural effusion.

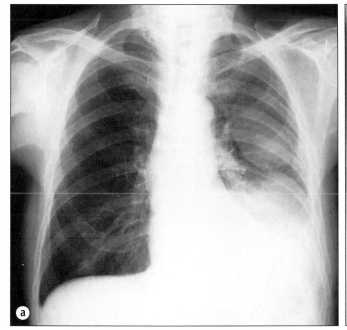
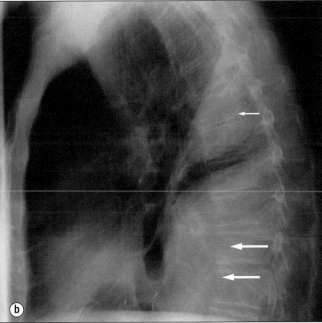

Fig. 1.80 (**a** and **b**) Loculated left pleural effusion. The lateral film (**b**) demonstrates fluid posteriorly (large arrows), with further loculations of fluid in the superior aspect of the left oblique fissure (small arrow).

PLEURAL THICKENING AND CALCIFICATION

Pleural thickening, which may be localized or generalized, unilateral or bilateral, is a common finding and results from a wide variety of diseases. Patients particularly susceptible to pleural thickening and calcification are those with previous tuberculosis or other infective empyema, haemothorax, or exposure to asbestos (**Fig. 1.81**).

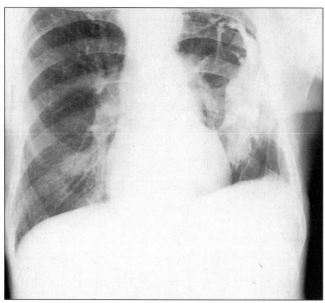

Fig. 1.81 *Widespread pleural calcification over the left hemithorax, with loss of volume of the left lung field, secondary to haemothorax after injury.*

PNEUMOTHORAX

Pneumothorax has been considered in detail above (*see* page 5).

NEOPLASTIC DISEASE

MALIGNANT TUMOURS

The most common malignant tumour of the pleura is secondary disease, often from primary breast carcinoma, or occasionally from abdominal and pelvic primaries. Although rare, the primary pleural tumour of most concern is mesothelioma, because of its relationship with exposure to asbestos, its increasing frequency, and its poor outlook. The interval between exposure to asbestos and the development of mesothelioma is often between 25 and 40 years. Local or widespread pleural thickening, often with an effusion and invasion of the chest wall, are the characteristic signs on chest radiograph or CT scans (**Figs 1.82** and **1.83**). Mesothelioma is one of the few tumours to seed itself along a biopsy tract, and biopsy should therefore be avoided if possible. Total pleuropneumonectomy is the only potential treatment, but prognosis is very poor.

BENIGN LESIONS

Lipomas and fibromas may arise from the pleural surface; both are rare, and the latter is particularly associated with HPOA.

INTERVENTIONAL PROCEDURES

Although a pleural effusion may be detected clinically, it is often prudent to obtain radiological images to show its position, size, and composition before drainage. A chest radiograph will reveal pleural fluid, but the position of the diaphragm may be unclear and, in such cases, ultrasonography or CT scanning should be performed. Drainage under ultrasound control is a relatively straightforward procedure, and allows placement of catheters of appropriate size, particularly in difficult cases.

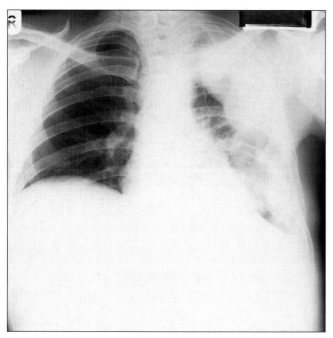

Fig. 1.82 *Mesothelioma, demonstrating lobulated opacities throughout the left pleural cavity.*

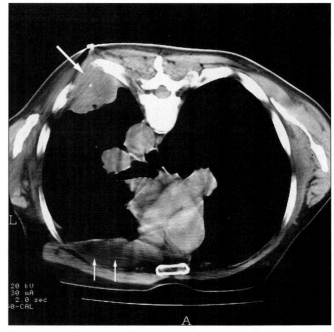

Fig. 1.83 *Mesothelioma affecting the posterior pleura, with destruction of the adjacent ribs and involvement of the chest wall (large arrow). Note the anterior effusion (small arrows).*

Part 3. Mediastinum

CONGENITAL ABNORMALITIES

There are a number of congenital cystic lesions that occur in the mediastinum and are related to various anatomical structures arising from the primitive foregut. Neuroenteric cysts and duplications have elements of neurogenic and intestinal tissue types, occur in the posterior mediastinum, and may be clinically silent. Bronchogenic cysts have already been mentioned (*see* page 2). Away from the foregut, the other well-known cystic lesion is the pericardial or springwater cyst (**Figs 1.84** and **1.85**). It is usually situated anteriorly, in the costophrenic recesses, and is often right-sided. These cysts are usually asymptomatic but, if very large, may cause compression of the heart.

TRAUMA

Rupture of the oesophagus, either as a result of instrumentation or by severe or prolonged vomiting, results in an intense inflammatory mediastinitis associated with considerable morbidity and mortality. Radiologically, oesophageal rupture can be shown by instillation of non-ionic contrast media through an oesophageal tube to reveal the site of leakage.

Aortic rupture, either partial or complete, typically occurs in deceleration road traffic accidents. If transection of the aorta is complete, 90% of patients may be expected to die rapidly, but if the lesion is diagnosed within the first 24 hours, surgical repair produces a good outcome. The aorta has three areas of attachment: the aortic root into the left ventricle, the site of the ligamentum arteriosus, and the hiatus of the diaphragm. The common site of damage is the middle attachment, and tears are often seen just distal to the ligamentum arteriosus. Partial rupture may later lead to the formation of a localized aneurysm at this characeristic site (**Fig. 1.86**).

INFECTION

ACUTE MEDIASTINITIS
Patients with acute mediastinitis are often severely ill, shocked, and have chest pain and fever. Causes include oesophageal perforation, spread of infection from the lungs, pleura, or surrounding structures, and postoperative median sternotomy. On a chest radiograph, the mediastinum may be seen to be widened and contain air; on a CT scan, collections of pus may be visible.

CHRONIC MEDIASTINITIS
Chronic inflammatory mediastinitis is rare, but can be caused by conditions similar to those that produce retroperitoneal fibrosis. The mediastinal pleura is thickened and mainly causes constriction of the superior vena cava, although the process can extend to involve the pulmonary veins.

INFLAMMATORY AND NEOPLASTIC CONDITIONS

Lymphadenopathy in the mediastinum is a common manifestation of diseases ranging from benign conditions such as sarcoidosis to widespread infiltration from any one of various primary malignancies. The differential diagnosis depends on the appearance of the nodes, the groups involved, the size, the patient's age and sex, and the presence of known systemic disease. Hodgkin's disease, in young people predominantly, may produce massive anterior mediastinal lymphadenopathy (*see* **Figs 1.64** and **1.65**). The radiograph may appear normal if the nodes involved are only slightly enlarged, and some nodes, such as those in the subcarinal area, may be difficult to see. CT provides excellent views of enlarged nodes and should be used to map the groups involved, particularly for follow-up after appropriate treatment.

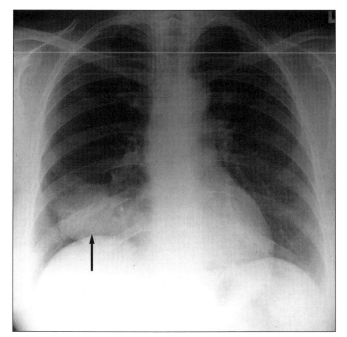

Fig. 1.84 *Pericardial cyst (springwater cyst): a well-defined soft-tissue lesion arising from the right cardiophrenic angle (arrow).*

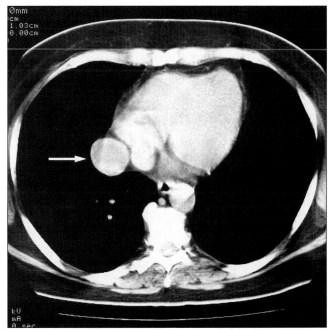

Fig. 1.85 *Pericardial cyst: a well-defined 3-cm cystic structure adjacent to the right atrium (arrowed).*

VASCULAR DISEASE

As a patient ages, the aorta loses its normal elasticity, dilates and elongates. The three fixation points described above (*see* page 29) enable this to be visualized on the posteroanterior chest radiograph: the ascending aorta produces a bulge to the right of the mediastinum, and the descending aorta produces one to the left. This is the so-called aortic unfolding, which can at times be very pronounced.

Aneurysms of the aorta are of various types, involve the ascending or descending sections, or both, and produce mediastinal masses on a chest radiograph.

When a patient has a suspected aortic dissection, it is important that the surgeon should know the entry and exit points, as management is different depending on which parts of the aorta are involved, and how far the internal tear extends. Angiography, ultrasound, MR imaging, transoesophageal echocardiography, and CT (**Fig. 1.87**) have all been used to demonstrate the aortic lumen in these patients. Often, local preference and expertise dictate which investigations are performed, and when.

Obstruction of the superior vena cava, either by nodal or malignant compression or by thrombosis, is a distressing condition for the patient, who presents with a swollen face, headache, and venous congestion. Relief can sometimes be obtained by the insertion of a vascular stent (**Fig. 1.88**) or by balloon angioplasty.

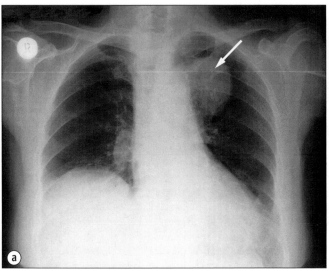

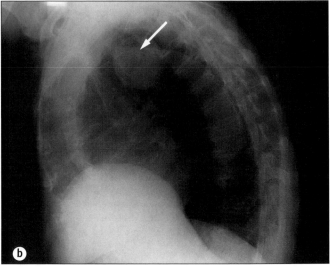

Fig. 1.86 (a and b) Traumatic aortic aneurysm. There is a well-defined cystic structure arising from the aortic arch (arrows), with calcification in the wall of the structure. Post-traumatic aortic aneurysm following partial aortic tear during previous deceleration injury.

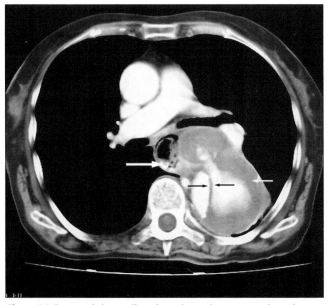

Fig. 1.87 Ruptured descending thoracic aortic aneurysm into the oesophagus. The CT scan demonstrates a large descending aortic aneurysm with intimal flap (black arrows), thrombus formation (white arrow), and contrast extending into the oesophagus (large arrow).

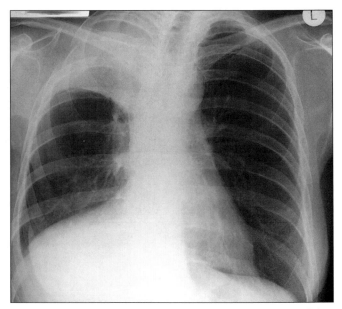

Fig. 1.88 Carcinoma of the right upper lobe, with destruction of the right 4th rib and venous occlusion. A vascular stent is in place in the left brachiocephalic vein and superior vena cava.

NEOPLASTIC DISEASE

THYROID

Extension of a goitre into the mediastinum may cause a considerable mass and tracheal compromise. The masses often contain calcifications, and may have been present for many years (**Fig. 1.89**). Sudden enlargement in a goitre may result from cystic degeneration or haemorrhage. Malignant thyroid lesions can also extend into the mediastinum, with either direct or metastatic spread.

THYMUS

Benign thymomas, sometimes associated with myasthenia gravis, thymic cysts, and malignant thymomas, cause anterior mediastinal masses that, if large enough, become visible on a chest radiograph (**Figs 1.90a** and **1.90b**). As for all mediastinal 'mass' lesions, CT (or MR imaging) is the best method of investigation.

TERATODERMOIDS

The spectrum of these embryonic rest tumours varies from a benign dermoid containing well-defined tissues such as fat, hair, cartilage, and teeth, to invasive, undifferentiated teratomas. Germ cell tumours secreting hormones such as alphafetoprotein and human chorionic gonadotrophin are malignant tumours (**Fig. 1.91**) and form part of the 'teratoma' group, according to some authorities.

POSTERIOR MEDIASTINAL TUMOURS

In the posterior mediastinum, the important group of tumours are those related to the nervous system, including the sympathetic chain. Neuroenteric cysts (**Figs 1.92a** and **1.92b**) are one of the recognized causes of posterior mediastinal masses. Neural tumours are closely related to the vertebrae, and may involve the spinal canal. A neurofibroma may be dumb-bell shaped, cause widening of its exit foramen, and splay the adjacent ribs (**Fig. 1.93**). A ganglion cell tumour—either a benign ganglioneuroma or its malignant counterpart, a neuroblastoma—may give rise to similar posterior mediastinal masses. A phaeochromocytoma can also, rarely, be situated in the posterior mediastinum.

INTERVENTIONAL PROCEDURES

The majority of anterior mediastinal mass lesions are accessible to biopsy via CT control, histological evidence often being preferable to fine-needle aspiration, particularly in the staging of lymphomas. Some central lesions, particularly in the subcarinal area, pose more problems, as access may be across a lung; nevertheless, cytological specimens are often obtainable even from these difficult areas.

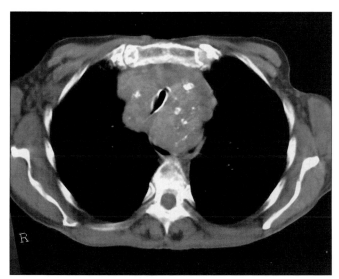

Fig. 1.89 *A thyroid mass, causing deviation and compression of the trachea in the upper mediastinum.*

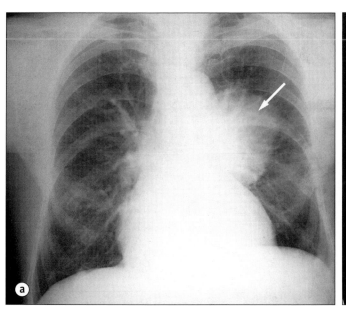
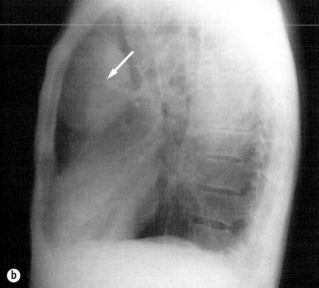

Fig. 1.90 (*a* and *b*) *Lobulated anterior mediastinal mass (arrows), biopsy-proven thymoma.*

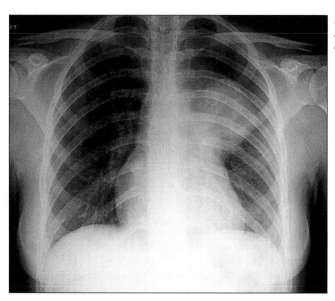

Fig. 1.91 Anterior mediastinal mass projected to the left side in a 23-year-old female patient. This was identified as a germ-cell tumour on biopsy.

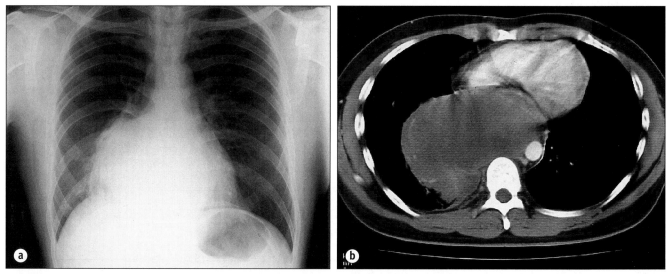

Fig. 1.92 (**a** and **b**) Posterior neuroenteric tumour: a soft-tissue mass projected over the right heart border. CT scan (**b**) shows a large, 15 × 10-cm cystic mass arising from the posterior mediastinum, displacing the opacified descending aorta to the left, and indenting the posterior aspect of the heart. Sarcomatous change in a neuroenteric cyst was proven histologically.

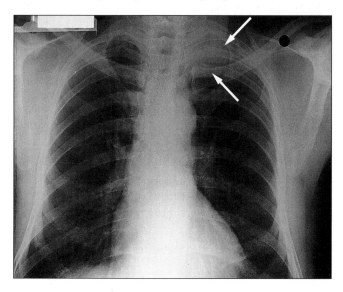

Fig. 1.93 Neurofibroma: a well-defined rounded opacity at the left apex (arrows).

chapter 2

Cardiovascular System

CONGENITAL ABNORMALITIES

DEFINITIONS

Some basic definitions help in the understanding of congenital heart disease:

- **Situs:** relating to the side or site.
- **Situs solitus:** the normal side for structures; e.g. in most people the heart is to the left, the spleen to the left, the liver to the right, etc. This term is rarely used today.
- **Situs inversus:** the mirror image of the normal. It may be total, or only certain organs may be affected; e.g. the heart may be on the right, but the liver in the normal position on the right also.
- **Laevocardia:** left-sided heart (normal).
- **Dextrocardia:** right-sided heart (abnormal).
- **Concordance:** correct relationship of structures and connections; e.g. the left atrium is connected to the left ventricle and the right atrium to the right ventricle.
- **Discordance:** structures incorrectly connected, e.g. left atrium to right ventricle (as in one form of transposition).

NEONATAL CIRCULATION

At birth, expansion of the lungs reduces the pulmonary vascular resistance, thereby causing an increase in pulmonary blood flow. The patent foramen ovale now closes because of the increased left atrial pressure. The ductus arteriosus also closes during the first 24 hours; this is secondary to increased oxygen saturation.

SHUNTS
Atrial septal defects

Three types of atrial septal defect (ASD) are recognized, depending on the position of the defect in the interatrial septum: secundum defects, primum defects, and sinus venosus abnormalities.

The size of the shunt is calculated depending on the amount of blood passing from the left side of the heart to the right. Classification of a shunt as '3 to 1' denotes that three times the amount of blood is pumped by the right heart than by the left heart. The bigger the defect, the larger the shunt.

Another important rule of cardiac physiology is that increased volume in a heart chamber causes that chamber to be dilated, whereas increased pressure causes hypertrophy. Thus, with an ASD, there is increased volume in the right heart and pulmonary arteries as a result of the left-to-right shunt at atrial level; an example is shown in **Fig. 2.1**. Eventually, increased flow in the pulmonary circulation leads to pulmonary arterial hypertension (*see* page 16). As the pulmonary pressure increases, it may become equal to or even greater than the systemic pressure, resulting in a reversed right-to-left shunt and hence cyanosis. This is known as Eisenmenger's complex, and may occur in any form of shunt (**Fig. 2.2**).

The various forms of shunt are very non-specific in appearance on chest radiographs, and other forms of imaging are required to demonstrate the internal cardiac anatomy. Echocardiography using non-invasive, high-frequency (3–10 MHz) ultrasound gives clear views of intracardiac anatomy and, combined with Doppler techniques, allows measurement of blood flow, velocity, and pressure within the heart and great vessels.

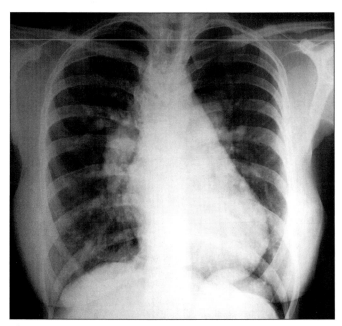

Fig. 2.1 Atrial septal defect. Cardiomegaly with marked dilatation of the main pulmonary arteries and peripheral pruning in a 24-year-old patient with a secundum atrial septal defect. Pulmonary artery pressure was only slightly increased.

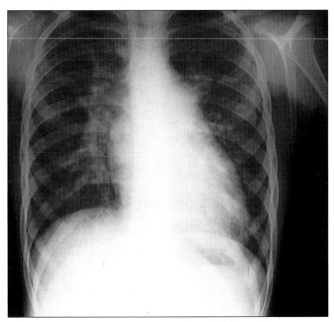

Fig. 2.2 Eisenmenger's complex. Atrial septal defect with severe pulmonary arterial hypertension. Pulmonary pressure equalled systemic pressure.

Ventricular septal defects

Ventricular septal defects (VSDs) are broadly divided into two types: those occurring in the membranous part of the septum at the base of the heart, and those in the muscular part of the septum. The chest radiograph appearances are often unremarkable, and may show only minor abnormalities.

Patent ductus arteriosus

Patent ductus arteriosus (PDA) represents the third main left-to-right shunt and is seen in particular in premature babies (**Fig. 2.3**). The drug indomethacin may be used to close the duct in babies, but surgery or interventional radiological techniques may also be necessary. Occasionally, a patent ductus arteriosus remains undetected in childhood and presents late in life, often with heart failure.

Atrioventricular septal defects

Atrioventricular septal defects (AVSDs) occur as large defects in both the atrial and ventricular septa, allowing communication between all four cardiac chambers, often with clefts in the atrioventricular valves, causing regurgitation (**Fig. 2.4**). This condition is seen commonly in babies with Down's syndrome.

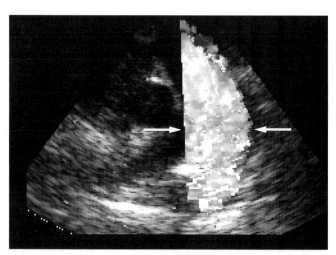

Fig. 2.3 *Patent ductus arteriosus shown by abnormal velocity jets in the main pulmonary artery (arrows).*

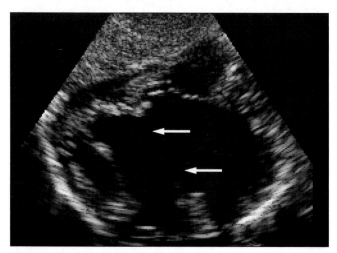

Fig. 2.4 *Echocardiogram demonstrating a large atrioventricular septal defect, with communication between all four cardiac chambers (arrows). Note the absence of the proximal interventricular septum and primum atrial septum. The tricuspid and mitral valves are separate.*

TETRALOGY OF FALLOT

Right ventricular hypertrophy, pulmonary stenosis, aortic over-ride, and a ventricular septal defect comprise the four features of tetralogy of Fallot. The chest radiograph shows pulmonary oligaemia, and an abnormally shaped heart (**Fig. 2.5**). Echocardiography confirms the defects.

TRANSPOSITION OF THE GREAT ARTERIES

If the aorta arises from the right ventricle and the pulmonary artery from the left ventricle, then transposition of the great arteries (TGA) exists. Unless there is either a congenital shunt defect or a man-made atrial defect (Rashind septostomy), TGA is incompatible with life, because two completely separate circulations exist. *In utero*, with the fetal circulation, the heart develops normally; the defect presents as an acute emergency a few hours after birth, when the ductus arteriosus closes.

HYPOPLASTIC LEFT-HEART SYNDROME

Underdevelopment of the entire left heart, including the ascending aorta and arch, results in the hypoplastic left-heart syndrome (HLHS). Most babies with this condition die within the first few days of life, after the ductus arteriosus has closed, as there is no significant systemic circulation.

CONDITIONS CAUSING CYANOSIS IN THE FIRST WEEK OF LIFE

Conditions associated with increased pulmonary vascularity include TGA, anomalous pulmonary venous drainage with obstruction, truncus arteriosus, single ventricle, and other rare forms of congenital heart disease. If the pulmonary vascularity is reduced, conditions such as pulmonary and tricuspid atresia may be present.

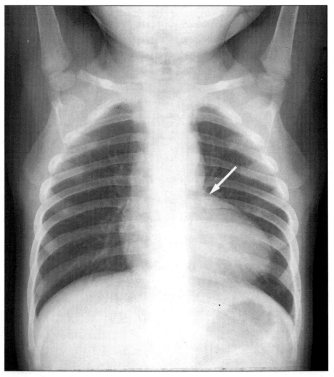

Fig. 2.5 *Tetralogy of Fallot. The heart is prominent and boot-shaped, with absent pulmonary conus and an increased angle at the aortopulmonary window in the upper left heart border (arrow). Pulmonary oligaemia is present.*

CONDITIONS CAUSING HEART FAILURE IN THE FIRST WEEK OF LIFE

HLHS, TGA, and critical aortic or pulmonary stenosis may result in early heart failure. Birth asphyxia with myocardial damage, and arrhythmias with tachycardia also present with heart failure early in life.

ELASTIC TISSUE DISORDERS

Ehlers–Danlos syndrome, cutis laxa, Marfan's cystic medial necrosis, and other disorders may cause abnormalities of the vascular tree, and are usually manifested by dilatation, with abnormal wall dynamics.

Marfan's disease causes dilatation of the ascending aorta with dissection that may be a presenting feature. Monitoring of the aortic diameter by ultrasound is recommended in patients with Marfan's syndrome and in members of their family.

COARCTATION OF THE AORTA

There are two forms of coarctation: preductal and postductal. Coarctation causes increased blood pressure in the ascending aorta and arch. The clinical condition and radiological signs depend on the severity of the coarctation. **Figure 2.6** shows examples of the condition. The MR images (**Figs 2.6a** and **2.6b**) are of a child and the chest radiograph (**Fig. 2.6c**) demonstrates an abnormal configuration of the aortic arch and bilateral rib notching. The notching is caused by reversed flow in dilated intercostal arteries, as a result of collateral circulation to the distal aorta.

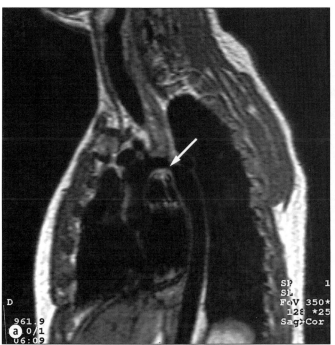

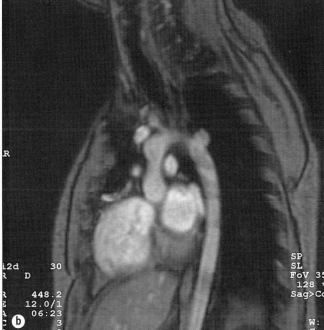

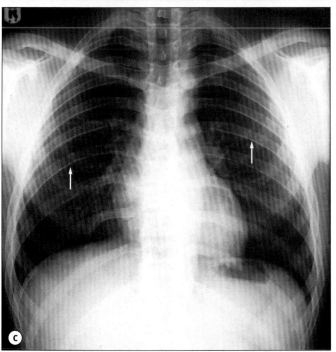

Fig. 2.6 (a) T1-weighted oblique sagittal MR image showing an aorta with coarctation (arrow). (b) Cine MRA of the same patient. (c) Chest radiograph of a patient with long-standing coarctation of the aorta. There is rib notching bilaterally (arrows), with an abnormal aortic knuckle and poststenotic dilatation distal to the coarctation.

TRAUMA

Deceleration injuries to the thoracic aorta are considered in the section on mediastinal disorders (*see* page 29). Blunt and penetrating injuries to the heart can occur, with cardiac rupture, acute haemorrhagic pericardial effusion, myocardial contusion, and valve damage. Direct stab wounds may lacerate the heart with immediate fatality but, occasionally, rapid surgical repair may be possible and life saving.

Direct injury to the peripheral vessels also may result from penetrating wounds from knives, bullets, or sharp objects (**Fig. 2.7**). The damage may cause laceration and haemorrhage, occlusion, false aneurysm formation, or arteriovenous fistulae. Arterial damage may occasionally be iatrogenic, after femoral artery catheterization, when all the above may occur. Some arterial damage, for example in pelvic trauma, may be so severe as to be potentially fatal; urgent arteriography and embolization may then be necessary.

Compression of vascular structures as a result of trauma may result in ischaemia to the area supplied. Such features are seen with displaced supracondylar fractures of the humerus with brachial artery compression, and in compartment syndromes in the lower leg.

INFECTION

CARDIAC INFECTION

Infection may affect the endocardium (endocarditis), the myocardium (myocarditis), or the pericardium (pericarditis).

Endocarditis

In endocarditis, vegetations usually form on the heart valves. Often, the aortic or the mitral valve is affected, but lesions on the right heart valves are being seen increasingly, particularly in drug abusers.

Lesions also occur at the site of congenital heart defects, and in patients with pacemakers, central venous catheters, and prosthetic heart valves. Diagnosis is made by echocardiography, often with transoesophageal techniques.

Myocarditis

Infections of the myocardium, often viral, cause reduced muscle function. This leads to a dilated cardiomyopathy and, if severe, to heart failure. Diagnosis is usually by echocardiography and measurement of viral titres, but cardiac biopsy is necessary occasionally. The chest radiograph shows a large heart, often with left ventricular failure, and pulmonary oedema.

BLOOD-VESSEL INFECTIONS
Syphilis

In syphilis, an endarteritis obliterans of the vasa vasorum results in destruction of the elastic tissue, causing dilatation of, in particular, the ascending aorta (**Fig. 2.8**). The aortic wall may calcify, and there is often aortic regurgitation.

Mycotic aneurysms

A rare complication of an aneurysm, often abdominal, is infection with *Staphylococcus*, *Streptococcus* or *Salmonella* (**Fig. 2.9**).

INFLAMMATORY CONDITIONS

CARDIAC (CARDIOMYOPATHIES)

Three main types of cardiomyopathy are recognized: hypertrophic, dilated (congestive), and restrictive. Some are inflammatory, but others are not. However, whatever the aetiology, the end results are similar, therefore the diseases will be considered together here.

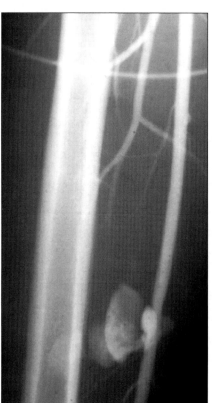

Fig. 2.7 *Laceration of the superficial femoral artery as a result of a stab wound.*

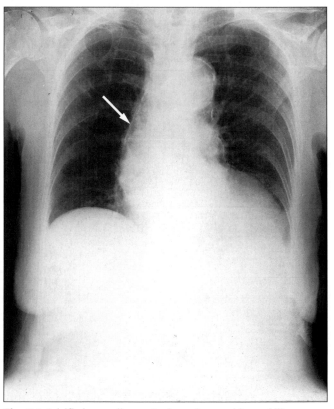

Fig. 2.8 *Calcified ascending aorta (arrow) caused by syphilis.*

Hypertrophic cardiomyopathy

The majority of cases of hypertrophic cardiomyopathy are familial, but sporadic cases do occur. The natural history of the disease is ill understood, and it may present at birth or as late as the eighth or ninth decade of life. Sudden death, often early in life, is one unfortunate method of presentation. Echocardiography reveals a hypertrophied septum, a slit-like left ventricle, abnormal mitral valve movements, and a variable degree of obstruction of the left ventricular outflow tract (**Fig. 2.10**).

Dilated cardiomyopathy

Dilated cardiomyopathy has a wide aetiology, ranging from infective myocarditis to connective tissue disorders, alcohol abuse, and neuro-muscular conditions such as Friedreich's ataxia. Whatever the cause, the heart dilates, cardiac output is reduced, and ventricular failure often intervenes. The chest radiograph may show cardiac enlargement with left heart failure. The echocardiogram shows bilateral ventricular

dilatation, global reduction in left ventricular function with a low ejection fraction, and atrioventricular valve regurgitation as a result of the ventricular dilatation.

Restrictive cardiomyopathy

Amyloid infiltration of the myocardium produces a restrictive cardio-myopathy—amyloidosis—characterized by a 'stiff' ventricle with reduced compliance, and poor ventricular filling on echocardiography. The amyloid deposits, particularly in the interventricular septum, produce bright echogenic 'spots' that are more or less characteristic (**Fig. 2.11**).

Other restrictive forms of cardiomyopathy occur in endomyo-cardial fibrosis (particularly affecting children in subtropical Africa), sarcoidosis, and Loeffler's eosinophilic endocarditis.

VASCULAR (VASCULITIDES)
Polyarteritis nodosa

Polyarteritis nodosa (PAN) is a necrotizing vasculitis of the small and medium-sized arteries, particularly of the kidney and gut. Arteriography may reveal multiple small aneurysms.

Churg–Strauss syndrome

Necrotizing vasculitis is the vascular feature that, together with respiratory features, characterizes the uncommon Churg–Strauss syndrome (*see* page 16).

Henoch–Schönlein purpura

The hypersensitivity reaction known as Henoch–Schönlein purpura, often seen in children, may be seen occasionally as haemorrhagic oedema in the bowel wall or in the colon on barium follow-through examination.

Takayasu's arteritis

Takayasu's arteritis is an inflammatory condition causing areas of narrowing of large blood vessels, particularly the aorta (**Fig. 2.12**). It is most commonly seen in girls or young women, and is variable in its extent and severity.

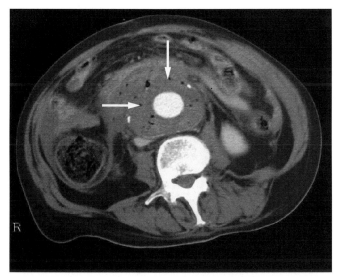

Fig. 2.9 *CT scan of an inflammatory aneurysm of the abdominal aorta. Multiple gas shadows are present throughout the inflammatory mass (arrows).*

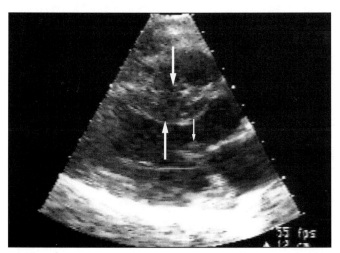

Fig. 2.10 *Hypertrophic obstructive cardiomyopathy. This long-axis echocardiogram through the left ventricle demonstrates increased septal thickening (arrows), with abnormal configuration of the anterior leaflet of the mitral valve (small arrow).*

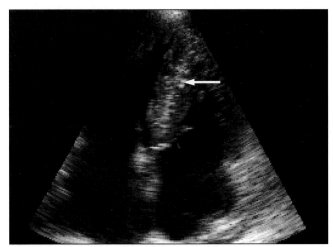

Fig. 2.11 *Amyloidosis, with increased echogenicity of the interventricular septum on echocardiography (arrow).*

Kawasaki's disease (mucocutaneous lymph-node syndrome)

The incidence of Kawasaki's disease in the western world is increasing. Its significance lies in one of its complications, the development of coronary artery aneurysms, that occurs in about 13% of all cases (**Fig. 2.13**).

Buerger's disease (thromboangiitis obliterans)

Buerger's disease is an occlusive peripheral vascular disorder, usually occurring in men younger than 40 years and related to smoking. Occlusion of the arteries, particularly in the legs, may require intravascular thrombolytic treatment or surgical intervention (thromboembolectomy or bypass procedures), or both. Occasionally, amputation of the limb is necessary.

VENOUS ABNORMALITIES
Deep venous thrombosis

Deep venous thromboses (DVTs) are very common, occurring in about 25% of all hospital surgical patients. They may be asymptomatic or symptomatic; the majority are limited to the calf veins and cause only minimal problems. The most important consequence of a DVT is pulmonary embolism, which is a major cause of morbidity and mortality.

The diagnosis of a DVT is often difficult clinically, but it can be reliably revealed by Doppler ultrasound or venography (**Figs 2.14a** and **2.14b**, respectively). Documentation of possible extensions of the thrombus into the thigh and on into the pelvis and abdomen is important when treatment is being considered, because the more proximal to the heart the thrombus becomes, the greater the danger of pulmonary embolism. If risk of pulmonary embolism is noted, one preventive measure is to introduce a caval stent (**Fig. 2.15**) to act as a filter preventing transmission of thrombi.

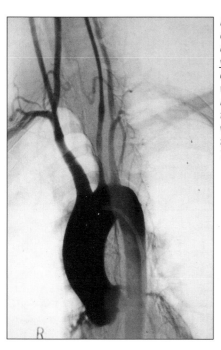

Fig. 2.12 Takayasu's arteritis. Oblique aortic arch angiogram in a young female demonstrating widespread areas of narrowing throughout the head and neck vessels consistent with the diagnosis of Takayasu's arteritis.

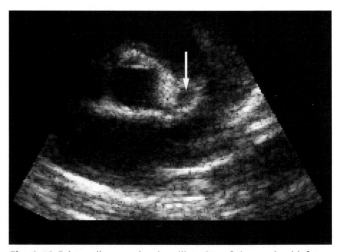

Fig. 2.13 Echocardiogram showing dilatation of the proximal left coronary artery (arrow) in a 4-month-old child who presented three weeks earlier with Kawasaki's disease.

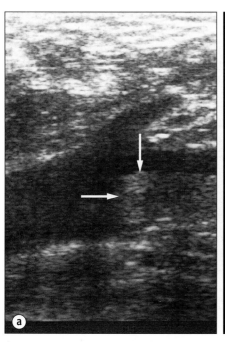
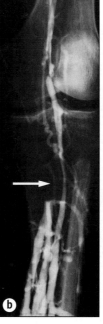
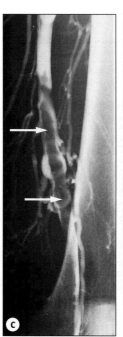
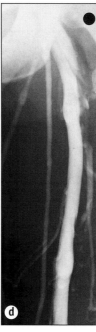

Fig. 2.14 Deep vein thrombosis. (a) Ultrasound image, showing femoral vein with no flow, distended with thrombus (arrows). (b–d) Lower limb venography demonstrates multiple filling defects in the calf veins and femoral vein (arrows).

NEOPLASTIC DISEASE

The most common myocardial tumours are secondary deposits from frequently occurring primary carcinomas such as those from the breast and the bronchus. They are rarely diagnosed during life, but are present in about 10% of patients who die from carcinomatosis. Secondary tumours that develop within the heart cavities are rare, more often affecting the right heart chambers than the left, and are produced by two different mechanisms. The first is either by direct growth of tumour along the systemic veins into the right heart chambers, or by direct invasion. The most common tumour spread in this way through the venous system is carcinoma of the kidney, which extends into the renal vein, thence through the inferior vena cava to the right atrium, and occasionally through to the right ventricle and beyond. Direct invasion into the left atrium may

occur with bronchial carcinoma. The second form of spread is by true metastatic disease; this also is usually confined to the right heart chambers. Germ-cell tumours are the most frequent of this rare form of secondary malignancy.

PRIMARY CARDIAC TUMOURS
Myxoma
Myxoma is the most common (but still rare) primary benign tumour of the heart, most frequently arising in the left atrium, from the left side of the interatrial septum (Fig. 2.16). This cardiac tumour may cause obstruction at atrial or valve level, thus acting as functional mitral stenosis. Patients may present with systemic manifestations such as fever, weight loss, and anaemia, or they may present with embolic phenomena.

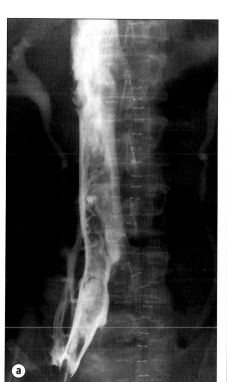 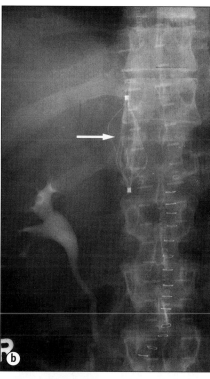

Fig. 2.15 (a) Inferior vena cavagram showing extensive thrombus from the right iliac vein extending to the proximal inferior vena cava. (b) Same patient after the positioning of an inferior vena caval filter (arrow).

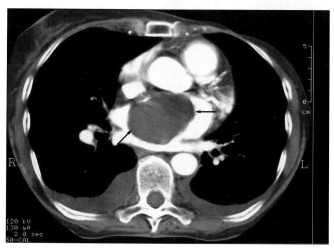

Fig. 2.16 This contrast-enhanced CT scan of a left atrial myxoma shows a large filling defect (small arrows) attached to the intra-atrial septum and filling most of the left atrium.

39

Rhabdomyoma

Rhabdomyomas are the most common primary cardiac tumour in children, 30% being associated with tuberous sclerosis. They may be single or multiple. They show on echocardiography as echo-bright lesions within the myocardium, intracavitary lesions being very rare (**Fig. 2.17**).

Fibroma

Fibromas are solitary tumours within the interventricular septum, sometimes associated with the naevoid basal-cell carcinoma syndrome.

Carcinoid diseases of the heart

Malignant gastrointestinal carcinoid tumours are associated with endocardial deposition of myofibromatous tissue, principally in the right heart valves, resulting in pulmonary and tricuspid stenoses.

Primary malignant cardiac tumours

Angiosarcomas and rhabdomyosarcomas account for the majority of primary malignant cardiac tumours; they comprise 20% of all primary cardiac tumours, the remaining 80% being the benign lesions as described above. There are no specific features to these tumours, which may metastasize and often are diagnosed only at autopsy.

BLOOD-VESSEL TUMOURS
Benign lesions
Haemangioma

Haemangiomas are the most common soft-tissue tissue tumours in childhood. They may be capillary, cavernous, arteriovenous, or venous. MR imaging is the best method of visualizing them.

Lymphangioma

Cystic hygromas occur mainly in the head and neck, are usually present at birth, and are associated with Turner's syndrome.

Maffucci's syndrome

The multiple enchondromatosis with soft-tissue tissue cavernous haemangiomas that represents Maffucci's syndrome shows characteristic bony lesions with soft-tissue masses containing calcified phleboliths (**Fig. 2.18**).

Klippel–Trenaunay syndrome

The overgrowth of the lower limb that occurs in Klippel–Trenaunay syndrome is associated with increased vascularity as a result of venous abnormalities and haemangiomas (**Fig. 2.19**).

Glomus tumour

Glomus tumour is a benign blood-vessel tumour often associated with the terminal phalanx of a finger.

Malignant lesions

All of the three following malignant tumours produce solid soft-tissue masses that have no specific features on imaging; the diagnosis often can be made definitively only by histological biopsy.

Haemangiopericytoma

Haemangiopericytoma is a variably aggressive tumour, often presenting in middle age, and affecting the lower limb and the retroperitoneum in the majority of cases.

Angiosarcoma

The rare but aggressive malignant lesion known as angiosarcoma occurs in a wide variety of sites, but is associated with chronic lymphoedema and thus may affect patients who have undergone mastectomy.

Kaposi's sarcoma

Kaposi's sarcoma is a soft-tissue tumour which, in one form, is associated with AIDS (**Fig. 2.20**).

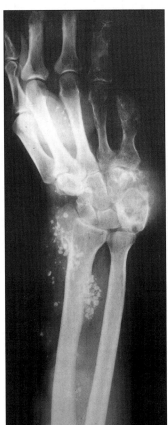

Fig. 2.18 Maffucci's syndrome. Multiple cartilage-based tumours in the hand and wrist associated with calcifications in the angiomatous malformations.

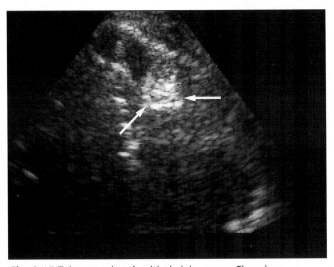

Fig. 2.17 Tuberous sclerosis with rhabdomyoma. There is an echogenic rhabdomyoma situated in the apex to the right ventricle in this child with tuberous sclerosis (arrows).

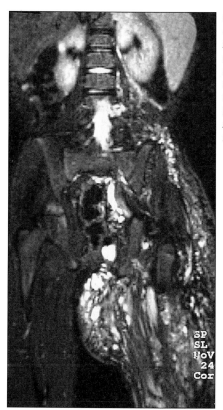

Fig. 2.19
Klippel–Trenaunay syndrome showing hypertrophy of the left lower limb and multiple dilated venous channels, revealed by coronal short tau inversion recovery MR imaging.

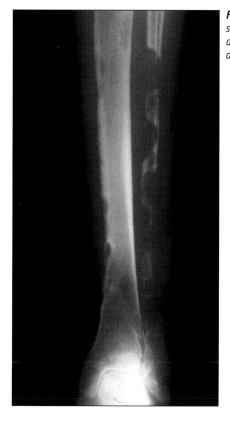

Fig. 2.20 *Kaposi's sarcoma, with multiple areas of bony destruction.*

DEGENERATIVE CONDITIONS

ATHEROSCLEROSIS
Ischaemic heart disease

Most of the imaging of ischaemic heart disease is concerned with the need to show the structure of the coronary arteries and their perfusion. The gold standard for coronary artery imaging (**Fig. 2.21**) remains the coronary arteriogram, radionuclide techniques being used for myocardial perfusion and function studies (**Fig. 2.22**). However, the technique of MR imaging of both coronary artery and coronary perfusion is developing rapidly and, being non-invasive, may eventually replace the more invasive investigations (**Fig. 2.23**).

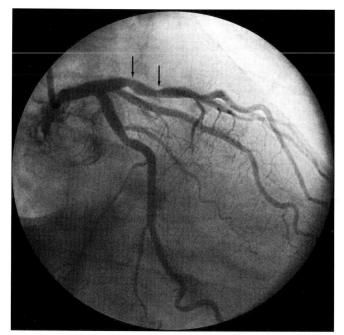

Fig. 2.21 *Coronary angiogram demonstrating areas of narrowing (arrows) in the left anterior descending artery.*

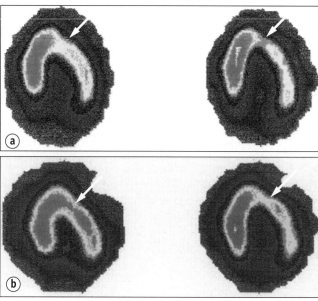

Fig. 2.22 *Cardiac nuclear medicine (radionuclide) scan. (a) Images acquired during stress show reduced perfusion of the lateral wall of the left ventricle (arrows) which resolves at rest (b) indicating reversible myocardial ischaemia.*

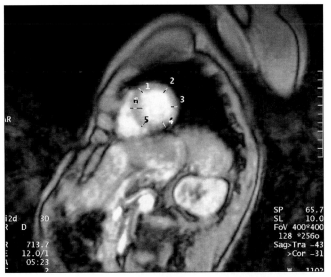

Fig. 2.23 *Cardiac MR image of the left ventricle wirth markers to assess wall thickness and movement during different phases of the cardiac cycle.*

Other imaging of ischaemic heart disease is concerned with demonstrating the consequences of the myocardial infarction that results from coronary artery disease. Complications, most of which are visible on either a chest radiograph or an echocardiogram, include left ventricular failure (**Fig. 2.24**), left ventricular dysfunction, mitral regurgitation, myocardial rupture either through the septum or into the pericardium, thrombus formation, and aneurysm. The autoimmune condition, Dressler's syndrome, develops between 1 and 6 weeks after an infarction; pericardial fluid may be visible on echocardiography.

Peripheral vascular disease

Atherosclerosis of the aorta and peripheral vessels causes atheromatous dilatation, leading to aneurysms (**Figs 2.25** and **2.26**) and areas of narrowing, with stenosis and occlusion. Clinically, these present with intermittent claudication, pain at rest, and gangrene. Investigation is by arteriography and Doppler ultrasound (**Figs 2.27** and **2.28**).

Aortic dissection

Aortic dissection is a life-threatening condition which occurs as a result of degeneration of the media of the aortic wall. An intimal tear allows arterial blood to track between the intima and adventitia, creating a false

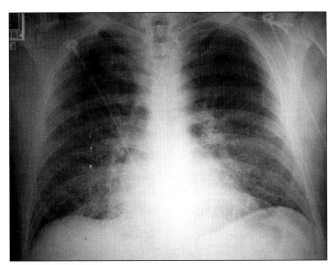

Fig. 2.24 *Chest radiograph of left ventricular failure, with cardiomegaly, upper lobe venous diversion, and interstitial pulmonary oedema.*

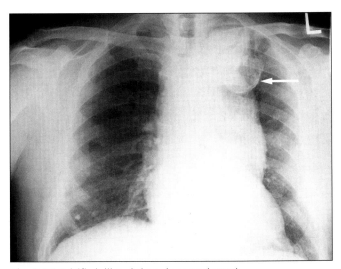

Fig. 2.25 *Calcified dilated thoracic aorta (arrow).*

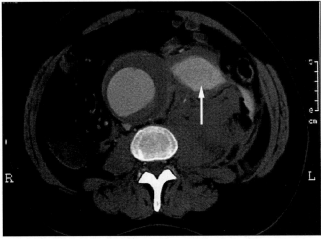

Fig. 2.26 *CT scan of a leaking abdominal aortic aneurysm, showing contrast extravasating into the retroperitoneal tissues (arrow).*

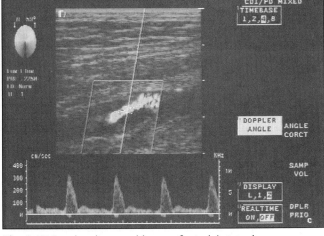

Fig. 2.27 *Doppler ultrasound image of arterial stenosis.*

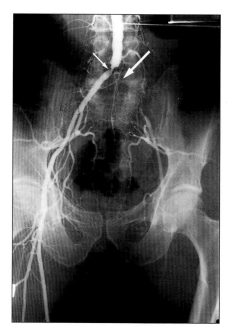

Fig. 2.28 Arteriogram demonstrating complete occlusion of the left common iliac artery (large arrow) and significant stenosis of the origin of the right common iliac artery (small arrow).

lumen (**Fig. 2.29**). Aortic dissections are classified as type I (dissection begins in the ascending aorta and extends round the arch to the descending aorta), type II (dissection is localized to the ascending aorta), or type III (dissection involves only the descending aorta). Arteries branching from the aorta may be occluded at their origins by a dissection.

VALVULAR HEART DISEASE
Aortic regurgitation

Aortic regurgitation (AI) may result from damage to the aortic leaflets or dilatation of the aortic valve ring in ascending aortic aneurysms. Whatever the aetiology, AI causes increased left ventricular end-diastolic volume and hence, sooner or later, left ventricular dilatation. The chest radiograph may show left ventricular enlargement.

Aortic stenosis

Aortic stenosis (AS) may be congenital or may be acquired, either after a rheumatic condition or in the elderly, by degeneration of the cusps, with commissural fusion. The resulting narrow valve causes an increase in left ventricular systolic pressure, resulting in hypertrophy. The early stages of hypertrophy are not visible on a chest radiograph, but can be measured accurately by echocardiography (**Fig. 2.30**); however, the chest radiograph may show poststenotic dilatation of the ascending aorta.

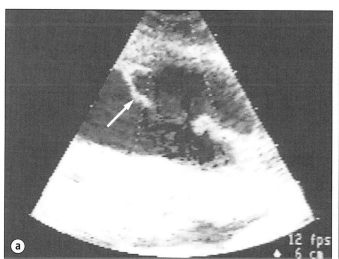

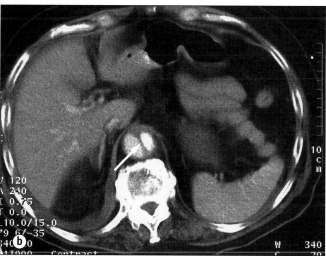

Fig. 2.29 (**a**) Transoesophageal echocardiogram of the proximal thoracic aorta, showing dissection flap (arrow). (**b**) CT scan, with contrast, of a dissection of lower thoracic and abdominal aortae. Both true and false lumens are shown, divided by an intimal flap (arrow).

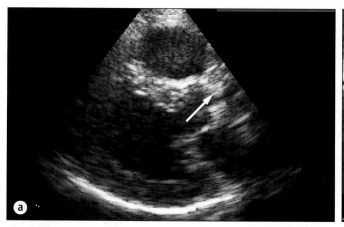

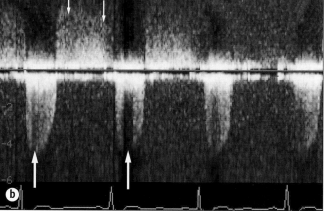

Fig. 2.30 Echocardiogram of aortic stenosis. (**a**) Long axis parasternal view of the left heart showing calcific aortic valve disease (arrow). (**b**) Doppler echocardiogram from the left ventricular apex demonstrating significant aortic stenosis with a high velocity jet into the ascending aorta, the gradient being 80 mmHg (large arrows). There is also evidence of some aortic regurgitation (small arrows).

Mitral regurgitation

Any dilatation of the atrioventricular valve ring results in mitral regurgitation. Other causes include prolapse of one or both leaflets, papillary muscle dysfunction and, rarely, chordal rupture. Depending on the severity of the condition, there is variable left ventricular and left atrial dilatation, best demonstrated on echocardiography. Chest radiography may show dilatation of both left heart chambers, together with pulmonary venous hypertension, which is a frequent accompaniment of mitral regurgitation (**Fig. 2.31**). In long-standing mitral valve disease, pulmonary hypertension can lead to the

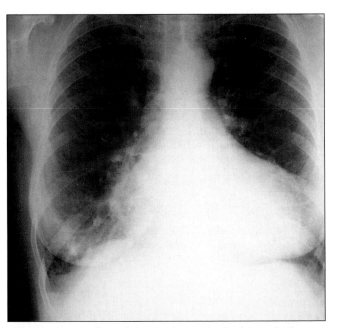

Fig. 2.31 Chest radiograph in a patient with mitral regurgitation, showing cardiac enlargement, upper lobe pulmonary venous diversion, and interstitial pulmonary oedema.

development of ossified nodules in the lungs (**Fig. 2.32**).

Mitral stenosis

The classical postrheumatic mitral stenosis is shown on the chest radiograph (**Fig. 2.33**) by subtle left atrial enlargement, often with upper lobe pulmonary venous blood diversion; the latter feature is a manifestation of pulmonary venous hypertension. On the echocardiograph, fusion of the commissures is seen to result in a reduced mitral valve orifice; this is shown on Doppler and by cross-sectional imaging.

Right heart valves

Valve lesions are less common in the right heart than the left, but have the same consequences as those described above. The causes of the valve diseases do vary, however, with inclusion of such conditions as carcinoid and drug-induced valve damage.

INTERVENTIONAL PROCEDURES

Catheters of varying sizes may be placed in the arterial system, most often through the femoral artery, for the purposes of injecting contrast medium for diagnostic arteriography, embolization, angioplasty, removal of intravascular foreign bodies, and thrombolytic therapy.

ANGIOPLASTY

Balloon angioplasty is a method of increasing the size of the lumen of an artery that is narrowed by atheroma or, occasionally, by other conditions such as fibromuscular hyperplasia. Inflation of the balloon under pressure dilates the vessel, but may cause tearing of the intima and localized dissection (**Fig. 2.34**).

STENTING

The insertion of metallic stents into arteries and veins has been practised for some years. Success rates for long-term patency are improving as a result of better stent technology and the availability of smaller stent delivery systems (**Fig. 2.35**).

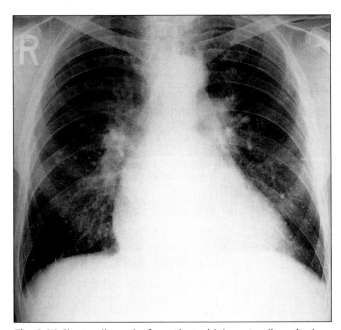

Fig. 2.32 Chest radiograph of a patient with long-standing mitral valve disease, with ossified pulmonary nodules.

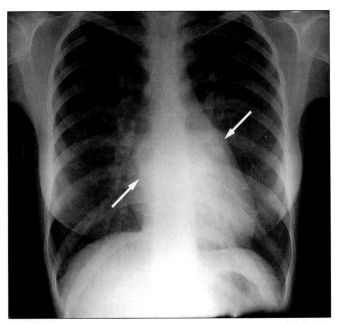

Fig. 2.33 Chest radiograph of a patient with mitral stenosis with left atrial enlargement (arrows), demonstrating upper lobe pulmonary venous diversion and mild interstitial pulmonary oedema.

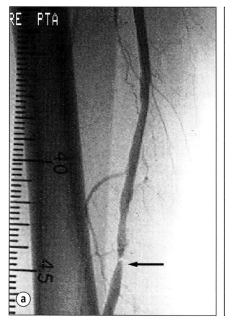

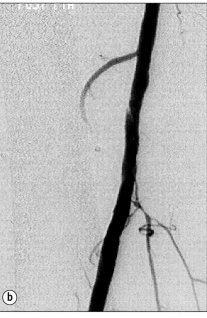

Fig. 2.34 (a) IADSA of a stenosed right superficial femoral artery *(arrow)*. *(b)* Appearance of the artery after angioplasty.

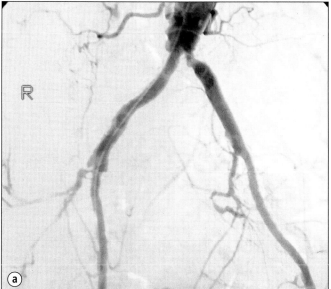

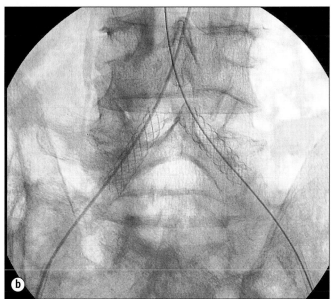

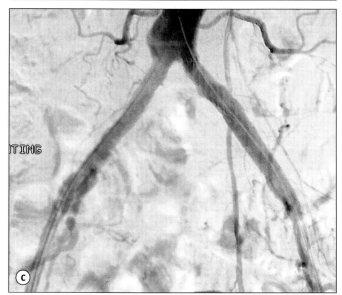

Fig. 2.35 IADSA of iliac arteries *(a)* before insertion of stents. *(b)* Position of common iliac stents bilaterally. *(c)* Post-stent angiogram demonstrating markedly improved flow and reduction in stenoses.

EMBOLIZATION

Embolization to stop bleeding or reduce tumour vascularity may involve the use of one of three types of agent: liquids such as alcohol; particulates such as gel foam (**Fig. 2.36**), and solids such as coils and balloons. Fistulae can also be closed with detachable coils or balloons, and a patent ductus arteriosus can be obliterated with an umbrella-like device (**Fig. 2.37**).

THROMBOLYSIS

Thrombus that is occluding an artery or vein can be lysed by the injection of drugs such as streptokinase, urokinase, or recombinant tissue plasminogen activator. Best results are obtained if the thrombus is fresh and the thrombolytic drug is injected directly into it through a carefully positioned catheter (**Fig. 2.38**).

DISEASES OF THE PERICARDIUM

CONGENITAL

Partial or complete absence of the pericardium may be associated with other congenital heart defects, or be an isolated finding.

Total absence of the pericardium is very rare, the most common lesion being a partial left-sided defect that may impart a characteristic shape to the heart on a chest radiograph (**Fig. 2.39**).

Benign pericardial (or springwater) cysts often are asymptomatic, occur at the right cardiophrenic angle, and cause problems only if they are large and compressive, or become infected (*see* Fig. 1.84).

PERICARDITIS AND PERICARDIAL EFFUSION

Inflammation of the pericardium, arising from infection or any one of

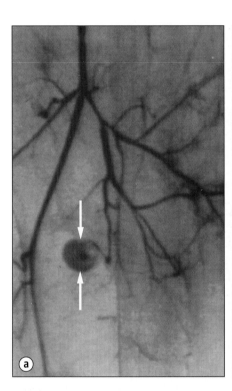
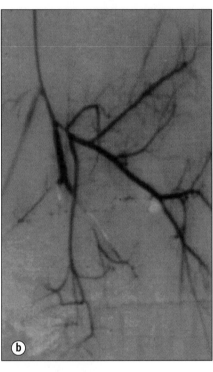

Fig. 2.36 *(a) False aneurysm arising from a branch of the profunda femoris artery as a result of a stab wound (arrows). (b) After embolization using a gelatine sponge, there is complete obliteration of the false aneurysm.*

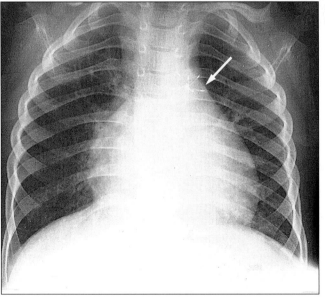

Fig. 2.37 *Closure of patent ductus arteriosus by means of an 'umbrella' device (arrow).*

a number of causes, results in abnormal pericardial surfaces, often with the production of fluid. Both acute and chronic infections may cause such pericarditis accompanied by pericardial effusion. Coxsackie B virus is one of the most common infections; tuberculous infection, although uncommon, is important because one of the long-term sequelae is chronic constrictive pericarditis.

Patients with pericarditis have a normal chest radiograph; even when considerable amounts of fluid are present in the pericardial sac, the heart shadow may, unhelpfully, appear normal. The diagnosis of a pericardial effusion is therefore made by echocardiography (**Fig. 2.40**), with which it is possible to gauge the amount of fluid present and, more importantly, its effect on the heart. However, very large pericardial effusions are visible on a chest radiograph, giving the cardiac outline a globular shape (**Fig. 2.41**).

Cardiac tamponade occurs when the pressure in the pericardial cavity is greater than the internal right heart pressure, causing compression of the right atrium and right ventricle, preventing systemic venous return, and so reducing cardiac output. Relief by aspiration and drainage is a relatively simple technique; it should be performed under direct ultrasonic guidance, to avoid complications. The development of tamponade depends not only on the amount of fluid present in the pericardial cavity, but also on the rate of accumulation of the fluid, the distensibility of the pericardium, and the presence or otherwise of underlying cardiac abnormality.

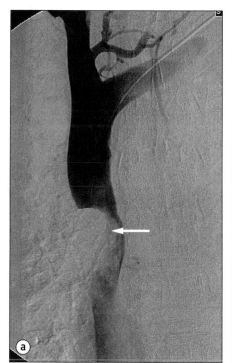
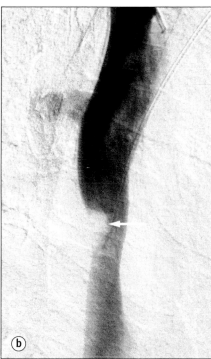

Fig. 2.38 (a) After small bowel resection this patient, who was receiving total parenteral nutrition via a central catheter, developed complete thrombosis of the superior vena cava (arrow), revealed on central venography. *(b)* After thrombolysis with streptokinase, the thrombus has significantly reduced in size (arrow), restoring venous return to the right side of the heart.

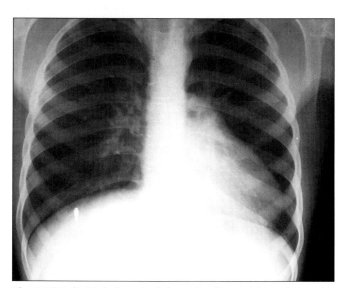

Fig. 2.39 Left-sided absence of the pericardium, with an abnormal contour to the left side of the heart.

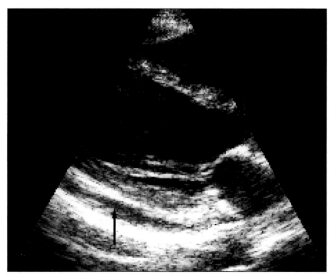

Fig. 2.40 Echocardiogram of a pericardial effusion (arrow).

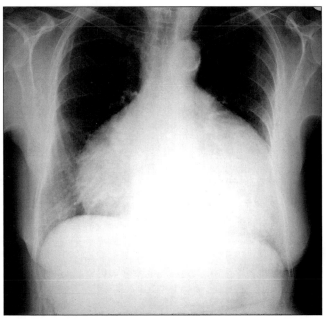

Fig. 2.41 Chest radiograph of a large pericardial effusion, showing the characteristic globular cardiac outline.

CHRONIC CONSTRICTIVE PERICARDITIS

When healing of an acute fibrous pericarditis occurs, or when a chronic pericardial effusion resolves, the pericardial space may become obliterated. The resulting fibrous sac envelops the heart, restricting its filling and contraction, which results in chronic cardiac impairment and right heart failure. The pericardium may be heavily calcified, as is seen particularly after tuberculous pericarditis but also in posthaemorrhagic conditions, radiation effects, postviral conditions and many other aetologies (**Fig. 2.42**). The method of choice for investigating the pericardium is now MR imaging, which has the ability to show minor degrees of pericardium thickening, not visible on any other imaging technique.

PERICARDIAL TUMOURS

The most common tumour involving the pericardial cavity is carcinoma of the bronchus with direct invasion. Secondary spread from breast, and bronchial malignancies may also occur, but primary tumours such as mesothelioma are rare. Most tumours, either primary or secondary, cause a pericardial effusion that is frequently heavily blood-stained, therefore cytological examination of any such aspirate is often diagnostic for malignancy.

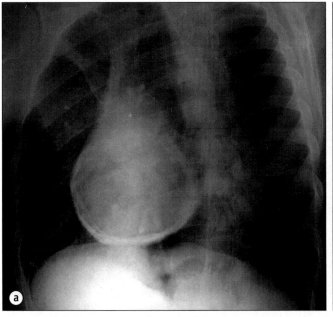

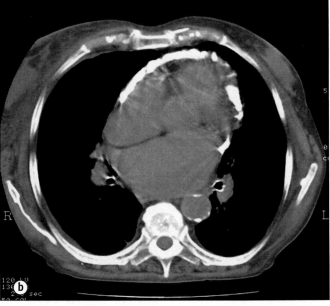

Fig. 2.42 (a) Oblique chest radiograph of chronic constrictive pericarditis, with heavy calcification of the pericardium. **(b)** CT scan of a patient with chronic constrictive pericarditis with anterior and lateral pericardial calcification.

chapter 3

Gastrointestinal System

Barium radiographic studies and endoscopy provide the main methods of investigating the gastrointestinal (GI) tract. Both have strengths and weaknesses and provide complementary information. Barium studies are relatively inexpensive and quick to perform, are better than endoscopy at demonstrating strictures and fistulae, but have the disadvantage of involving ionizing radiation. Endoscopy gives better visualization of the mucosa, and enables biopsy of any pathology. Endoscopic treatment is possible sometimes; for example, removal of polyps and injection sclerotherapy of oesophageal varices are both performed endoscopically.

Plain films are important in the diagnosis of GI obstruction and perforation. Ultrasound is used in the diagnosis of certain GI abnormalities in childhood, particularly pyloric stenosis, and can show ascites and peritoneal abscesses. CT scanning is used widely in staging of GI malignancies, and is being applied increasingly in the investigation of elderly patients for cancer of the colon.

CONGENITAL AND NEONATAL ABNORMALITIES

ATRESIAS
Oesophageal atresia

Oesophageal atresia can be diagnosed antenatally (*see* Chapter 6) in the 30% of cases in which there is polyhydramnios and absence of a fluid-filled stomach. Postnatally, the infants exhibit choking during feeding, drooling, and respiratory distress as a result of aspiration; they usually have at least one associated tracheo-oesophageal fistula (TOF). Neonatal surgery is required.

Oesophageal atresia is classified into different types according to the presence or absence of a TOF, and its site. Chest radiographs show an oblong lucency in the superior mediastinum, which is the dilated oesophagus proximal to the atretic segment; contrast studies are required to demonstrate the site of a TOF. The most common type, accounting for about 80% of cases, is oesophageal atresia with a TOF to the distal oesophagus. Plain films show gas within the GI tract when there is a TOF to the distal oesophagus or an H-shaped fistula to both proximal and distal oesophageal segments (**Fig. 3.1**). In the absence of a TOF, or when the fistula is to the proximal oesophagus, there is no abdominal gas.

Duodenal atresia

One-third of cases of duodenal atresia are associated with Down's syndrome; a further 20% of cases of duodenal stenosis or atresia are associated with an annular pancreas. The diagnosis can be suspected antenatally if a dilated and fluid-filled stomach and proximal duodenum are seen. Postnatally, this 'double bubble' sign can be seen on a plain film, with gas filling the dilated stomach and proximal duodenum (**Fig. 3.2**).

Small bowel atresia

Duodenal and ileal atresia or stenosis can be multiple; patients present with abdominal distension and vomiting. Plain films show various degrees of small bowel dilatation, depending on the site of the atresia (**Fig. 3.3**).

Imperforate anus

This is a complex group of congenital anomalies which are divided broadly into high and low types. The high type of imperforate anus involves rectal atresia above the level of the levator ani muscles, whereas with the low type the rectum extends inferior to the levator

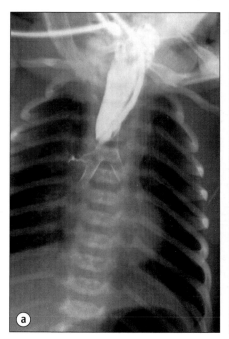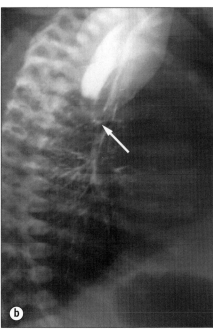

Fig. 3.1 (**a**) *Oesophageal atresia and tracheo-oesophageal fistulae (anteroposterior view). Contrast outlines the proximal oesophageal segment as far as the level of the atresia. A tracheo-oesophageal fistula is present. Because there is gas in the stomach, there must also be a fistula to the lower oesophageal segment.* (**b**) *Lateral view in the same patient, showing the site of the tracheo-oesophageal fistula (arrow).*

muscles. There may be associated fistulae into the urethra in boys or the vagina in girls. The differentiation between high and low types is important in determining the type of surgery undertaken: high types require a defunctioning colostomy before corrective surgery later in infancy, whereas the low type can be managed with an anoplasty.

Plain films may reveal a dilated colon and rectum. A lateral film is taken with the infant prone, the anal skin identified with a radio-opaque marker, and the pelvis elevated (**Fig. 3.4**). Ultrasound can demonstrate echogenic meconium in the distal rectal pouch. If this is less than 10 mm from the anal skin, then the lesion is a low type, but if the distance from the skin to the rectal pouch is greater than 10 mm, the lesion is likely to be a high type and further imaging is required. MRI is useful in evaluating the levator muscle sling, and can

help predict whether surgical reconstruction is likely to achieve continence. Water-soluble contrast studies are performed to identify the sites of fistulae.

Gastric and colonic atresias are rare.

OTHER CAUSES OF NEONATAL GASTROINTESTINAL OBSTRUCTION
Midgut malrotation

During normal embryological development, the midgut herniates out of the fetal abdomen and, as it returns, undergoes a complex rotational procedure, effectively rotating anticlockwise by 270° around the axis of the superior mesenteric artery. Thus the normal final position of the midgut has the duodenal loop on the right side of the abdomen, with the duodenojejunal flexure in the left upper quadrant, the caecum in the right lower quadrant, and the root of the mesentry extending from the duodenojejunal flexure to the ileocaecal valve. Failure of this normal rotation can result in several abnormalities (**Fig. 3.5**).

Midgut volvulus

Midgut volvulus occurs around the short, abnormal mesenteric base; it causes duodenal obstruction, and can result in midgut infarction. An upper GI contrast study will reveal an abnormal position of the duodenojejunal junction, which lies to the right of midline and may show characteristic spiralling of the obstructed small bowel.

Ladd's bands

Ladd's bands are abnormal peritoneal bands that extend from the liver, across the malrotated duodenum, to the caecum. They can cause extrinsic duodenal compression, which has a presentation similar to that of duodenal atresia.

Meconium ileus

The majority of cases of this condition occur in babies with cystic fibrosis. It is caused by abnormally viscous small bowel contents (meconium), which result in distal small bowel obstruction. Plain films show dilated loops of small bowel that may have a 'foamy' appearance because of the mixture of air with the abnormal

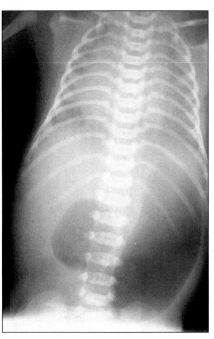

Fig. 3.2 *Supine abdominal radiograph in a neonate with duodenal atresia. The stomach and duodenum are distended with gas, giving rise to the 'double bubble' sign.*

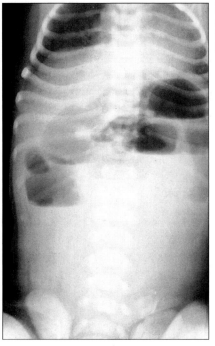

Fig. 3.3 *Abdominal radiograph in an infant with small bowel atresia.*

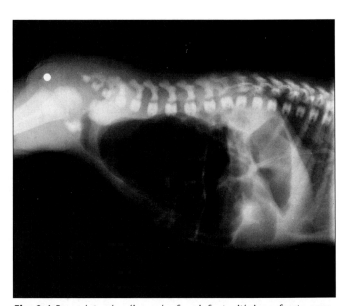

Fig. 3.4 *Prone lateral radiograph of an infant with imperforate anus (high type). The radio-opaque marker is taped to the skin at the site where the anus should be. There are dilated gas-filled loops of bowel, ending at the level of the sacrum.*

meconium; there may be focal areas of calcification, or evidence of perforation. A water-soluble contrast enema (**Fig. 3.6**) will show a small, unused colon. Occasionally, because of the hydrostatic effect of the contrast refluxing into the terminal ileum, a contrast enema may relieve the obstruction; however, surgery is usually required.

Meconium plug syndrome/neonatal small left colon
Meconium plug syndrome and neonatal small left colon are related conditions that may co-exist. In meconium plug syndrome, there is delayed passage of meconium, the child has abdominal distension, and plain films show dilated loops of bowel. A water-soluble enema is usually effective in relieving the obstruction.

Small left colon syndrome usually occurs in infants of diabetic mothers and has the same clinical presentation as meconium plug syndrome. A contrast enema will show an abrupt change in calibre of the colon in the region of the splenic flexure. Biopsy is required to distinguish this condition from Hirschprung's disease.

Hirschprung's disease
Hirschprung's disease can present in the neonatal period, with signs of large bowel obstruction, or can become apparent later in childhood. It is due to a lack of normal ganglion cells in the bowel wall, causing functional obstruction, typically in the rectosigmoid colon (**Fig. 3.7**), but it can involve a more extensive segment of bowel, from the anus proximally. Diagnosis is made by biopsy, to establish absence of ganglion cells.

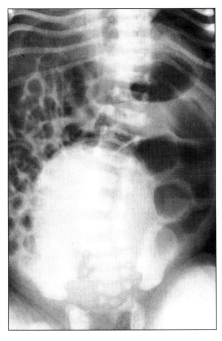

Fig. 3.5 Midgut malrotation. All the small bowel lies on the right side of the abdomen.

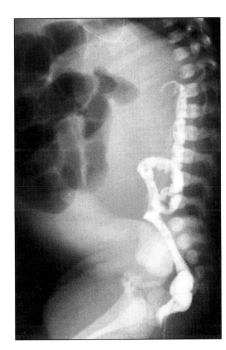

Fig. 3.6 Lateral view of a water-soluble contrast enema in an infant with meconium ileus. This child has cystic fibrosis.

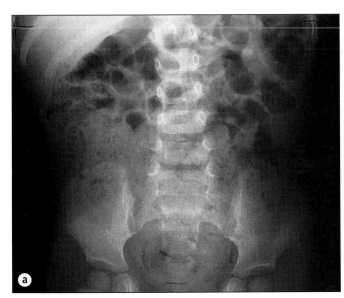

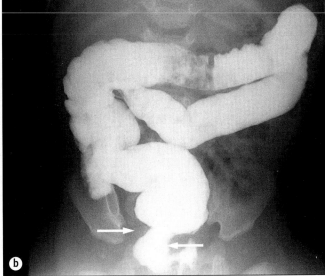

Fig. 3.7 (a) Supine abdominal radiograph showing marked faecal loading in the colon of a child with Hirschprung's disease. *(b)* Water-soluble contrast enema examination in the same child, demonstrating an abrupt change in calibre of the distal sigmoid colon (arrows), typical of Hirschprung's disease.

Necrotizing enterocolitis

Necrotizing enterocolitis is an acquired, life-threatening condition of babies that is seen most often in premature infants in special-care baby units. It usually occurs in infants receiving enteral feeding, and is believed to be caused by a combination of infection and bowel ischaemia. Plain films reveal a typical appearance of dilated loops of bowel containing intramural gas (**Fig. 3.8**). The gas may extend into the portal venous system, and the bowel can perforate. Late complications include malabsorption, stricture formation, and peritoneal abscesses.

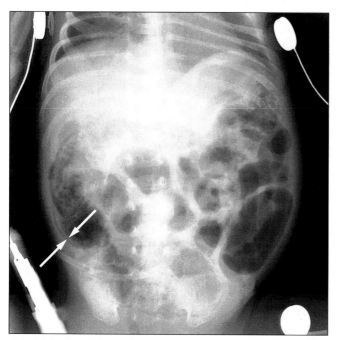

Fig. 3.8 *Supine abdominal radiograph in a premature neonate with necrotizing enterocolitis. Intramural gas can be seen (arrows).*

Hypertrophic pyloric stenosis

Hypertrophic pyloric stenosis can present in neonates, but it is most commonly diagnosed in infants more than 4 weeks old. It is most commonly seen in males, and presents with projectile vomiting. Ultrasound is the investigation of choice, and reveals the hypertrophied antral and pyloric muscles (**Fig. 3.9**).

Intussusception

Intussusception is said to occur when a proximal part of the bowel passes into a more distal segment of bowel; it is defined according to the segments of bowel involved. In children, intussusception is most common between the ages of 3 months and 2 years and is more common in boys than in girls. In the majority of these patients, the terminal ileum intussuscepts into the colon (ileocolic intussusception) and there is no identifiable underlying abnormality. Outside the above age range, however, intussusception is more often caused by an underlying abnormality such as a Meckel's diverticulum, lymphoma, haemangioma, or a duplication cyst. Clinically, children with intussusception have abdominal pain, vomiting, and sometimes rectal bleeding.

Plain films show small bowel obstruction (**Fig. 3.10a**), but sometimes there is surprisingly little bowel dilatation, as a result of vomiting. Plain films are occasionally diagnostic, showing the intussuscepted bowel outlined by air. Ultrasound can also be diagnostic, and shows a kidney-shaped mass surrounded by concentric layers of mucosa.

Treatment by enema is indicated, using barium (**Fig. 3.10b** and **3.10c**), water-soluble contrast, or air. This hydrostatic reduction of the intussusception should be attempted only when there is no evidence of peritonitis or perforation, and when the child is haemodynamically stable.

Hydrostatic reduction is successful in more than 67% of patients, although it may require up to three attempts; if the third attempt is unsuccessful, surgery is indicated.

ABDOMINAL WALL DEFECTS

Gastroschisis and omphalocele are described in Chapter 6.

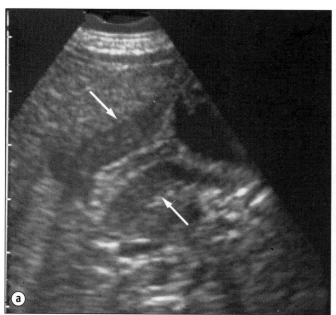

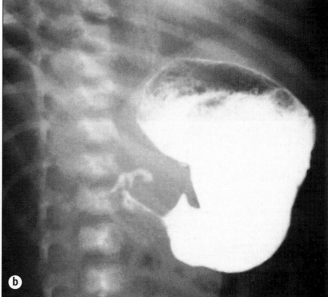

Fig. 3.9 (a) *Ultrasound image in pyloric stenosis, showing marked hypertrophy of the pyloric muscle (arrows).* **(b)** *Barium meal in the same patient.*

GASTRO-OESOPHAGEAL REFLUX

Gastro-oesophageal reflux is a normal finding in neonates and the most common cause of infantile vomiting. The diagnostic role of imaging is not to demonstrate reflux, but to exclude GI obstruction, in an infant in whom conservative management (upright posture and thickening feeds) fails, or in whom there are other signs of obstruction (**Fig. 3.11**).

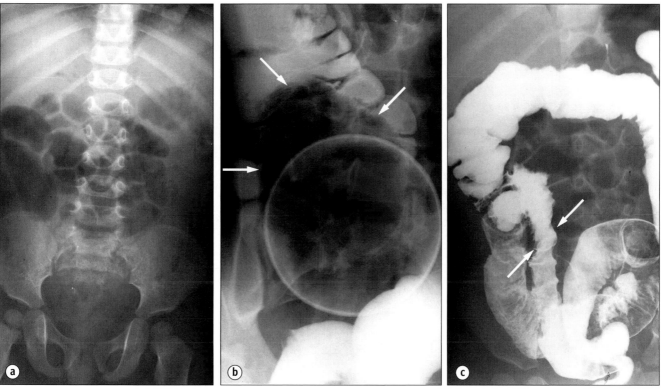

Fig. 3.10 (a) Supine abdominal radiograph of a child with ileocolic intussusception, demonstrating dilated loops of small bowel. (b) Ileocolic intussusception in an adult during hydrostatic reduction. The intussuscipiens is seen as a filling defect in the ascending colon (arrows). (c) Appearance after successful hydrostatic reduction of ileocolic intussusception in the patient shown in (a). Barium has refluxed freely into the terminal ileum, which shows mucosal oedema (arrows).

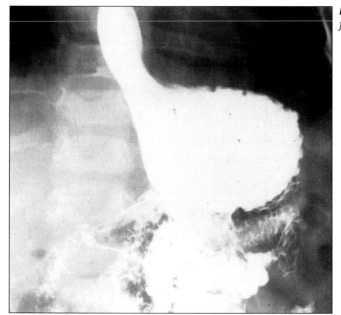

Fig. 3.11 Infantile gastro-oesophageal reflux. There is reflux of barium from the stomach to the oesophagus.

TRAUMA

Traumatic perforation of the gastrointestinal tract may be iatrogenic or accidental. Intrumentation of the pharynx and oesophagus during endoscopy can result in perforation of these structures, particularly if biopsy is performed. Perforation can also follow impaction of a foreign body, such as a fish bone. Spontaneous oesophageal perforation (Boerhaave's syndrome) can occur as a result of increased intraoesophageal pressure, for example during coughing, vomiting, weight lifting, and childbirth.

Plain films reveal subcutaneous (surgical) emphysema, with or without mediastinal emphysema (**Fig. 3.12a**); in the case of thoracic oesophageal perforation, there is frequently a pleural effusion. Contrast studies can be used to identify the site of perforation (**Fig. 3.12b**).

Accidental trauma

Stab wounds can perforate any part of the GI tract; most frequently, the small bowel, colon, or cervical oesophagus are involved. Blunt trauma can result in rupture of the duodenum because of its retroperitoneal, fixed position; this is a recognized complication in road traffic accidents and non-accidental injury in childhood.

Rectal perforation

Rectal instrumentation at proctoscopy or barium enema can result in rectal perforation. Barium enema should not be performed within 3 days of a mucosal biopsy taken with the aid of a flexible colonoscope, or within 7 days of a rigid sigmoidoscopic biopsy.

INFECTION

INFECTION RELATED TO ACQUIRED IMMUNODEFICIENCY SYNDROME

The GI tract is a common site for AIDS-related infection (**Fig. 3.13**). In most cases, the diagnosis is based on clinical presentation and microbiological findings, but in some cases there are specific radiological appearances (**Figs 3.14** and **3.15**).

OTHER GASTROINTESTINAL INFECTIONS WITH TYPICAL RADIOLOGICAL APPEARANCES
Tuberculosis

Tuberculosis remains common, and in the GI tract the most common site is the terminal ileum. A small bowel study, or barium enema, will show deformity of the caecum and terminal ileum, with bowel wall thickening; the features may be very similar to those of Crohn's disease (**Fig. 3.16**).

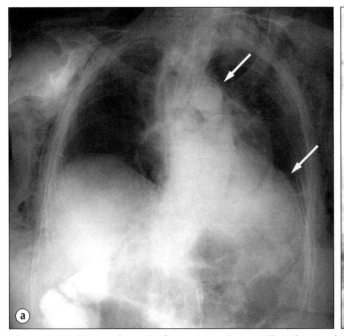
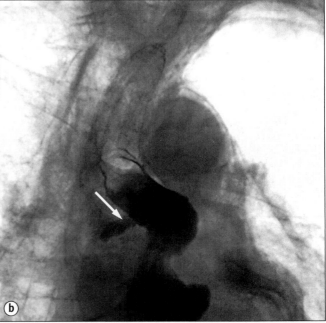

Fig. 3.12 *(a) Chest radiograph after recent endoscopy. There is extensive gas in the soft tissues of the neck and chest (surgical emphysema). A pneumomediastinum, with gas outlining the borders of the heart and aortic arch (arrows), is also apparent. (b) Water-soluble contrast swallow in the same patient, demonstrating the site of oesophageal perforation (arrow). The patient has a large hiatus hernia.*

Yersiniosis

Yersiniosis can present clinically like acute appendicitis, because of acute inflammation in the terminal ileum, caecum, and adjacent mesentery. Imaging shows thickening and ulceration of the small bowel mucosa that can resemble the appearance of Crohn's disease.

Actinomycosis

Actinomycosis is a rare condition that is predisposed to by previous surgery, poor oral hygiene, diabetes, and steroid treatment. A chronic appendix abscess forms, and there is a tendency for fistulae to develop between the small bowel, skin, bladder, or colon.

Gastrointestinal infections associated with AIDS	
Site	**Infective agent**
Oesophagus	*Candida albicans* (see **Fig. 3.14**) *Herpes simplex* Cytomegalovirus (CMV)
Stomach	CMV (occasionally)
Small bowel	*Cryptosporidium* *Mycobacterium tuberculosis* (MTB) *Mycobacterium avium intracellulare* (MAI) CMV (rarely)
Colon	CMV (commonly) (see **Fig. 3.15**) Caecal MTB and MAI

Note: Ileocaecal disease may be complicated by intussusception, appendicitis, or perforation.

Fig. 3.13 *Gastrointestinal infections associated with AIDS.*

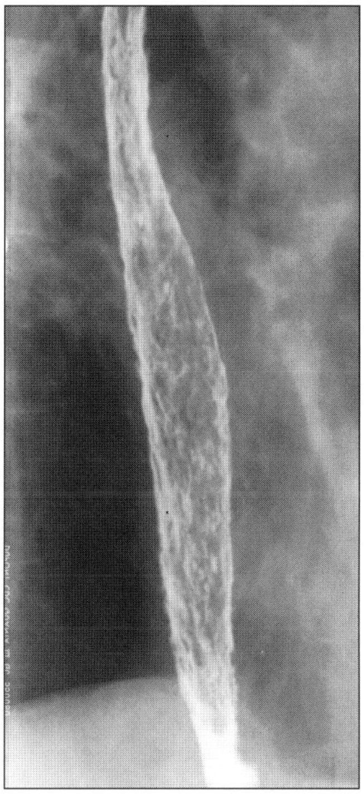

Fig. 3.14 *Barium swallow in a patient with AIDS who has oesophageal candidiasis. Note the extensive mucosal irregularity, with ulceration.*

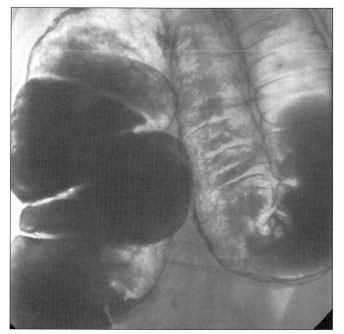

Fig. 3.15 *Double-contrast barium enema in cytomegalovirus colitis, showing diffuse mucosal ulceration in the ascending colon and proximal transverse colon.*

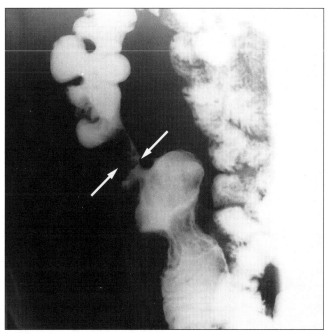

Fig. 3.16 *Small-bowel study in a patient with tuberculosis of the caecum, demonstrating deformity of the terminal ileum and scarring of the caecum (arrows).*

Giardiasis

The diagnosis of giardiasis is usually made clinically, or by stool culture. Imaging can show thickening of mucosal folds in the duodenum and proximal small bowel.

Worms

Roundworm infestation (ascariasis) can lead to small bowel obstruction, particularly in children. Plain films show dilated loops of small bowel, and may also demonstrate worms coiled within the gut lumen (**Fig. 3.17**). Tapeworms are usually present as a single long worm in the small bowel of asymptomatic adults; they can be seen on barium studies.

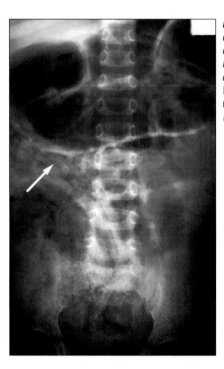

Fig. 3.17 Supine abdominal radiograph of a child with small-bowel obstruction caused by ascariasis. Worms can be seen within the gut lumen (arrow).

Pseudomembranous colitis

Bacterial overgrowth of *Clostridium difficile* after treatment with certain antiobiotics can cause pseudomembranous colitis. If the diagnosis is not obvious clinically, the inflammatory pseudomembrane that is produced in the rectum and colon in this condition can be demonstrated on a double-contrast barium enema.

Typhlitis

Typhlitis is found in children and adults who are neutropenic, usually as a result of leukaemia, aplastic anaemia, or treatment with immuno-suppressive drugs. It is an inflammatory process involving the caecum, terminal ileum, and appendix, and can result in bowel wall thickening and necrosis. It is believed to be the result of a combination of infection and infarction.

INFLAMMATORY CONDITIONS

Increased production of gastric acid, and/or reduced mucosal protection from acid destruction, are implicated in a variety of common disorders in the upper GI tract. Ingested irritants such as alcohol, oral steroids, and non-steroidal anti-inflammatory drugs (NSAIDs) can cause mucosal inflammation and ulceration. Infection with *Helicobacter pylori* is common in the population and its prevalence increases with age. It is now known to cause peptic ulcer disease and gastritis. Current guidelines recommend that patients who test positive for *H. pylori* on gastric mucosal biopsy, carbon urea breath test, or serology, and who have a proven benign gastric ulcer, duodenal ulcer, gastritis, or certain types of gastric lymphoma, should receive treatment with antibiotics and a proton-pump inhibitor, to eradicate this organism.

PEPTIC OESOPHAGITIS

Reflux of gastric acid into the lower oesophagus, leading to peptic oesophagitis, can occur in isolation; the risk is increased if there is a hiatus hernia. The stratified squamous mucosa of the lower oeso-phagus becomes inflamed and may ulcerate and bleed, sometimes leading to iron deficiency anaemia. One long-term complication of

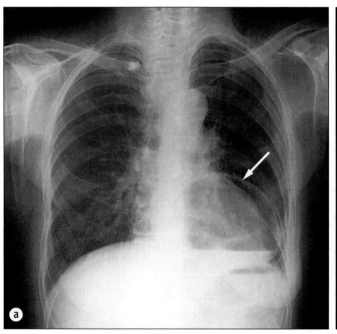

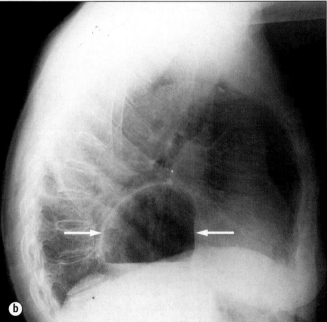

Fig. 3.18 Posteroanterior (a) and lateral (b) chest radiographs showing a large hiatus hernia (arrows).

reflux is the formation of a benign oesophageal stricture, causing dysphagia. Another complication of long-standing reflux is a change in the mucosa lining the distal oesophagus, from squamous to columnar epithelium. This is called Barrett's oesophagus, and is associated with an increased risk of adenocarcinoma.

A barium swallow will demonstrate gastro-oesophageal reflux (*see* Fig. 3.71a) and a hiatus hernia (**Figs 3.18** and **3.19**), and a stricture is also easily demonstrated (**Fig. 3.20**). Signs that suggest a benign stricture include short length, smooth contour, and lack of the mucosal 'shoulder' that is typical of adenocarcinoma of the oesophagus (*see* page 63); nevertheless, biopsy is required to exclude malignancy. Oesophagitis is best diagnosed on endoscopy.

GASTRITIS

Inflammation of the gastric mucosa can be associated with superficial erosions and can be caused by ingestion of alcohol, steroids, and NSAIDs; *H. pylori* infection is associated with antral gastritis. Erosions can be focal, with surrounding oedema (**Fig. 3.21**). Endoscopy is the best method of investigation of gastritis, and enables biopsy of the gastric mucosa. Radiographic appearances after a barium meal can be non-specific, and include poor coating of the mucosa with barium and thickening of the gastric rugae; the latter feature is sometimes described as hypertrophic gastritis.

Ménétrier's disease is an extreme form of hypertrophic gastritis, with marked rugal thickening in the fundus and greater curvature. Biopsy

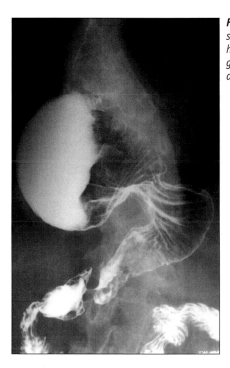

Fig. 3.19 Barium meal showing a large hiatus hernia, with the gastric fundus lying above the diaphragm.

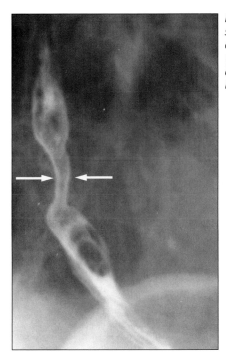

Fig. 3.20 Barium swallow of a benign oesophageal stricture (arrows), proximal to a sliding hiatus hernia.

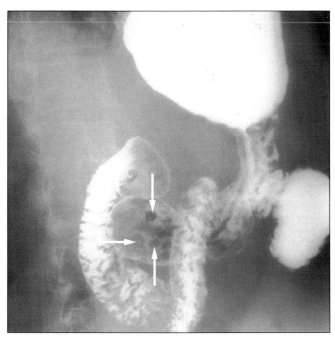

Fig. 3.21 Barium meal in a patient with gastritis, showing multiple superficial gastric erosions, with surrounding mounds of oedema (arrows).

is required to distinguish this from gastric cancer or lymphoma.

In elderly patients, thinning of the gastric mucosa with loss of rugal folds can be seen. This is termed atrophic gastritis, and is associated with gastric ulcers (despite reduced production of acid) and gastric cancer.

GASTRIC ULCER

The most common sites for benign gastric ulcers are along the lesser curve of the stomach and gastric antrum. A barium meal will show a persistent barium-filled ulcer crater, which may be deep and project beyond the stomach wall, with surrounding radiating folds caused by mucosal scarring (**Fig. 3.22**). Benign gastric ulcers are characteristically round or oval, with a smooth 'collar' of surrounding mucosa that has been undermined by the ulcer. Any irregularity to the ulcer should raise the suspicion of an ulcerated gastric cancer; endoscopy is indicated to exclude malignancy.

DUODENITIS AND DUODENAL ULCER

Duodenitis and duodenal ulcer are common abnormalities and can result in various radiographic abnormalities revealed by barium studies, ranging from prominent mucosal folds and superficial erosions (**Fig. 3.23**) to giant ulcers (>2 cm). Most ulcers develop in the first part of the duodenum, also known as the duodenal bulb (**Fig. 3.24**); postbulbar ulcers in the second part of the duodenum are less common. Multiple ulcers should raise the suspicion of Zollinger–Ellison syndrome. This rare syndrome is due to a gastrin-secreting tumour of the pancreatic islet cells which results in multiple ulcers of the oesophagus, stomach, duodenum, and jejunum.

Double-contrast barium radiography with the use of an intravenous smooth muscle relaxant (glucagon or hyoscine), or upper GI endoscopy are the investigative techniques of choice.

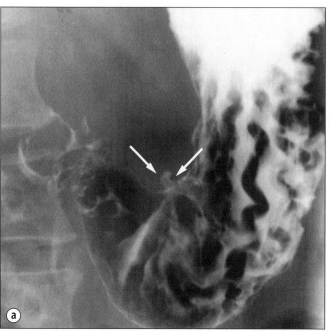
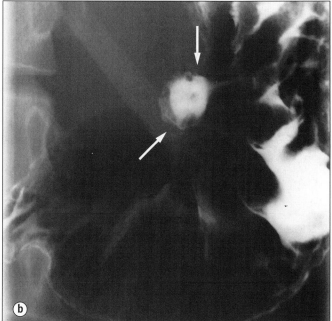

Fig. 3.22 Two examples of benign gastric ulcers. **(a)** An ulcer with surrounding radiating mucosal folds produced by scarring, at the typical site on the lesser curvature (arrows). **(b)** A large, benign gastric ulcer, projecting beyond the line of the lesser curvature (arrows).

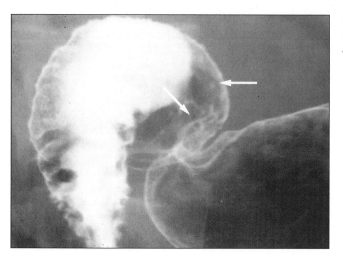

Fig. 3.23 Double-contrast barium meal in duodenitis, showing multiple small superficial erosions on the superior aspect of the first part of the duodenum (arrows).

COMPLICATIONS OF PEPTIC ULCERATION

Gastric and duodenal ulcers may perforate, bleed, erode into adjacent structures, or cause stenosis and gastric outlet obstruction. Perforation causes peritonitis and an 'acute abdomen'. An erect chest radiograph and a supine abdominal radiograph will show a pneumoperitoneum with gas beneath the hemidiaphragms and outside the bowel wall (**Fig. 3.25**). Bleeding from an ulcer cannot be diagnosed radiologically; the investigation of choice in a patient with haematemesis or melaena is upper GI endoscopy. Gastric outlet obstruction is evident when in spite of fasting, a patient nevertheless has food residue in the stomach and there is delayed gastric emptying on a barium meal.

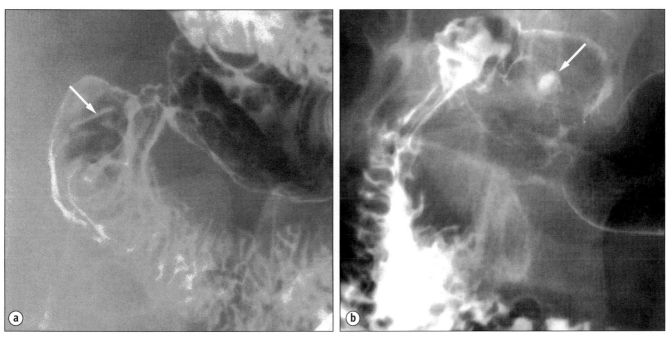

Fig. 3.24 *Two examples of duodenal ulcers. (**a**) A linear ulcer (arrow), surrounded by mucosal oedema. (**b**) An obvious ulcer of the first part of the duodenum (arrow).*

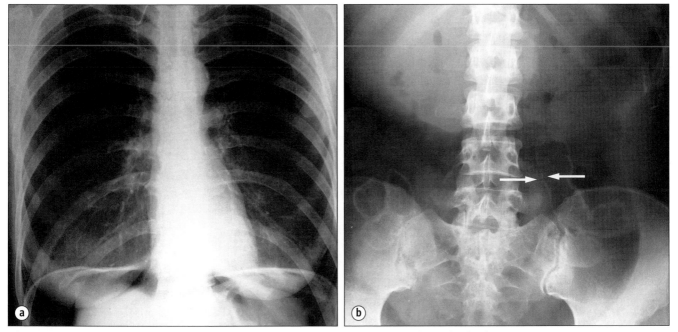

Fig. 3.25 *Pneumoperitoneum caused by a perforated duodenal ulcer. (**a**) Erect chest radiograph, showing free gas beneath both hemidiaphragms. (**b**) Supine abdominal radiograph, showing gas outlining both sides of the bowel wall (arrows), indicating free air in the peritoneal cavity.*

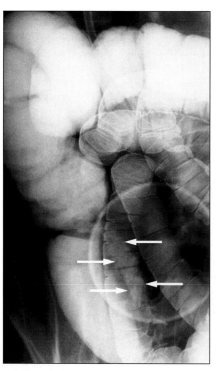

Fig. 3.26 Crohn's disease involving the terminal ileum (arrows), shown on a small bowel enema. This is a compression view, taken using a ball to displace loops of bowel from the area of interest.

INFLAMMATORY BOWEL DISEASE
Crohn's disease

Crohn's disease is a chronic inflammatory disease of unknown cause that can affect any part of the GI tract from the mouth to the anus. The most common site of involvement is the terminal ileum (**Fig. 3.26**), and Crohn's disease is the most common disease of the small bowel in Europe and North America. The clinical presentation is usually abdominal pain, and can include diarrhoea, weight loss, poor growth, and anaemia.

Inflammation and ulceration of the gut wall can give rise to several different imaging appearances (**Fig. 3.27**).

A small bowel enema may reveal mucosal nodules in the jejunum (**Fig. 3.28**) or ileum. 'Cobblestoning' (**Fig. 3.29**) is a term used to describe the appearance produced by mounds of normal mucosa distributed between linear ulcers. 'Pseudodiverticula' are outpouchings of the bowel wall between areas of scarring. The term 'skip lesion' refers to abnormal segments of bowel separated by normal segments. Strictures may be multiple and long, giving rise to the 'string sign of Kantor' (**Fig. 3.30**). Fistulae (between diseased segments of bowel and adjacent structures) and sinuses (between diseased segments of bowel and skin)are typical of Crohn's disease (**Fig. 3.31**); perianal disease is characteristic, with multiple fistulae and skin tags.

Crohn's disease of the colon can give radiographic images similar to those of ulcerative colitis (**Fig. 3.32**).

Radiological appearances of Crohn's disease	
Site	**Radiological appearance**
Oesophagus	Superficial ulceration
Stomach	Superficial ulceration Thickened rugal folds
Duodenum	Superficial ulceration Thickened mucosal folds Strictures
Small bowel	Ulceration, superficial and deep linear Thickened mucosal folds and nodules (*see* **Fig. 3.28**) 'Cobblestoning' (*see* **Fig. 3.29**) Bowel wall thickening Strictures (*see* **Fig. 3.30**) Skip lesions Pseudodiverticula Fistulae and sinuses (*see* **Fig. 3.31**)
Colon	Ulceration, superficial and deep fissuring (*see* **Fig. 3.32**) Bowel wall thickening Asymmetric involvement Skip lesions Pseudodiverticula Fistulae, especially anal Relative rectal sparing

Fig. 3.27 Radiological appearances of Crohn's disease.

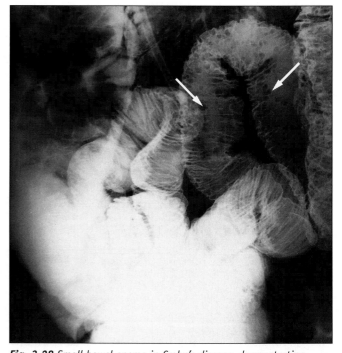

Fig. 3.28 Small-bowel enema in Crohn's disease, demonstrating multiple mucosal nodules in the jejunum (arrows).

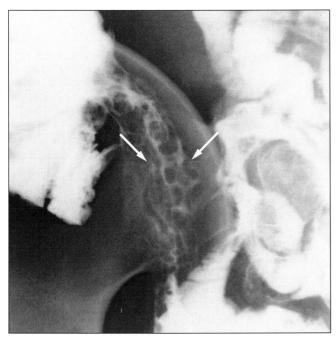

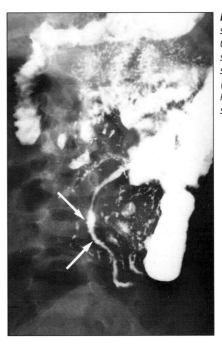

Fig. 3.30 *Small-bowel study in a child with Crohn's disease, showing a long stricture of ileum (arrows); this is known as the 'string sign of Kantor'.*

Fig. 3.29 *'Cobblestoning' of the terminal ileum in Crohn's disease (arrows).*

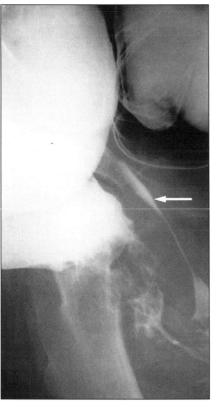

Fig. 3.31 *Barium enema in a patient with Crohn's colitis. Barium has entered the vagina (arrow) through a colovaginal fistula.*

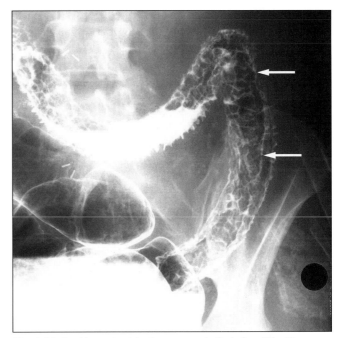

Fig. 3.32 *Double-contrast barium enema in Crohn's colitis. There are multiple deep and linear ulcers (arrows).*

Ulcerative colitis

Ulcerative colitis is an inflammatory disease limited to the rectum and colon, apart from occasional associated 'backwash ileitis', with total colitis. Ulcerative colitis is more common than Crohn's disease and, typically, presents with diarrhoea and rectal bleeding. The disease always involves the rectum, with a variable extent of colonic involvement, always in continuity; thus skip lesions are not seen in ulcerative colitis. Features of a barium enema that help distinguish ulcerative colitis from Crohn's colitis are rectal involvement (**Fig. 3.33**), continuous disease (**Fig. 3.34**), and bowel shortening. However, appearances in ulcerative colitis and Crohn's colitis may be identical and rectal biopsy is usually required to distinguish the two; results are always abnormal in ulcerative colitis.

Nuclear medicine studies using radioisotope-labelled white blood cells can help identify sites of active disease in both Crohn's disease and ulcerative colitis (**Fig. 3.35**).

Complications of colitis

Toxic megacolon

Fulminant acute colitis produces the condition known as toxic megacolon, which is seen on a plain abdominal film as dilatation of the colon (usually the transverse colon) to >5 cm, with islands of mucosa resulting from extensive mucosal ulceration (**Fig. 3.36**). The bowel wall is extremely friable, and perforation is likely. Toxic megacolon is usually caused by ulcerative colitis, but can occur in Crohn's disease and other forms of colitis.

Carcinoma

Patients who have ulcerative colitis for more than 10 years have an increased risk of carcinoma of the colon. Regular double-contrast barium enema or colonoscopy is indicated, to identify suspicious lesions.

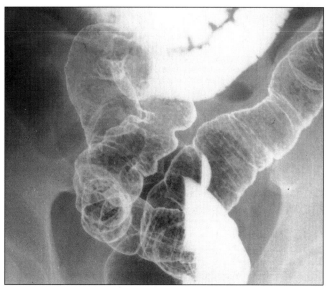

Fig. 3.33 Double-contrast barium enema in early ulcerative colitis, showing granularity of the rectal and sigmoid mucosa.

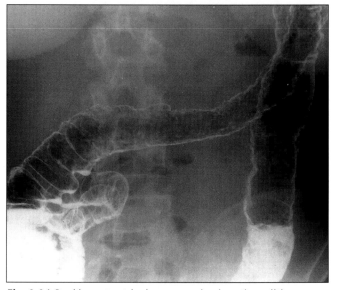

Fig. 3.34 Double-contrast barium enema in ulcerative colitis, revealing continuous disease as far as the hepatic flexure.

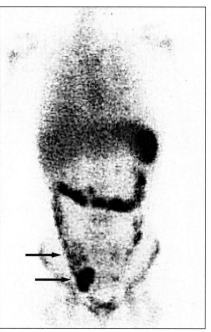

Fig. 3.35 Radioisotope-labelled white cell scan in Crohn's colitis, showing disease activity in the caecum, ascending colon (arrows), and transverse colon, and a skip lesion in the descending colon.

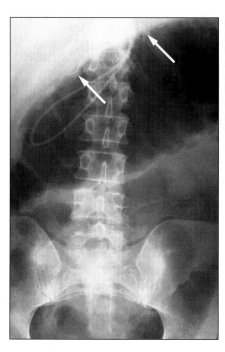

Fig. 3.36 Supine abdominal radiograph of toxic megacolon, demonstrating gross dilatation of the transverse colon, with islands of mucosa visible (arrows).

NEOPLASTIC DISEASE

The three most common tumours of the GI tract are cancers of the oesophagus, stomach, and colon.

OESOPHAGEAL CANCER

There are two main types of oesophageal cancer: squamous carcinoma and adenocarcinoma. The incidence of oesophageal carcinoma is increasing and, although it accounts for only about 1% of all malignancies, it has a very poor survival rate.

The initial investigation of choice in a patient with dysphagia is a barium swallow, followed by endoscopy, and biopsy of any suspicious abnormality. Early tumours can appear as polyps or irregular plaques, but rarely cause symptoms and so are seen less often than large tumours. The most common finding in a patient with progressive dysphagia is an obvious, irregular stricture (**Fig. 3.37**) that appears polypoid or shouldered (**Fig. 3.38**).

CT scanning is currently the method of choice for staging

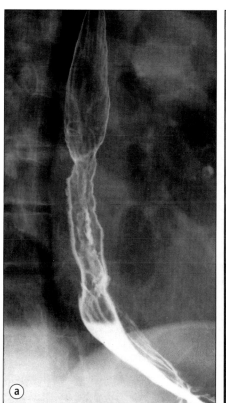
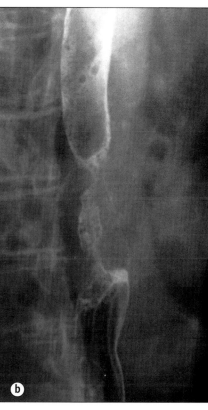

Fig. 3.37 Two examples of strictures associated with oesophageal carcinoma. (*a*) A long, irregular stricture. (*b*) A more extensive stricture is seen in this patient, who had mediastinal invasion at the time of diagnosis.

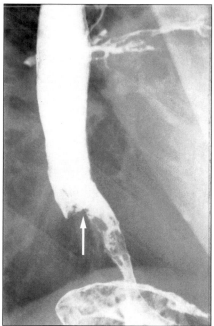

Fig. 3.38 Barium swallow appearance of a carcinoma of the lower third of the oesophagus, showing typical 'shouldering' (arrow).

oesophageal cancer (**Fig. 3.39**). The role of MRI is increasing; this technique is probably superior at demonstrating local invasion of tumour. Endoscopic ultrasound gives excellent depiction of the local extent of tumour and the degree of invasion through the oesophageal wall.

Squamous carcinoma of the oesophagus

Factors predisposing to squamous carcinoma of the oesophagus include smoking, use of alcohol, head and neck tumours, coeliac disease, caustic

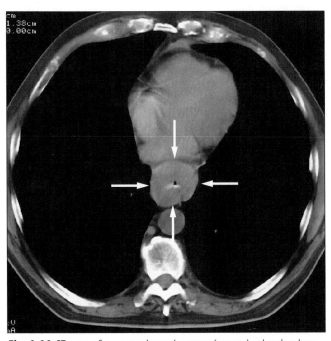

Fig. 3.39 *CT scan of an oesophageal cancer (arrows), showing how close the lesion lies to the left atrium (anteriorly) and the thoracic aorta (posteriorly).*

strictures of the oesophagus, achalasia, and Paterson–Kelly–Brown syndrome (this is also known as Plummer–Vinson syndrome, and consists of iron-deficiency anaemia, dysphagia, glossitis, and a post-cricoid web). These tumours can occur throughout the oesophagus; they are most common in the middle third. Patients present initially with dysphagia for solids; this progresses to complete dysphagia.

By the time the tumour is diagnosed, most patients have local, and sometimes distant, spread. The tumours spread initially by direct invasion of adjacent structures such as the pericardium, trachea, bronchial tree, diaphragm, and occasionally the aorta. Fistulae from the oesophagus to the airways occur in 5–10% of cases. There is early lymphatic spread to the mediastinal, neck, epigastric, and retrocrural nodes. Blood-borne (haematogenous) spread to the liver, lungs, adrenals, and bones is seen with advanced disease.

Adenocarcinoma of the oesophagus

Adenocarcinomas occur in the lower third of the oesophagus. They arise in Barrett's mucosa, that is at sites of gastric metaplasia, where the normal squamous epithelium has been replaced by columnar epithelium. The incidence of these tumours is increasing. They are predisposed to by Barrett's oesophagus and scleroderma.

Spread of adenocarcinoma is the same as that of squamous carcinoma, except that adenocarcinoma often spreads distally into the stomach.

Other oesophageal cancers

Other less common malignancies of the oesophagus are lymphoma, leiomyosarcoma, spindle-cell sarcoma, malignant melanoma, and Kaposi's sarcoma. The oesophagus may be directly invaded by adjacent tumours of the stomach, bronchus, neck, or lymph nodes.

GASTRIC CANCER

The incidence of gastric cancer is decreasing, but the prognosis in most countries remains poor. In Japan, where the incidence is high, early detection by screening with barium meal and endoscopy,

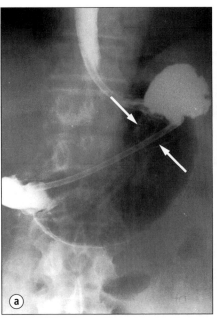
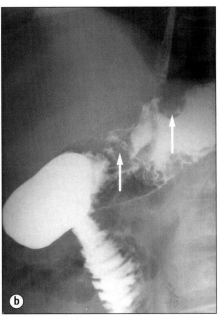
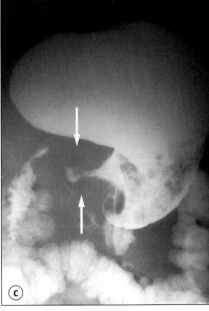

Fig. 3.40 *Barium meal examinations, demonstrating the variety of appearances of gastric carcinoma.*
(a) Small polypoid tumour near the gastro-oesophageal junction (arrows). (b) Irregular tumour involving the gastric fundus and lesser curvature (arrows). (c) Large antral tumour (arrows), causing gastric outlet obstruction; there is food residue in the distended stomach.

combined with radical surgical techniques, have improved the outcome for patients. Factors that are believed to predispose to gastric cancer include atrophic gastritis, adenomatous polyps, pernicious anaemia, partial gastrectomy, Ménétrier's disease, and dietary nitrates.

Clinically, patients present with epigastric pain, weight loss, anaemia, early satiety, and vomiting. Most gastric cancers have invaded locally and to local lymph nodes by the time of diagnosis. Direct spread can occur to the distal oesophagus, duodenum, liver, pancreas, spleen, and transverse colon. Lymphatic spread is common and is to the perigastric, coeliac, left gastric, hepatic, and splenic nodes. Spread to left supraclavicular nodes is also common. Haematogenous spread to the liver is common and is followed by later spread to the lungs, adrenals, bones, and brain. Peritoneal spread may cause ascites; bilateral ovarian metastases (Krukenberg tumours) are a well-recognized complication.

The initial investigation is usually a barium meal, which can show various abnormalities in gastric cancer (**Fig. 3.40**). Changes range from the subtle, with distortion of rugal folds or an irregular ulcer, to

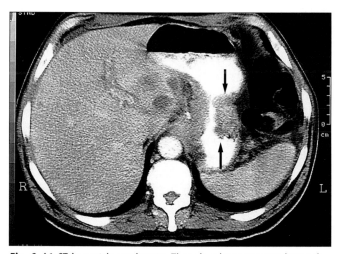

Fig. 3.41 *CT in gastric carcinoma. There is a large tumour (arrows) arising from the greater curvature with epigastric and retrocrural lymphadenopathy.*

an obvious polypoid mass or diffuse infiltration of the stomach wall. Endoscopy and biopsy are indicated for any suspicious lesion found on barium meal. Staging of gastric cancer is by CT scan (**Fig. 3.41**) to assess direct invasion, local and regional lymph nodes, and liver metastases; laparoscopic ultrasound also has been used in staging. As with oesophageal cancer, endoscopic ultrasound has a role in assessing the local extent of the tumour.

Other malignant tumours that arise in the stomach include lymphoma, Kaposi's sarcoma, leiomyosarcoma, and carcinoid tumour. Direct invasion can occur from tumours of the oesophagus, colon, pancreas, kidney, or the very rare duodenal carcinoma. Haematogenous spread of breast cancer and melanoma can cause submucosal metastases.

COLORECTAL CANCER

Colorectal cancer is the most common malignancy of the GI tract and, as a cause of death, is second only to breast cancer in women and lung cancer in men. It is particularly common in Europe and North America, especially in northern countries.

It is believed that almost all colorectal cancers occur as a result of malignant change in a pre-existing adenomatous polyp; thus an important role of imaging is the detection of colonic polyps. Polyps are common and are found in about 10% of double-contrast barium enema examinations (**Figs 3.42** and **3.43**). Their incidence increases with age. The risk of malignant change in a polyp increases with size—50% of those larger than 2 cm in diameter will be malignant; those larger than 1 cm in diameter should be removed because of this risk. Inflammatory and hyperplastic polyps are benign, but cannot always be differentiated from adenomatous polyps on imaging. Most polyps occur in the left side of the colon, over 60% being in the rectosigmoid region.

More than 50% of large bowel tumours arise in the sigmoid colon and rectum, and can therefore be seen at direct examination by flexible sigmoidoscopy. The remainder are evenly distributed in the rest of the colon.

Conditions that predispose to colorectal cancer include polyposis syndromes (*see* Fig. 3.53), adenomatous polyps, long-standing ulcerative

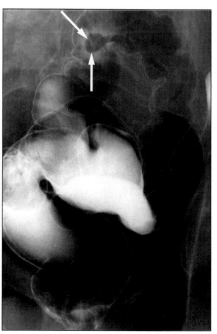

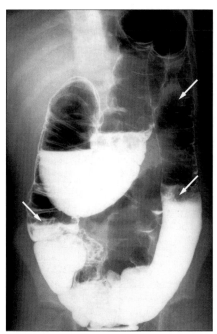

Fig. 3.42 *Double-contrast barium enema, showing a pedunculated polyp in the sigmoid colon (arrows).*

Fig. 3.43 *Double-contrast barium enema in a patient with multiple colonic polyps (arrows).*

colitis, and, probably, a low fibre/high animal fat diet. In addition, some families have a genetic predisposition to colorectal cancer (in the absence of a hereditary polyposis syndrome), and in some of these there is clustering of other tumours of the breast, ovary, and endometrium. In these families, colorectal cancer tends to arise at an earlier age.

Presenting features are altered bowel habit (constipation or diarrhoea), rectal bleeding, anaemia (especially with caecal tumours), weight loss, and intestinal obstruction. In some countries, screening for colorectal carcinoma is now recommended, with regular faecal occult blood testing and sigmoidoscopy.

Spread of colorectal cancer occurs initially through the bowel wall. Tumour then involves local and regional lymph nodes, followed by spread via the portal venous system to the liver. Invasion locally

into adjacent structures can involve the bladder, prostate, seminal vesicles, uterus, vagina, small bowel, or stomach, and can result in the development of fistulae into these organs. Bony involvement can be caused by local invasion of the pelvic bones or haematogenous spread.

The methods of diagnosis of colorectal cancer are double-contrast barium enema, flexible sigmoidoscopy, and colonoscopy. Barium enema may show early cancer as a polyp (**Fig. 3.44**) but, more commonly, an advanced cancer is seen, as a large polypoid mass or 'apple-core' stricture (**Figs 3.45** and **3.46**). Patients who present with large-bowel obstruction should undergo a single-contrast enema using water-soluble contrast, because of the risk of barium peritonitis if perforation occurs (**Fig. 3.47**).

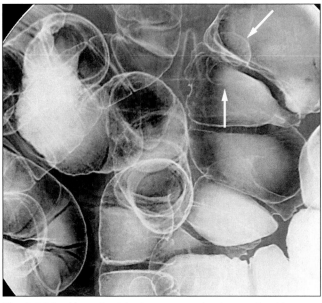

Fig. 3.44 *Double-contrast barium enema, showing a polypoid mass in the descending colon (arrows). This was an early colonic carcinoma.*

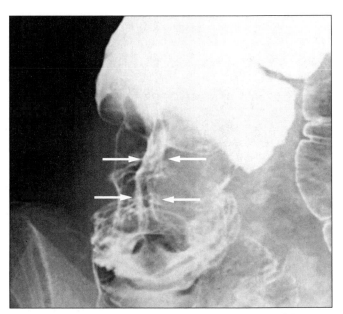

Fig. 3.45 *Double-contrast barium enema of a carcinoma of the ascending colon that has a typical 'apple-core' appearance (arrows).*

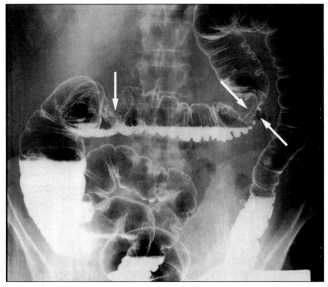

Fig. 3.46 *Double-contrast barium enema in a patient with multiple colonic polyps and carcinomas (arrows).*

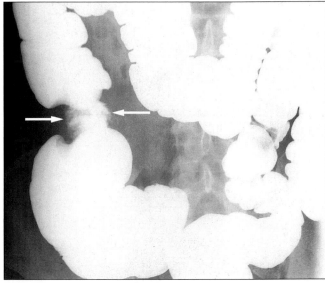

Fig. 3.47 *Single-contrast enema examination using water-soluble contrast, in a patient who presented with large bowel obstruction caused by this carcinoma of the ascending colon.*

Endorectal ultrasound is accurate in staging local invasion of rectal cancers. CT and, more recently, MRI are used in staging of colorectal cancer, and CT also has a role in the primary diagnosis of colorectal cancer (**Fig. 3.48**). The staging method for colorectal cancer remains Duke's classification, which is surgical and pathological (**Fig. 3.49**). Imaging, other than endorectal ultrasound, cannot determine the layers of bowel wall invasion and therefore gives a modified staging, on the basis of invasion into adjacent organs, enlarged lymph nodes, and distant metastases.

Other malignancies that can involve the colon are lymphoma, carcinoid, Kaposi's sarcoma, and stromal tumours. Direct spread can occur from primary tumours of the ovary, prostate, stomach, cervix, kidney and gall bladder. Haematogenous metastases from breast and other primaries can cause subserosal masses in the colon.

SMALL-BOWEL TUMOURS

Unlike the upper GI tract and the colon, in the small bowel, primary tumours are uncommon and benign tumours are seen almost as often as malignant tumours. Symptoms from small-bowel tumours are often vague, non-specific abdominal pain being the most common. This often leads to delay in diagnosis. Occasionally, small-bowel tumours cause bleeding or intussusception.

The investigation of choice for evaluating the small bowel is a small-bowel enema. This is an uncomfortable examination, which involves passing a tube from the mouth to the duodenojejunal flexure and infusing a large volume of dilute barium, followed by water or methyl cellulose, to obtain double-contrast images. A small bowel study is a single-contrast examination with images of the small bowel taken after a large volume of oral barium. It is neither as sensitive nor specific as a small-bowel enema.

Benign small-bowel tumours
Adenoma
Adenomas of the small bowel can be single or multiple and may be part of a polyposis syndrome. They are usually asymptomatic, unless they bleed or give rise to intussusception. Adenomas can also develop in the stomach and colon.

Leiomyoma
These are the most common benign small-bowel tumours, and can also occur in the oesophagus, stomach (**Fig. 3.50**), and colon. They are vascular tumours that, on imaging, are well-defined soft-tissue masses, often with superficial ulceration.

Other benign small-bowel tumours include lipomas, haemangiomas, and neurogenic tumours.

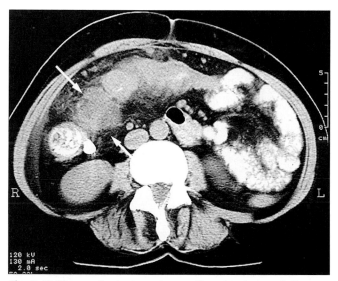

Fig. 3.48 *CT scan of colonic carcinoma. There is a large soft-tissue mass in the transverse colon (arrows).*

Duke's classification	
A	Tumour limited to mucosa
B	Extension through wall but no nodes
C	Positive nodes
D	Distant metastases

Stages B and C have subdivisions

Fig. 3.49 *Duke's classification.*

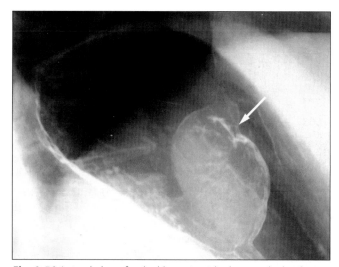

Fig. 3.50 *Lateral view of a double-contrast barium meal, showing a large, smooth mass in the body of the stomach, with central ulceration (arrow). This is a leiomyoma.*

Malignant small bowel tumours

Lymphoma

Intestinal lymphoma is non-Hodgkin's in type; involvement of the gut may be primary or it may be secondary to disseminated lymphoma. The small bowel is the second most common site for intestinal lymphoma in the GI tract, after the stomach. Imaging shows bowel wall thickening, with an infiltrating mass (**Fig. 3.51**), which can be multifocal.

Carcinoid tumours

The appendix is the most common site for carcinoid tumours of the small bowel, with approximately one-third arising in the ileum (**Fig. 3.52a**). They can cause a characteristic desmoplastic reaction, with strands of fibrosis extending into the mesentery (**Fig. 3.52b**). They all have malignant potential. Small carcinoids are usually asymptomatic; the carcinoid syndrome usually develops only when liver metastases are present, and comprises intermittent symptoms of skin flushing,

diarrhoea, and bronchospasm. The syndrome is caused by secretion of serotonin by tumour cells, and urinary 5-hydroxyindoleacetic acid levels are increased. Symptoms can be relieved by embolization of liver metasteses (see page 94).

Adenocarcinoma

The duodenum is the most frequent site of adenocarcinoma of the small bowel. There is a predisposition to these unusual tumours in coeliac disease, Crohn's disease, and some polyposis syndromes (*see* Fig. 3.53).

Kaposi's sarcoma

Kaposi's sarcoma occurs most commonly as part of AIDS, and is a vascular tumour that can arise in the mouth, oesophagus, stomach, small bowel, or colon. In the small bowel, these tumours must be distinguished from non-Hodgkin's lymphoma, infection with *Mycobacterium avium intracellulare*, and lymphadenopathy of the AIDS-related complex.

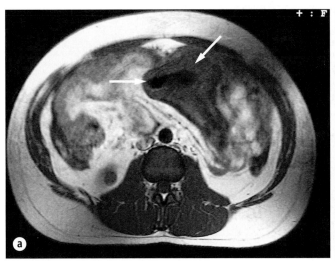
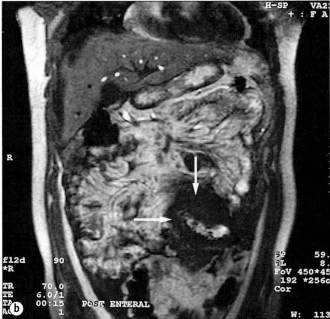

Fig. 3.51 Non-Hodgkin's lymphoma of the small bowel is seen as extensive bowel wall thickening and a necrotic soft-tissue mass (arrows). (**a**) T1-weighted axial MR image. (**b**) Coronal gradient echo MR image.

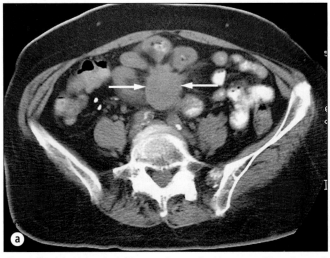
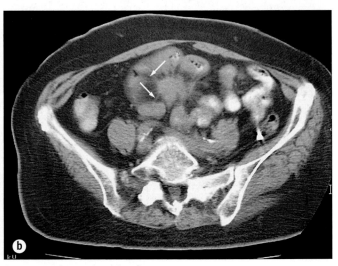

Fig. 3.52 (**a**) Abdominal CT scan of a carcinoid tumour. There is a soft-tissue mass (arrows) arising from the ileum. (**b**) A section 10 mm inferior to that in (**a**) shows the typical desmoplastic reaction in the mesentery, with fibrosis tethering adjacent loops of small bowel (small arrows).

Leiomyosarcoma
Malignant transformation of a benign leiomyoma may lead to the development of a leiomyosarcoma. Typically, these tumours are visible as bulky masses on CT, and grow eccentrically.

Small-bowel metastases
Small bowel involvement with metastases may be extrinsic as a result of peritoneal seedings, or intrinsic as a result of haematogenous spread, usually from a melanoma or bronchial carcinoma.

POLYPOSIS SYNDROMES

Several syndromes with multiple polyps in the GI tract have been identified (**Fig. 3.53**). The polyps may be adenomatous, and therefore have a malignant potential, or they may be hamartomatous. The most common site is the colon (**Fig. 3.54**).

Gardener's syndrome and Turcot's syndrome are probably subtypes of familial adenomatous polyposis syndrome. They have the additional features of osteomas, sebaceous cysts, abnormal teeth, desmoid tumours, and periampullary carcinomas (Gardener's syndrome) or malignant tumours of the central nervous system (Turcot's syndrome).

VASCULAR DISORDERS

GASTROINTESTINAL HAEMORRHAGE

There are many causes of GI bleeding. Those most frequently encountered in clinical practice are listed in **Figure 3.55**.

Polyposis syndromes		
Syndrome	**Main site of polyps**	**Type of polyps**
Familial adenomatous polyposis	Colon, rectum	Adenomatous
Gardener's syndrome	Colon, rectum	Adenomatous
Turcot's syndrome	Colon, rectum	Adenomatous
Peutz-Jegher's syndrome	Stomach, small bowel, (colon)	Hamartomatous
Juvenile polyposis	Colon	Hamartomatous
Metaplastic polyposis	Rectum (colon)	Hamartomatous
Canada–Cronkhite syndrome	Diffuse	Hamartomatous

Fig. 3.53 Polyposis syndromes.

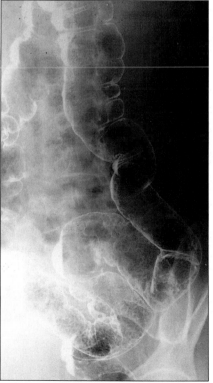

Fig. 3.54 Barium enema in familial adenomatous polyposis coli, showing multiple small polyps carpeting the colon.

Causes of gastrointestinal (GI) haemorrhage	
Upper GI tract	Oesophagitis
	Mallory–Weis tear
	Oesophageal varices
	Peptic ulcer
	Gastritis/duodenitis
	Neoplasms, esp. leiomyoma
	Arteriovenous malformations
Lower GI tract	Haemorrhoids
	Neoplasms
	Diverticular disease
	Small-bowel ulceration (NSAIDs)
	Caecal angiodysplasia
	Ischaemic colitis
	Inflammatory bowel disease

Fig. 3.55 Causes of gastrointestinal haemorrhage.

Chronic GI blood loss, whether from the upper or lower GI tract, presents with anaemia.

Upper GI bleeding may present as haematemesis of fresh blood or altered blood ('coffee ground' vomit), or as melaena. Upper GI endoscopy is the investigation of choice; barium studies are not helpful, as it is not possible to identify the lesion that is bleeding.

Lower GI bleeding may present as fresh rectal bleeding, or the passage of dark, altered blood if the bleeding site is in the small bowel or proximal colon. Proctoscopy, sigmoidoscopy, and colonoscopy are the investigations of choice.

If the investigations mentioned above are negative in the presence of continued bleeding, mesenteric angiography is indicated. The coeliac, superior mesenteric, and inferior mesenteric arteries are catheterized in turn to identify extravasation of contrast (**Figs 3.56** and **3.57**). If the source of blood loss remains occult, a nuclear medicine study using radiolabelled red cells may reveal accumulation of the cells at the site of bleeding.

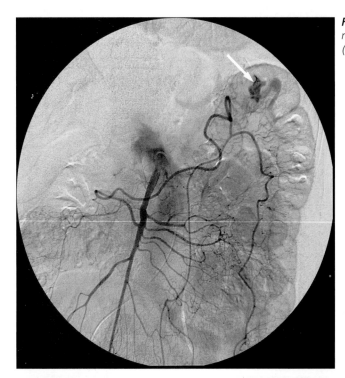

Fig. 3.56 *Superior mesenteric angiogram in a patient with profuse rectal bleeding. Note the extravasation of contrast in the splenic flexure (arrow), as a result of a bleeding diverticulum.*

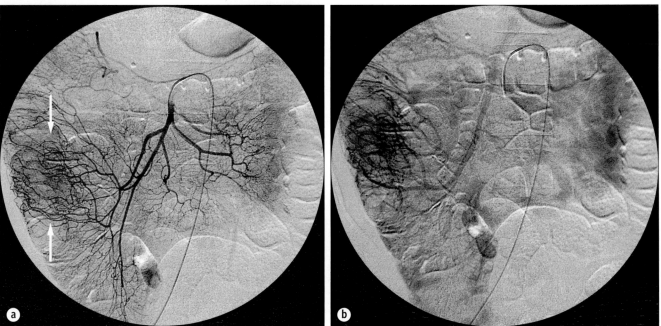

Fig. 3.57 *(a) Superior mesenteric angiogram in a patient with rectal bleeding. Colonscopy was possible only as far as the hepatic flexure, where fresh blood was seen. Note the increased vascularity in the middle ascending colon (arrows). (b) Later films from the same patient, showing contrast extravasation and early venous drainage which was due to a carcinoma of the colon.*

INTESTINAL ISCHAEMIA

The most common cause of small bowel ischaemia is occlusion of the superior mesenteric artery by thrombosis or embolism. Any torsion of the gut, such as a strangulated hernia or volvulus, also will result in ischaemia.

Plain film signs in small bowel ischaemia are often minimal compared with the severity of the patient's illness. Small bowel dilatation and intramural gas tend to be late signs (**Fig. 3.58**). Plain film signs of ischaemic colitis are more obvious, mucosal oedema giving a characteristic 'thumb print' pattern in the acute stage (**Fig. 3.59**). Chronic colonic ischaemia results in strictures (**Fig. 3.60**); the typical sites for these are the splenic flexure and proximal descending colon, at the watershed between the arterial supplies from the superior and inferior mesenteric arteries.

There are many other causes of intestinal ischaemia, involving small vessels (**Fig. 3.61**). Typically, these give rise to strictures.

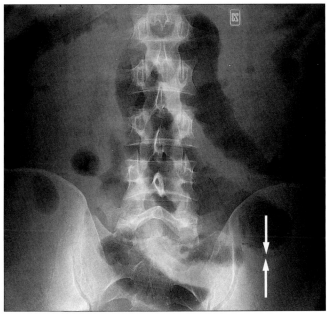

Fig. 3.58 *Supine abdominal radiograph of small bowel ischaemia. There are dilated loops of small bowel with intramural gas (arrows). At laparotomy, the small bowel was found to be infarcted.*

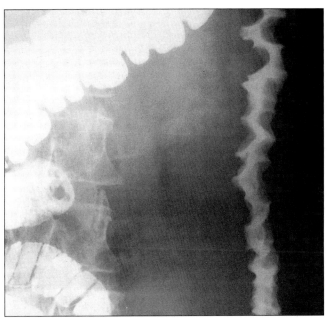

Fig. 3.59 *Water-soluble contrast enema in acute ischaemic colitis. There is extensive mucosal oedema, giving a 'thumb printing' pattern.*

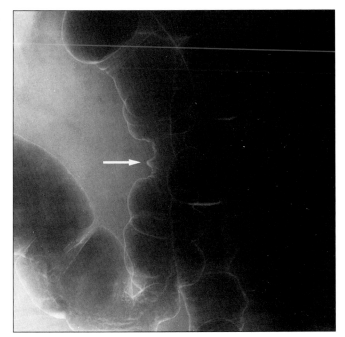

Fig. 3.60 *Double-contrast barium enema in chronic ischaemic colitis, showing a focal, smooth stricture (arrow).*

Causes of intestinal ischaemia	
Occlusive	Arterial thrombosis/embolism
	Dissecting abdominal aortic aneurysm
	Trauma
	Intussusception
	Volvulus
	Strangulated hernia
	Ischaemic colitis
Non-occlusive	Radiotherapy
	Systemic lupus erythematosus
	Polyarteritis nodosa
	Thrombangiitis obliterans

Fig. 3.61 *Causes of intestinal ischaemia.*

INTESTINAL LYMPHANGIECTASIA

Intestinal lymphangiectasia is a rare condition that may be primary, as a result of a congenital abnormality of the lymphatics, or secondary to lymphatic obstruction. It gives rise to malabsorption. On a small bowel examination, there is generalized thickening and nodularity of the mucosal folds of the small bowel (**Fig. 3.62**).

DEGENERATIVE CONDITIONS

PHARYNGEAL DYSMOTILITY

A variety of diseases affecting pharyngeal innervation (e.g. stroke and bulbar palsy) or muscles can result in pharyngeal dysmotility. Aspiration can occur, and patients are at risk of aspiration pneumonia. Video fluoroscopy of swallowing allows dynamic examination of swallowing abnormalities. Barium of different consistencies is used, to mimic normal diet and determine if it is safe for the patient to continue oral feeding, or if an alternative route such as a gastrostomy should be used.

OESOPHAGEAL SPASM

Oesophageal spasm is common in elderly patients and is caused by non-propulsive contraction of the oesophageal circular muscle (tertiary contractions). Clinically, it can present with chest pain and intermittent dysphagia. A barium swallow shows multiple transient strictures giving the oesophagus a 'corkscrew' appearance (**Fig. 3.63**).

DIVERTICULA

Diverticula can occur throughout the GI tract, but those at the following sites are the most common.

Pharyngeal pouch

A pharyngeal pouch arises at a congenitally weak point in the pharyngeal wall, between the superior and middle pharyngeal constrictors (Killean's dehiscence). If large, they collect food debris and cause dysphagia. A pharyngeal pouch can sometimes be seen on a plain film of the neck, and is obvious on a barium swallow (**Fig. 3.64**).

Duodenal diverticulum

Duodenal diverticula are most often found on the medial aspect of the second part of the duodenum in the region of the ampulla, where they may make cannulation of the common bile duct and pancreatic duct impossible at endoscopic retrograde cholangiopancreatography.

Jejunal diverticula

Multiple jejunal diverticula can become colonized by bacteria; bacterial overgrowth results in malabsorption (**Fig. 3.65**).

Colonic diverticular disease

Colonic diverticular disease is very common in the western world, and rare in Africa. It is believed to be caused by a low-residue diet, resulting in increased intracolonic pressure, with hypertrophy of the circular smooth muscle; mucosa and submucosa then herniate between bands of hypertrophied circular muscle at points of natural weakness. The sigmoid colon is the most common site for diverticular disease, but diverticula can occur throughout the colon (**Fig. 3.66**).

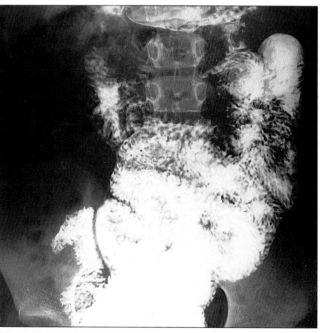

Fig. 3.62 Intestinal lymphangiectasia on a small bowel study, demonstrating the characteristic diffuse thickening and nodularity of the mucosal folds.

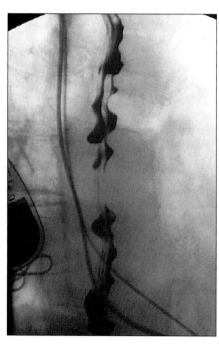

Fig. 3.63 Barium swallow in an elderly patient with diffuse oesophageal spasm. The oesophagus has a 'corkscrew' appearance. The patient has a permanent pacemaker.

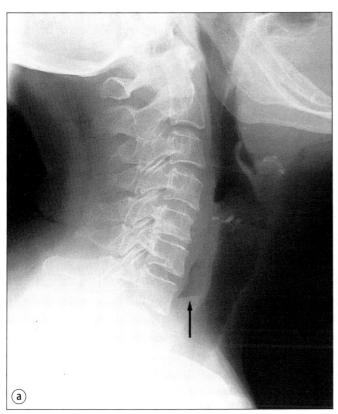

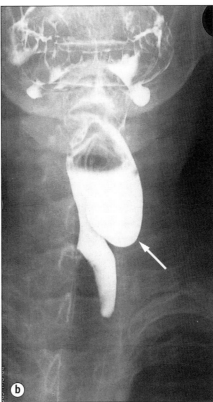

Fig. 3.64 (a) Lateral soft-tissue view of the neck in a patient with a pharyngeal pouch. An air–fluid interface is seen anterior to the cervical spine (arrow). (b) Barium swallow of the same patient, showing the pharyngeal pouch (arrow) filled with barium.

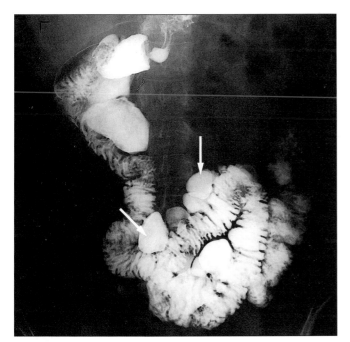

Fig. 3.65 Small-bowel study demonstrating multiple diverticula arising from the jejunum (arrows) in a patient with jejunal diverticulosis.

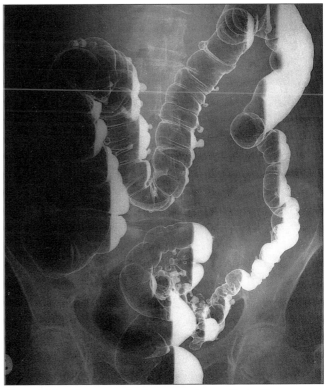

Fig. 3.66 Double-contrast barium enema in a patient with diverticular disease. There are multiple diverticula, which are most numerous in the sigmoid colon.

Complications of diverticular disease include diverticulitis (which presents like a left-sided appendicitis), pericolic abscess (**Fig. 3.67**), perforation, strictures, fistulae into adjacent organs (**Fig 3.68**), and haemorrhage. The presence of diverticular disease on a barium enema makes the exclusion of polyps and small tumours more difficult.

PELVIC FLOOR ABNORMALITIES AND RECTAL PROLAPSE

Abnormalities of the pelvic floor present with constipation or faecal incontinence. The most common group of patients with these abnormalities are middle-aged women who have suffered pelvic floor trauma during childbirth.

The radiological examination that evaluates the pelvic floor and abnormalities of defaecation is called evacuation proctography. Abnormal descent of the perineum, rectoceles (outpouchings of the rectal wall) and rectal prolapse can be diagnosed by this means.

METABOLIC AND TOXIC CONDITIONS

MALABSORPTION

Malabsorption can be caused by abnormal digestion in chronic pancreatitis, biliary obstruction, or Zollinger–Ellison syndrome, or following ileal resection. In these diseases the small bowel appears normal.

There are many diseases of the small bowel that can result in failure of normal absorption of dietary nutrients. Clinically, malabsorption presents with growth failure (in children), weight loss, anaemia, and steatorrhoea (loose, pale stools that float because of their high fat content). Some of the more common causes and their radiological appearances are listed in **Figure 3.69**.

A small bowel enema is the best radiological investigation of the small bowel, although appearances are often non-specific.

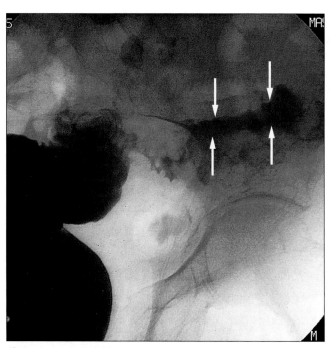

Fig. 3.67 *Water-soluble contrast enema demonstrating a pericolic abscess. Contrast is seen to track into a collection (arrows) adjacent to the diseased sigmoid colon.*

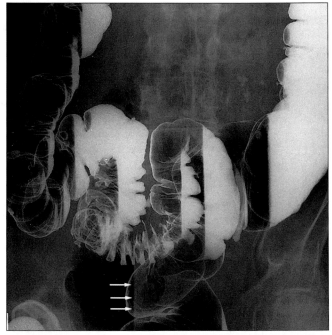

Fig. 3.68 *Double-contrast barium enema in a patient with a vesicocolic fistula secondary to diverticular disease. This film was taken with a horizontal X-ray beam and the patient lying on their left side; it shows an air–fluid interface in the urinary bladder (arrows).*

Coeliac disease

Coeliac disease is the most common cause of malabsorption in northern Europe, and can occur at any age. It is caused by an immunological reaction to the α-gliadin factor in gluten. The diagnosis is made on a combination of clinical features and subtotal villous atrophy revealed on jejunal biopsy. The mucosal abnormality should resolve on a gluten-free diet, and recur after a gluten challenge.

Complications of coeliac disease are non-Hodgkin's lymphoma of the small bowel, carcinoma of the duodenum, and ulcerative jejunoileitis. Related conditions are dermatitis herpetiformis and hyposplenism.

DRUG TOXICITY IN THE GASTROINTESTINAL TRACT

Drugs known to be toxic in the gastrointestinal tract include slow-release potassium tablets, which can cause oesophageal ulceration and stricture formation, and NSAIDs, which can cause ulceration in the stomach, duodenum, and small bowel, and small bowel strictures.

Small-bowel diseases causing malabsorption, and their appearances on small-bowel enema examination (SBE)	
Disease	**SBE appearance**
Coeliac disease	Dilatation of the jejunum Reduced mucosal folds in jejunum Increased mucosal folds in ileum Complications (*see above*)
Crohn's disease	Thickened mucosal folds and nodules (*see* **Figs 3.26–3.32**) Ulceration and 'cobblestoning' Bowel wall thickening Strictures, fistulae, and sinuses Skip lesions and pseudodiverticula
Systemic sclerosis	Lumen dilatation Crowding of mucosal folds Sacculations of antimesenteric border
Jejunal diverticulosis	Multiple jejunal diverticula (*see* **Fig. 3.65**)
Short-bowel syndrome	Dilatation of remaining small bowel Increased number and thickness of mucosal folds
Whipple's disease	Multiple mucosal nodules
Amyloidosis	Thickened mucosal folds and nodules
Eosinophilic gastroenteritis	Mucosal thickening in gastric antrum and small bowel
Intestinal lymphangiectasia	Thickened mucosal folds and tiny nodules (*see* **Fig. 3.62**)
Mastocytosis	Bowel wall thickening and large nodules

Fig. 3.69 *Small-bowel diseases causing malabsorption, and their appearances on small-bowel enema examination.*

GASTROINTESTINAL TRACT ABNORMALITIES IN DIABETES MELLITUS

Diabetic autonomic neuropathy can cause a variety of GI tract abnormalities, as a result of parasympathetic dysfunction (Fig. 3.70). Radiological manifestations of autonomic neuropathy are listed in Figure 3.71.

MISCELLANEOUS CONDITIONS

ACHALASIA

Achalasia is a primary motility disorder of the oesophagus that affects young adults. There is failure of relaxation of the lower oesophageal sphincter, and absence of normal peristalsis. A barium swallow shows a dilated oesophagus, which often contains food residue, and tapered narrowing to the lower oesophageal sphincter (Fig. 3.72).

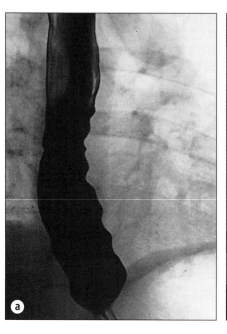

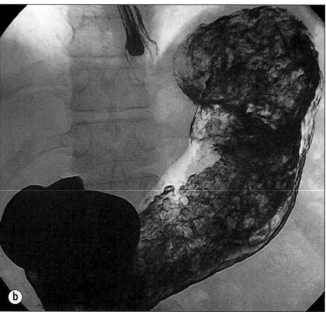

Fig. 3.70 Barium swallow and meal in a 24-year-old patient with diabetic autonomic neuropathy. (*a*) Gastro-oesophageal reflux and tertiary contractions of the oesophagus. (*b*) A large amount of solid food residue remains in the stomach, despite a 12-hour fast.

| \multicolumn{2}{c}{Gastrointestinal tract manifestations of autonomic neuropathy} ||
Site	Radiological manifestation
Oesophagus	Tertiary contractions Gastro-oesophageal reflux
Stomach	Solid residue in stomach after overnight fast Delayed gastric emptying on nuclear medicine studies No evidence of mechanical obstruction Elongated, sausage-shaped stomach Acute gastric dilatation
Small bowel	Dilatation and delayed transit
Colon	Faecal residue and delayed transit

Other metabolic abnormalities, such as hypokalaemia and hepatic coma, can result in gastric dilatation and ileus.

Fig. 3.71 Gastrointestinal tract manifestations of autonomic neuropathy.

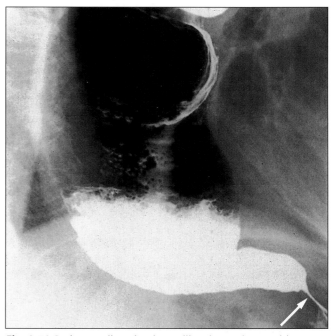

Fig. 3.72 Barium swallow showing a dilated oesophagus with a tapered stricture (arrow) at its lower end; this is typical of achalasia.

DILATATION OF THE GASTROINTESTINAL TRACT

Plain films often show a dilated small bowel, colon, or both. There are many causes, both obstructive and non-obstructive, which are listed in **Figure 3.73**.

Paralytic ileus

Paralytic ileus is a term which means dilated bowel due to lack of normal peristalsis. It is common, and is seen with peritonitis (caused by any inflamed viscus; e.g. appendicitis, cholecystitis, pancreatitis) and after laparotomy. The plain film findings may be identical to those of obstruction.

Adhesions

Adhesions are the most common cause of small-bowel obstruction (**Fig. 3.74**). They are fibrous bands that occur between the peritoneal surfaces of loops of bowel, secondary to previous laparotomy or laparoscopy. In the absence of a history of previous surgery, an obstructed hernia should be suspected. It is important, therefore, to include the hernial orifices on any plain film of the abdomen when obstruction is suspected.

Volvulus

Volvulus is a twisting of the gut that can affect any part of the GI tract that has a mesentery. The typical sites are the stomach, small bowel (associated with congenital malrotation), caecum, and sigmoid colon (**Fig. 3.75**).

PNEUMOPERITONEUM

Gas in the peritoneal cavity, termed pneumoperitoneum, can occur as a result of perforation of a viscus, or can be seen after laparotomy. The most common cause is a perforated peptic ulcer, but tumours and diverticula can also perforate. An erect chest radiograph and a supine abdominal radiograph are the investigations of choice. The former will show free gas beneath the diaphragm, and the latter will show gas on both sides of the bowel wall, indicating intraluminal and intraperitoneal gas (*see* Fig. 3.25).

INTRA-ABDOMINAL ABSCESSES

Intra-abdominal abscesses are localized collections of pus that arise either as a complication of surgery, or by extension of inflammation and infection from a bowel abnormality such as diverticulitis, appendicitis, or Crohn's disease. Ultrasound and CT scanning will show

Causes of intestinal dilatation	
Obstructive	Postoperative adhesions
	Tumour
	Hernia
	Intussusception
	Volvulus
	Gall-stone ileus
Non-obstructive	Postoperative
	Peritonitis
	Pancreatitis
	Trauma
	Diabetic autonomic neuropathy
	Hypokalaemia
	Hepatic coma
	Mesenteric infarction
	Toxic dilatation in colitis

Fig. 3.73 *Causes of intestinal dilatation.*

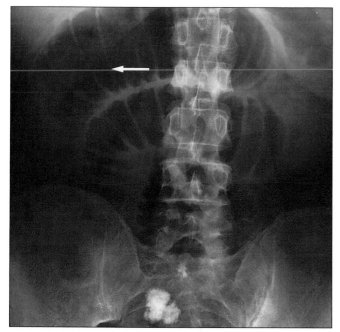

Fig. 3.74 *Supine abdominal radiograph in small bowel obstruction. The multiple, dilated loops are of small bowel; they can be distinguished from large bowel because the mucosal folds (arrow) cross the full width of the dilated small bowel, unlike colonic haustra.*

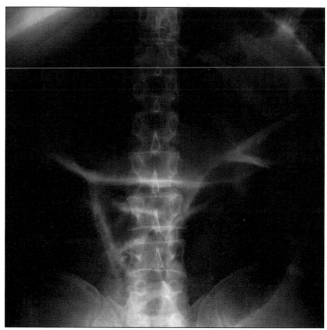

Fig. 3.75 *Supine abdominal radiograph showing an enormously dilated colon as a result of sigmoid volvulus.*

these abscesses. If these investigations are negative, an [111]indium-labelled white cell nuclear medicine scan is often helpful in locating the source of sepsis in a pyrexial patient (**Fig. 3.76**).

INTRAPERITONEAL FLUID

Free intraperitoneal fluid (ascites) is best seen on ultrasound. With the patient in the supine position, fluid collects in the pelvic peritoneal cavity, and is seen on ultrasound to outline pelvic organs and loops of bowel (**Fig. 3.77**).

PNEUMATOSIS COLI

Pneumatosis coli is an uncommon condition in which blebs of gas collect in the wall of the colon (**Fig. 3.78**). It usually occurs in patients with chronic obstructive pulmonary disease. Occasionally, a bleb may rupture, causing a pneumoperitoneum.

BEZOAR

A bezoar is a collection of solid material in the stomach. It can occur in children as a result of ingestion of foreign bodies or hair chewing (a trichobezoar), or in diabetic patients with gastric autonomic neuropathy.

POSTOPERATIVE APPEARANCES

Figures **3.79** to **3.82** show some characteristic appearances after GI surgery.

INTERVENTIONAL PROCEDURES

OESOPHAGEAL STENTING

Stenting of the oesophagus using expandable metallic stents is now the palliative treatment of choice for inoperable oesophageal cancer (**Fig. 3.83**).

OESOPHAGEAL BALLOON DILATATION

Benign oesophageal strictures can be dilated with a balloon catheter (**Fig. 3.84**). This procedure can be performed repeatedly if the stricture recurs.

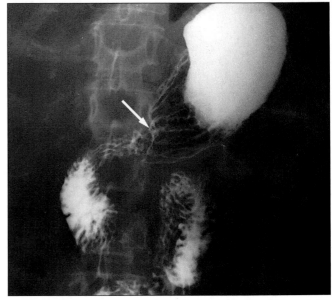

Fig. 3.76 [111]Indium-labelled white cell scan, showing the site of an intra-abdominal abscess (arrow). The normal spleen is also apparent.

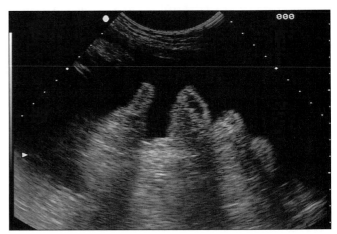

Fig. 3.77 Ultrasound image showing free intraperitoneal fluid (black areas) surrounding loops of bowel, in a patient with ascites.

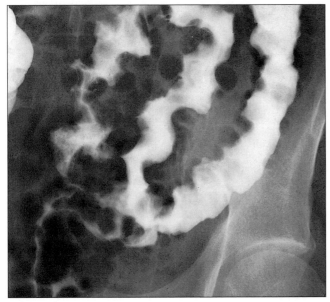

Fig. 3.78 Barium enema in pneumatosis coli. Note the multiple gas-filled blebs in the wall of the rectum, sigmoid and descending colon.

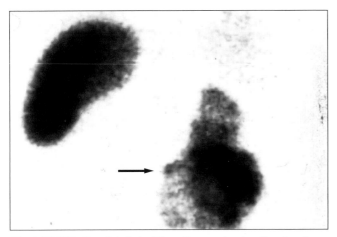

Fig. 3.79 Barium meal in a patient who has had a previous partial gastrectomy (Bilroth I). There has been resection of the gastric antrum and pylorus, with gastroduodenal anastomosis (arrow).

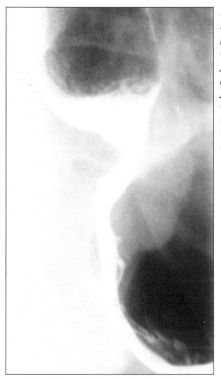

Fig. 3.80 *Barium swallow, showing the postoperative appearances after fundoplication. This procedure is performed for severe gastro-oesophageal reflux, and the gastric fundus is wrapped around the lower oesophagus.*

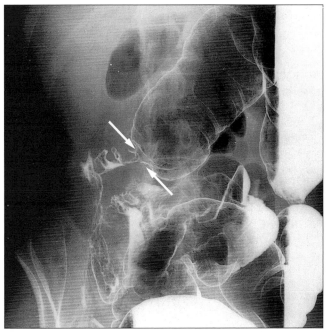

Fig. 3.81 *Barium enema after right hemicolectomy for Crohn's disease. There has been recurrence of disease at the ileocolic anastomosis (arrows).*

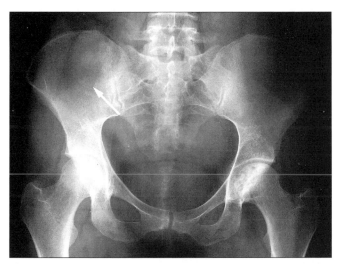

Fig. 3.82 *Pelvic radiograph in a patient with Crohn's disease who has undergone total colectomy and ileostomy. The plastic ring of the stoma bag is faintly radio-opaque (arrow). Note the absence of the usual colonic and rectal gas, and avascular necrosis of the left femoral head secondary to steroid treatment.*

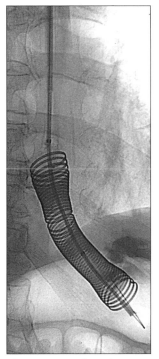

Fig. 3.83 *Oesophageal stent in situ. This patient had an inoperable carcinoma of the lower third of the oesophagus, and had complete dysphagia before insertion of the stent. After the procedure, he was able to manage a soft diet. The stent delivery system can be seen within the stent lumen.*

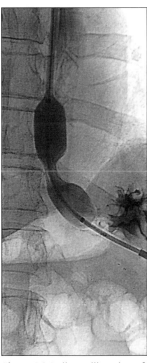

Fig. 3.84 *Balloon dilatation of a benign oesophageal stricture. The site of the stricture is seen at the waist of the balloon. With successful dilatation, the waist of the balloon disappears.*

GASTROSTOMY

In patients who are unable to swallow safely, usually because of stroke or other neurological disease involving the pharyngeal muscles, direct feeding into the stomach can be carried out through a gastrostomy. The gastrostomy tube can be inserted radiologically, by direct puncture of the distended stomach (**Fig. 3.85**), or endoscopically.

COLONIC STENTING

Benign or malignant strictures of the colon can be stented in patients who are not suitable for surgical resection.

EMBOLIZATION OF VASCULAR ABNORMALITIES

In a patient with profuse GI haemorrhage, it is sometimes possible to embolize the bleeding lesion to prevent further haemorrhage. This may be a temporary procedure such as embolization of a vascular tumour before surgical resection, or a definitive treatment of, for example, a bleeding arteriovenous malformation.

Care must be taken to ensure that embolization in the mesenteric circulation does not result in bowel infarction. Because of collateral circulation, it is also important that all branches supplying an abnormality are identified and occluded, otherwise haemorrhage may continue.

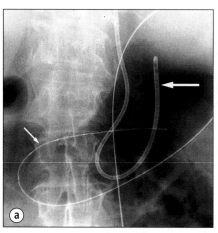
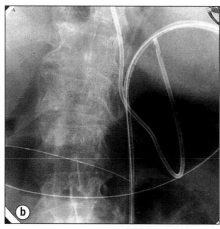
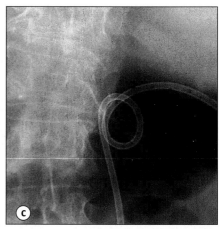

Fig. 3.85 Percutaneous gastrostomy. (*a*) The patient's stomach is distended with air through a nasogastric tube (large arrow), the anterior wall of the stomach is punctured percutaneously, and a guidewire is inserted (small arrow). (*b*) The gastrostomy tube is fed over the guidewire. (*c*) The guidewire and nasogastric tubes are withdrawn, and the retaining 'pigtail' of gastrostomy tube is formed.

chapter 4

Liver, Biliary System, Pancreas, and Spleen

Part 1. Liver

CONGENITAL ABNORMALITIES

Many inherited metabolic diseases, for example glycogen storage diseases, cystic fibrosis, and Gaucher's disease, have associated liver disease—often cirrhosis. Polycystic kidney disease may be associated with congenital hepatic fibrosis in neonates or, more commonly, with multiple hepatic cysts in adults (Fig. 4.1).

TRAUMA

Both blunt and direct trauma may affect the liver, causing laceration and haemorrhage that, if not contained within the liver capsule, may result in a large intraperitoneal bleed. CT with intravenous contrast reveals the damage sustained by the liver, and its relationship to the porta hepatis, the capsule, and the surrounding structures (Fig. 4.2).

INFECTION

Viral hepatitis
In viral hepatitis, the liver may appear diffusely enlarged and hypoechoic on ultrasound; however, these changes are non-specific.

Liver abscess
Most liver abscesses are pyogenic, a few are amoebic or fungal, and some are caused by hydatid disease; this last cause is particularly common in areas of the world where hydatid disease is endemic, such as the Middle East. The diagnosis of liver abscess is made on either ultrasound or CT (Fig. 4.3).

Pyogenic abscesses, if left undiagnosed or untreated, are fatal; their presentation is often late, because of their insidious onset and non-specific symptoms. If an abscess is found, aspiration for diagnostic purposes, followed by catheter drainage percutaneously, is the treatment of choice, combined with appropriate antibiotics.

Amoebic abscesses in the liver occur after colonic infestation, are usually single, and occur in the right lobe of the liver. They may rupture into the peritoneum, superiorly through the diaphragm into the pleural space or, rarely, into the pericardial space.

World wide, hydatid cysts in the liver are the most common infective cyst of the liver. On CT, they show a characteristic appearance, with a large cyst often surrounded by daughter cysts (Fig. 4.4). Calcification may occur around the cyst. Other complications include secondary infection and rupture of the cyst.

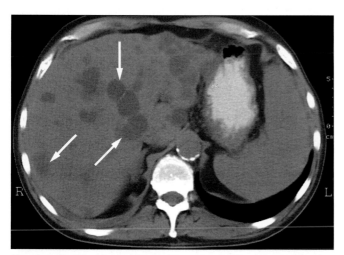

Fig. 4.1 CT of liver in a patient with autosomal dominant polycystic kidney disease with multiple hepatic cysts (arrows).

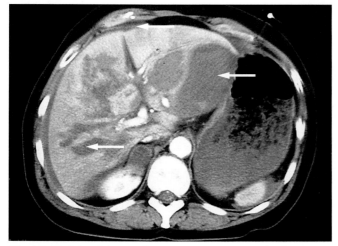

Fig. 4.2 CT of the abdomen after trauma. There is extensive liver laceration, resulting in intrahepatic and peritoneal bleeding (arrows).

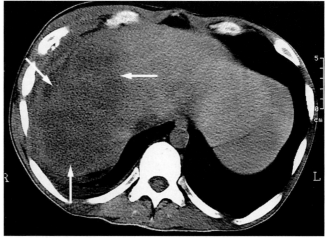

Fig. 4.3 Unenhanced CT scan, showing an extensive low-density area in the right lobe of the liver (arrows); this is a hepatic abscess.

Schistosomiasis

Schistosomiasis is a common tropical disease with liver involvement seen in two forms of the disease, caused by *Schistosoma mansoni* and *Sch. japonicum*. The worms, and later their eggs, enter the portal venous system; after repeated infestation, this causes the chronic form of the disease, with marked periportal fibrosis, portal hypertension, and varices (*see* Fig. 4.7).

INFLAMMATORY CONDITIONS

Non-infective hepatitis

Hepatitis can be caused by alcohol and drugs, and may occur in autoimmune conditions. In common with infective hepatitis, it can have non-specific appearances on imaging, with a generally bright echo pattern on ultrasound.

Cirrhosis

Cirrhosis is the end result of many chronic liver diseases. The most common cause is alcoholic liver disease. Fatty infiltration occurs after the stage of hepatitis, but before cirrhosis (**Fig. 4.5**), and is diagnosed on CT by low attenuation of the liver parenchyma compared with the normal blood vessels. Later, cirrhosis develops and the liver has an irregular shape, becomes shrunken, and has a variable echo pattern on ultrasound (**Fig. 4.6**) and variable attenuation on CT. The features of portal hypertension, namely varices, ascites, and splenomegaly, may then develop (**Fig. 4.7**). Regenerating nodules in cirrhotic livers may pose a diagnostic problem on both CT and ultrasound, but can be differentiated from malignancy by their uptake on radionuclide technetium–sulphur colloid scans (**Fig. 4.8**).

The haemodynamic effects of cirrhosis can be demonstrated by ultrasound, to reveal the liver texture, complemented by Doppler studies of the systemic arterial and venous systems and of the portal venous system.

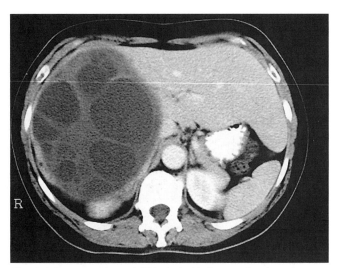

Fig. 4.4 *Contrast-enhanced CT in hydatid disease, showing a large cystic lesion occupying most of the right lobe of the liver, with multiple smaller daughter cysts.*

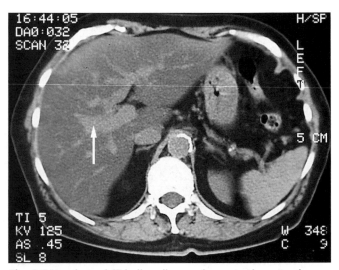

Fig. 4.5 *Unenhanced CT in liver disease, demonstrating extensive fatty change. Most of the liver parenchyma is hypodense because of fatty infiltration, making the normal blood vessels (arrow) hyperdense in comparison.*

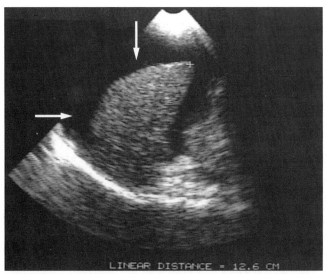

Fig. 4.6 *Longitudinal right upper quadrant ultrasound image in cirrhosis. The liver is shrunken and of irregular echogenicity and contour, and surrounding ascites can be seen (arrows).*

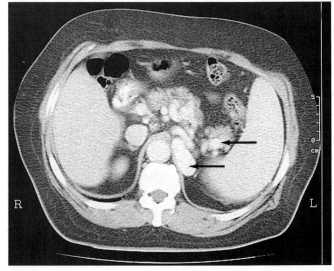

Fig. 4.7 *Contrast-enhanced CT showing the features of portal hypertension, including multiple varices (arrows) and splenomegaly.*

Hepatic disease associated with inflammatory bowel disease

Abnormal liver function tests are present in about 5% of patients with inflammatory bowel disease. Chronic active hepatitis, cirrhosis, and amyloidosis can occur in patients with Crohn's disease and ulcerative colitis; they are probably related to genetic immunological abnormalities affecting both the liver and the bowel.

NEOPLASTIC DISEASE

MALIGNANT LIVER TUMOURS
Metastases

At autopsy, about 50% of patients with malignant disease will show evidence of secondary metastatic tumour in the liver; this is by far the most common liver malignancy. Diagnosis of liver metastases is important in the initial staging of malignancy, assessment of response to treatment, and detection of recurrent disease. CT without contrast and ultrasound are comparable in their accuracy rates for diagnosing metastatic liver disease, some tumours having characteristic appearances.

The ultrasound appearances may vary considerably, from echo-bright lesions common in colonic metastases to echo-poor, almost cystic, lesions (Fig. 4.9). Correlation between the origin of the primary tumour and the liver appearances is often poor. On CT, images of metastases (Fig. 4.10) may be delineated more clearly by contrast enhancement, but the timing of scanning after contrast is important as, depending on the vascularity of the tumour, metastases may be isodense with liver, either on unenhanced scans or during certain phases of contrast enhancement.

On plain abdominal radiographs, calcification in the liver may be seen in deposits from colonic tumours; however, it also occurs in thyroid and carcinoid metastases, and the sign is therefore non-specific (Fig. 4.11).

MR imaging with new specific contrast agents is as yet unproven for this application, but early trials are encouraging, particularly in the diagnosis of early small metastases (Fig. 4.12).

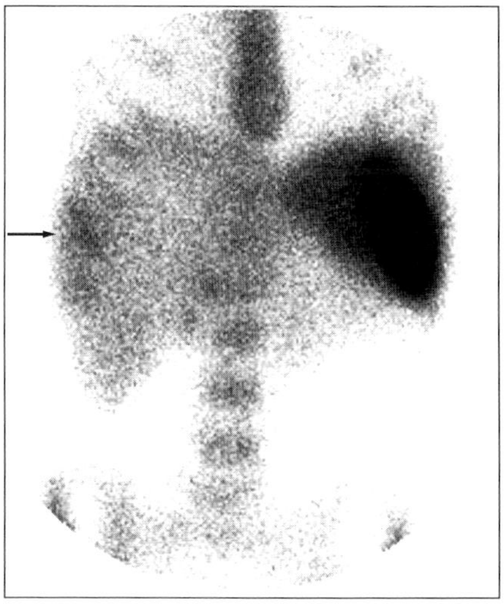

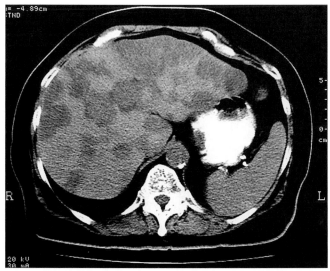

Fig. 4.8 Radionuclide ^{99m}technetium–sulphur colloid scan in a patient with cirrhosis. The liver has an irregular contour, and there is radionuclide uptake into a cirrhotic nodule (arrow).

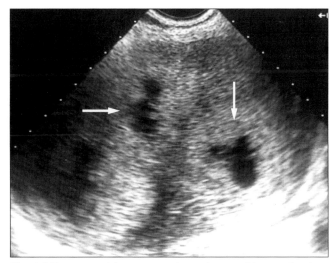

Fig. 4.9 Transverse right upper quadrant ultrasound image, showing multiple metastases (arrows).

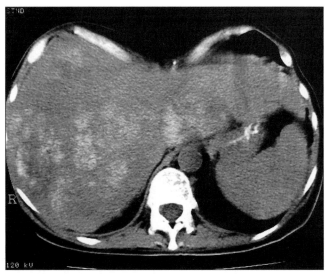

Fig. 4.10 Unenhanced CT image, showing multiple hypodense hepatic metastases in both right and left lobes of the liver.

Fig. 4.11 Unenhanced CT image, showing multiple hepatic metastases that are hyperdense because of calcification. These were from a primary colon cancer.

Hepatocellular carcinoma

Hepatocellular carcinoma (HCC) is the most common primary tumour of the liver in adults. There is a low incidence in the western world, mainly related to the low incidence of hepatitis B infection, but in the Far East, where chronic hepatitis B is much more common, the incidence of HCC is also greater. There is also an increased incidence of HCC in patients with cirrhosis and haemochromatosis. More than 50% of non-cirrhotic patients with HCC have high levels of alpha fetoprotein; the percentage increases among those with cirrhosis.

Radiologically, ultrasound, CT (**Fig. 4.13**), and MR imaging can all be used to demonstrate a focal liver mass. Further assessment of the hepatic artery by angiography is necessary when treatment options are considered that include resection, embolization, and intra-arterial chemotherapy.

Hepatoblastoma

The peak incidence of hepatoblastoma occurs in infancy; it is the third most common intra-abdominal childhood malignancy, after neuro-blastoma and nephroblastoma. The tumour has rapid growth and is highly invasive, metastazing to the lungs and abdominal lymph nodes.

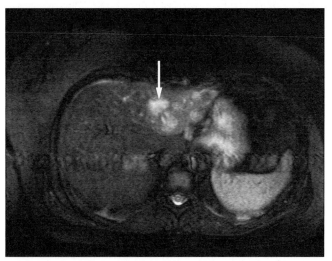

Fig. 4.12 *T2-weighted axial MR image, showing multiple high-signal metastases in the left lobe of the liver.*

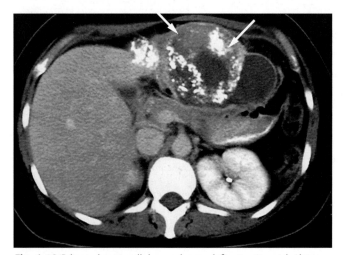

Fig. 4.13 *Primary hepatocellular carcinoma (after treatment by intra-arterial chemotherapy) in the left lobe of the liver (arrows).*

BENIGN TUMOURS
Haemangioma

The use of ultrasound for the routine scanning of the liver in a variety of conditions has led to the recognition of the high percentage of normal patients (about 5%) who have an asymptomatic, single, <3 cm, echo-bright peripheral lesion that is characteristic of a haemangioma. If there is doubt as to the diagnosis, it may be confirmed on CT, by the delayed uptake of intravenous contrast into the lesion, which slowly infills towards the centre over the course of a few minutes; the slow uptake occurs in the abnormal vascular spaces that comprise the tumour. Whereas the majority of haemangiomas are small and single, multiple lesions can exist, and their size may be considerable (**Fig. 4.14**). The α fetoprotein concentration is always normal in these cases, distinguishing them from HCC.

Adenoma

Liver-cell adenoma has the potential for malignant change, and may be difficult to differentiate from HCC on imaging alone. It is associated with use of oral contraceptives, and may present with bleeding. The size of the tumour varies from 6 cm to approximately 15 cm.

Focal nodular hyperplasia

Focal nodular hyperplasia is a benign, hamartomatous, well-defined liver mass that, on imaging and pathologically, shows a stellate configuration with radiating septae and a central scar. It is usually an incidental finding, and debate continues as to what, if any, treatment should be given. As with other hamartomas, there is no malignant potential.

VASCULAR SYSTEM

NORMAL VASCULAR ANATOMY

There is a wide variation in the arterial supply of the liver, which comes totally from the coeliac axis, in the conventional form, in only 70% of patients. In the remaining 30% of patients, the right hepatic artery may arise from the superior mesenteric artery (**Fig. 4.15**), which may occasionally also provide the total hepatic arterial supply. Variations in the origins of the intrahepatic arteries are also common.

The liver has a dual blood supply, the other major component being the portal venous system, formed primarily from the superior mesenteric and splenic veins. The liver vasculature drains into the inferior vena cava through the three hepatic veins.

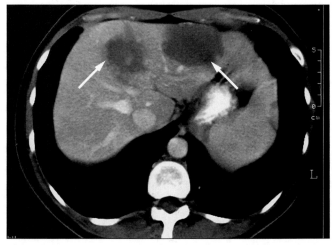

Fig. 4.14 *Contrast-enhanced CT of two large cavernous haemangiomas (arrows), showing early peripheral contrast enhancement.*

VASCULAR ABNORMALITIES
Arterial flow
Increased arterial flow is present in patients who have cirrhosis and in whom the portal venous flow is reduced, absent, or retrograde, and in patients with benign and malignant nodular disease, with which a pathological circulation may exist.

Portal venous hypertension
An increase in portal venous pressure as a result of obstruction will cause the extensive collateral circulation to carry portal blood into the systemic circulation. Such portosystemic shunts lead to hepatic encephalopathy, septicaemia, haemorrhage, and other circulatory problems. There are four main groups of venous collaterals involved:

- The para-umbilical veins open up to form 'caput medusae' (**Fig. 4.16**).
- The retroperitoneal vessels dilate and become tortuous (*see* Fig. 4.7).
- The left renal vein provides a route for shunting.
- Anastomoses that exist around the cardia of the stomach and the anus become grossly dilated.

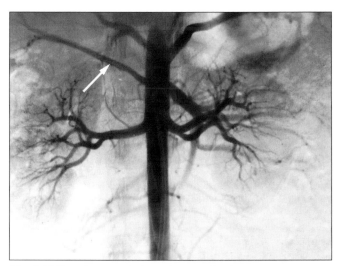

Fig. 4.15 *Superior mesenteric angiogram, showing a common anatomical variation, with the hepatic artery (arrow) arising from the superior mesenteric artery rather than the coeliac artery.*

Gastric varices are best diagnosed endoscopically; they may be seen on barium swallow examination, but this is a relatively insensitive technique, does not delineate a site of bleeding, if present, and correlates poorly with severity of the disease.

CT and ultrasound can delineate the portal venous system and assess its patency, size, and structure. With the latter technique, additional Doppler information on flow, velocity, and pressure can be obtained (**Fig. 4.17**). The portal venous system can also be shown on delayed images after injection of contrast into the coeliac axis and superior mesenteric artery, and this technique has now largely replaced the direct needle puncture of the spleen necessary for spleno-portography.

Budd–Chiari syndrome
Occlusion of the hepatic veins between their origin in the liver parenchyma and the entrance into the inferior vena cava results in the Budd–Chiari syndrome. High inferior vena cava occlusion as a result of thrombosis, tumour, or a web (seen in Japan) may also cause the syndrome. Clinically, patients develop hepatosplenomegaly, ascites, and, ultimately, portal hypertension. Contrast-enhanced CT or ultrasound may demonstrate hepatic vein or inferior vena cava occlusion, often with sparing of the caudate lobe because of its direct drainage through small veins into the inferior vena cava. Direct catheterization of the hepatic veins confirms the diagnosis.

METABOLIC CONDITIONS

Haemochromatosis
Hepatomegaly, with the development of cirrhosis, occurs in the genetic or acquired disease known as haemochromatosis. One in three patients with this form of cirrhosis develop hepatocellular carcinoma. CT of the liver demonstrates high attenuation, because of iron deposition.

Wilson's disease
Wilson's disease is an autosomal recessive disease that results in deposition of copper, often in the liver, kidneys, and basal ganglia of the brain. Progression to chronic active hepatitis, cirrhosis, and portal hypertension is common. There are no specific appearances of the disease on CT or ultrasound.

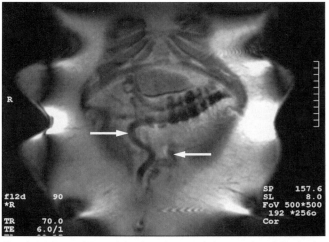

Fig. 4.16 *Coronal T1-weighted MR image of the anterior abdominal wall. There are multiple dilated veins (arrows) around the umbilicus—a 'caput medusae'.*

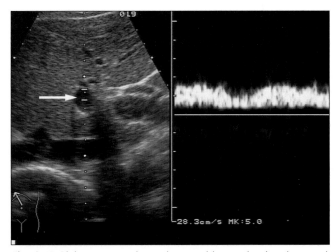

Fig. 4.17 *Right upper quadrant ultrasound image showing the portal vein (arrow); the corresponding Doppler venous wave form is shown on the right.*

Part 2. Biliary system

CONGENITAL ABNORMALITIES

There is a marked variability in the junctional anatomy of the bile ducts, and particularly of the anastomosis of the cystic duct with the bile duct, the latter being important to surgeons undertaking laparoscopic cholecystectomy.

Choledochal cyst
A choledochal cyst is formed by a segmental dilatation of part of the extrahepatic bile duct system, resulting in a cystic mass that may compress the surrounding structures, produce jaundice, or be a source of infection (**Fig. 4.18**). These cysts usually present by the time the patient is 10 years of age.

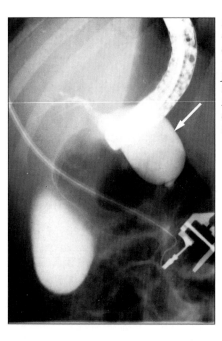

Fig. 4.18 ERCP in a 4-year-old child with a choledochal cyst (arrow). Note the focal dilatation of the bile duct. The other structure filling with contrast is the gall bladder.

Caroli's disease
Caroli's disease comprises familial cystic dilatation of the intrahepatic bile ducts, resulting in stasis, stone formation, and cholangitis.

TRAUMA

The majority of trauma to the bile ducts is iatrogenic, after surgery. Tearing of the extrahepatic ducts results in severe biliary peritonitis. Surgical ligatures, incorrectly applied, may cause stenosis or even occlusion of the common hepatic or common bile ducts leading to obstructive jaundice. Rupture of the gall bladder can occur, but is usually secondary to infection plus obstruction.

INFECTION

Acute cholecystitis is a common condition that results usually from cystic duct blockage caused by a stone. Plain abdominal radiography may reveal the presence of calcified biliary stones, a sentinel loop of bowel caused by local inflammation, or a paralytic ileus.

If an empyema develops, a mass may be visible; rarely, gas in the wall of the gall bladder produces the condition of emphysematous cholecystitis.

Ultrasound is the imaging modality of choice in these conditions. It enables visualization of gall-bladder wall thickening and oedema (**Fig. 4.19**) and assessment of the bile ducts, and reveals the presence or absence of biliary sludge, gall stones, and localized abscess formation.

INFLAMMATORY CONDITIONS

Gall stones
About 30% of gall stones are calcified and hence radio-opaque. There are three main types of stone: pigment stones that contain calcium salts of bilirubin, phosphate, and carbonate, and 50% of which are radio-opaque; non-opaque cholesterol stones; and a mixed variety, which are the most common and are multiple and faceted, 15% being radio-opaque (**Figs 4.20 and 4.21**).

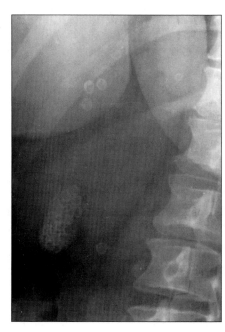

Fig. 4.20 Plain film of the right upper quadrant, showing multiple radio-opaque, faceted gall stones within the gall bladder, cystic duct, and common bile duct.

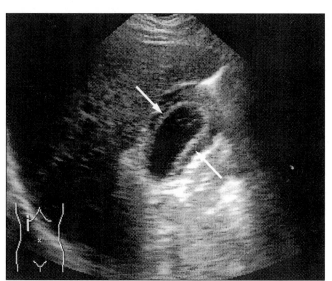

Fig. 4.19 Ultrasound of the gall bladder in a patient with acute cholecystitis, demonstrating extensive thickening and oedema of the gall bladder wall (arrows).

Chronic cholecystitis

Chronic cholecystitis is the most common disease to affect the gall bladder, and is almost invariably associated with gall stones. The bile is thick, the term biliary sludge often being used to describe it; when it also contains a high concentration of calcium, it becomes sufficiently radio-opaque to be seen on a plain abdominal radiograph—the so-called 'limey bile' (**Fig. 4.22**). Occasionally, the thick-walled gall bladder becomes calcified, forming the 'porcelain gall bladder'.

Sclerosing cholangitis

Sclerosing cholangitis is a condition of unknown cause, characterized by inflammatory fibrosis of the intra- or extrahepatic bile ducts, or both; it is best shown by endoscopic retrograde cholangiopancreatography (ERCP) (**Fig. 4.23**). The disease may occur in isolation, or in patients with inflammatory bowel disease.

Biliary parasites

Roundworms (*Ascaris lumbricoides*) are a common infestation in certain parts of the world. They inhabit the gut (*see* Fig. 3.17) and, when there is heavy involvement of the duodenum, they may also invade the bile ducts. Infective cholangitis, liver abscesses, strictures, and obstruction are some of the associated complications.

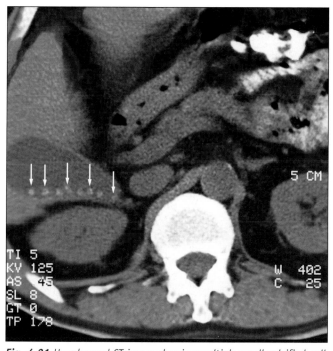

Fig. 4.21 Unenhanced CT image showing multiple small calcified gall stones in the gall bladder (arrows).

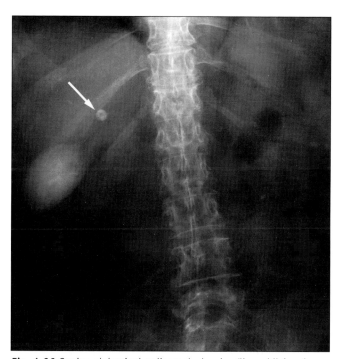

Fig. 4.22 Supine abdominal radiograph showing 'limey bile' and a calculus in the cystic duct (arrow), caused by chronic cholecystitis.

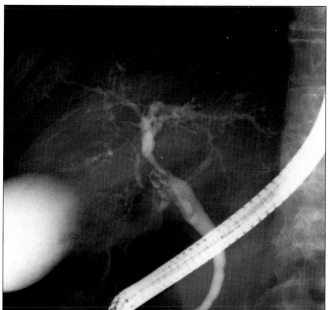

Fig. 4.23 ERCP in a patient with sclerosing cholangitis. There are multiple strictures of the intra- and extrahepatic biliary tree, giving the bile ducts a beaded appearance.

NEOPLASTIC DISEASE

MALIGNANT TUMOURS
Cholangiocarcinoma

The cholangiocarcinoma, or Klatskin tumour, causes a malignant stricture of either the intrahepatic or the extrahepatic bile ducts, best shown by percutaneous transhepatic cholangiography (PTC) (**Fig. 4.24**) or ERCP (**Fig. 4.25**). There is an increased risk of this tumour in patients with sclerosing cholangitis, congenital anomalies of the biliary system, and inflammatory bowel disease. Surgery is often difficult and only palliative. Radiological intervention includes balloon dilatation of the stricture, with either internal stenting or external catheter drainage, to relieve the obstructive jaundice (*see* page 93).

Gall-bladder carcinoma

The fairly rare gall-bladder carcinoma is associated with chronic inflammation and calcification. Ultrasound or CT may demonstrate a soft-tissue mass arising from the gall bladder, but the diagnosis is difficult to make before operation.

BENIGN BILE-DUCT AND GALL-BLADDER TUMOURS

Adenomas are premalignant, and must be differentiated from adenomyomas, as found in adenomyomatosis, which are benign. Adenomas are usually single and measure up to 2 cm in size; adenomyomas are small, multiple, and may have appearances similar to cholesterol deposits. The presence of Rokitansky–Aschoff sinuses in the gall-bladder wall confirms the diagnosis of adenomyomatosis (**Fig. 4.26**).

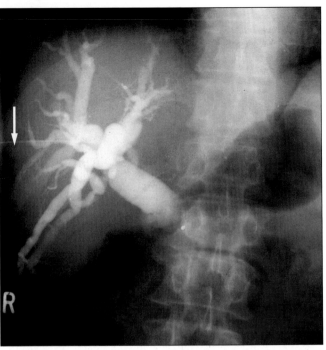

Fig. 4.24 PTC showing complete occlusion of the common hepatic duct as a result of a cholangiocarcinoma. Contrast has been introduced through a transhepatic needle (arrow) into a dilated intrahepatic bile duct.

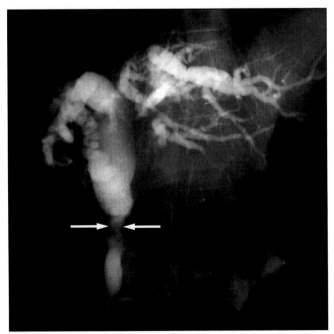

Fig. 4.25 ERCP in a patient with a cholangiocarcinoma of the common bile duct (arrows). The tumour is not causing complete obstruction, and contrast was introduced by cannulating the ampulla at ERCP. The endoscope has been removed.

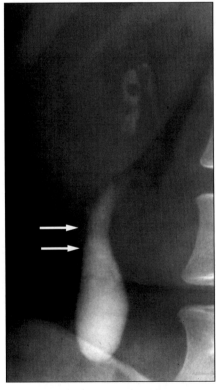

Fig. 4.26 Oral cholecystogram, showing multiple Rokitansky–Aschoff sinuses (arrows) in adenomyomatosis of the gall bladder.

Part 3. Pancreas

CONGENITAL ABNORMALITIES

Annular pancreas
The pancreas originates from two segments, ventral and dorsal, that normally unite after duodenal rotation. If rotation fails, the two parts of the pancreas remain separate, and the pancreatic ducts have anomalous openings. The resultant annular pancreas may obstruct the duodenum. Most cases present in the neonatal period or in infancy.

Pancreas divisum
If the ventral and dorsal buds of the pancreas do not fuse, the accessory and main pancreatic ducts do not unite, resulting in pancreas divisum. Most of the pancreas then drains through the accessory duct (of Santorini), only a small segment draining through the main duct (of Wirsung). This is a fairly common anomaly, and is associated with an increased incidence of pancreatitis. ERCP is the method of choice for diagnosing this condition.

TRAUMA
By virtue of its anatomical position, almost in the centre of the abdomen, the pancreas is protected from most penetrating injuries. However, damage similar to that seen in the duodenum can result from blunt trauma associated with lap-strap or steering-wheel injuries in road traffic accidents. If the duct is torn, acute pancreatitis may result. It is best shown by CT (**Fig. 4.27**) supplemented by ERCP.

INFLAMMATORY CONDITIONS

Acute pancreatitis
Plain abdominal radiography in acute pancreatitis may show a localized paralytic ileus, often with involvement of the transverse colon, but the appearances are often unreliable. Ultrasound shows generalized pancreatic enlargement, with decreased echogenicity if there is severe oedema. CT is the investigative modality of choice in most institutions, as it shows retroperitoneal structures so clearly, delineating the spreading oedema often accompanying acute pancreatitis (**Fig. 4.28**) and also, with intravenous contrast, assessing the severity of pancreatic damage and necrosis. CT also demonstrates the complications of phlegmon (tissue necrosis), abscess, haemorrhage, and spreading collections of fluid in the paracolic gutters, the retroperitoneum, and many other areas.

Pseudocysts occur where collections of fluid encyst—in the pancreas, in the peripancreatic tissues (**Fig. 4.29**), or remotely—and form when pancreatic enzymes escape from the duct and destroy tissue. They may be small or large, single or multiple, and may drain spontaneously into surrounding structures such as the stomach or colon. They are usually echo-free on ultrasound, but may contain debris and can become infected, and thus echo-dense. Surgery may be required to decompress or remove them.

Acute relapsing pancreatitis can cause progressive damage and fibrosis, leading to chronic pancreatitis.

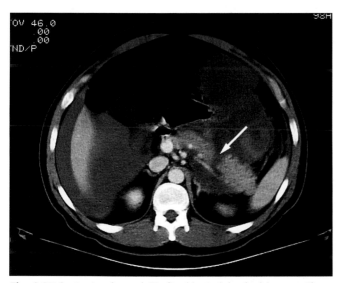

Fig. 4.27 *Contrast-enhanced CT after blunt abdominal trauma. There has been traumatic division of the body of the pancreas (arrow), and traumatic pancreatitis, with free intraperitoneal fluid, can be seen.*

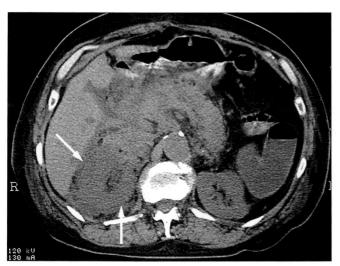

Fig. 4.28 *Unenhanced CT in acute pancreatitis. Note the diffuse swelling of the pancreas, with oedema extending into surrounding tissues, including the right pararenal space (arrows).*

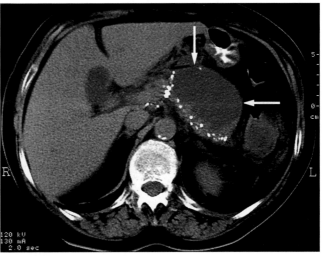

Fig. 4.29 *Unenhanced CT of a pancreatic pseudocyst (arrows) in a patient with pre-existing chronic pancreatitis.*

Chronic pancreatitis

Alcohol is the most common cause of chronic pancreatitis. On a plain abdominal film, calcification may be seen within the area of the pancreas in about 50% of cases (**Fig. 4.30**). Most calcifications lie within the pancreatic ducts, but occasionally they exist in the parenchyma. The parenchyma may be severely damaged, with fat necrosis, reduction in size of the gland, and atrophy, or it may be apparently little affected. The pancreatic duct is often dilated and this implies disease, seen on either CT or ultrasound and confirmed by ERCP (**Fig. 4.31**).

NEOPLASTIC DISEASE

Neuroendocrine tumours (apudomas)

The two important neuroendocrine tumours in this group are the gastrinoma producing the Zollinger–Ellison syndrome, and the insulinoma. Gastrinomas are often multiple; most are benign, but malignant foci may be present. Insulinomas are usually solitary, and in some patients are part of the multiple endocrine neoplasia syndrome. These neoplasms may be difficult or impossible to find by the standard imaging of ultrasound and CT, and superselective angiography of the pancreatic arterial supply may be necessary to show the hypervascularity with which they are associated.

Pancreatic carcinoma

Most pancreatic carcinomas are adenocarcinomas; their incidence is increasing steadily. Cystic tumours do occur, but are rare. The three main symptoms of pancreatic carcinoma are jaundice, weight loss, and pain; the jaundice is caused by obstruction of the common bile duct by carcinomas that occur in the head of the pancreas (**Fig. 4.32**), where over 50% originate. Diabetes mellitus is frequently associated with pancreatic carcinoma, but its relationship to the tumour is unclear.

Imaging of pancreatic carcinoma is essentially by ultrasound and CT, ERCP being the next investigation of choice. Percutaneous biopsy can be performed under either ultrasound or CT control.

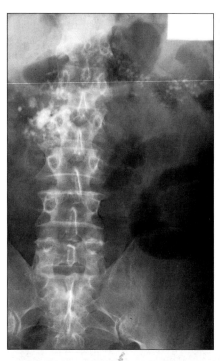

Fig. 4.30 Supine abdominal radiograph in a patient with severe chronic pancreatitis. There is extensive calcification throughout the pancreas.

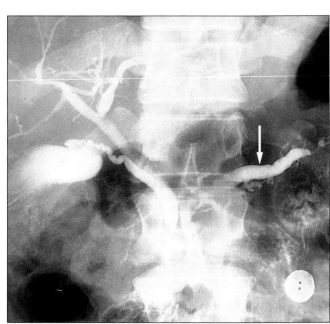

Fig. 4.31 ERCP in chronic pancreatitis. The main pancreatic duct is dilated (arrow), and contrast has filled the dilated side branches.

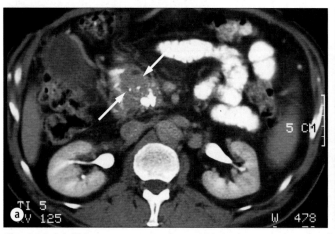
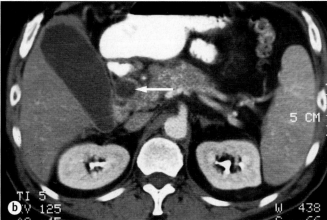

Fig. 4.32 (a) CT image, contrast-enhanced by the intravenous and oral routes, showing a mass in the head of the pancreas (arrows). The patient has chronic pancreatitis with calcification. **(b)** Same patient showing evidence of biliary obstruction, namely a dilated common bile duct (arrow) and gall bladder.

Part 4. Spleen

CONGENITAL ABNORMALITIES

There are complex congenital heart syndromes that are associated with situs anomalies and involve the spleen. Bilateral right-sidedness is associated with a transverse liver, asplenia, two right atria, and two 'right' lungs. Bilateral left-sidedness has absent gall bladder, polysplenia, two 'left' lungs, and different forms of congenital heart disease.

Small accessory areas of splenic tissue are called 'splenunculi'; they are encountered commonly on ultrasound and CT, sometimes being misdiagnosed as solid masses. If present, they may enlarge progressively if the patient undergoes splenectomy.

TRAUMA

Both direct injury and blunt trauma may damage the spleen. Subcapsular haemorrhage and rupture, either acute or delayed, may be seen on ultrasound or, perhaps better, with CT (**Fig. 4.33**). Spleen preservation, if it possible, is now the treatment of choice, because of the risk that severe pneumococcal septicaemia may occur in patients after splenectomy.

INFECTION AND INFLAMMATORY CONDITIONS

Calcified lesions within the spleen can result from previous tuberculosis or histoplasmosis infection. Haematomas may also calcify. Diseases such as malaria and kala-azar that are common world wide cause significant splenomegaly, but have no specific imaging features.

NEOPLASTIC DISEASE

Secondary metastatic disease may affect the spleen, but it is usually asymptomatic (**Fig. 4.34**); primary malignancies are exceedingly rare. The most significant splenic involvement in malignant disease occurs in lymphomas, but both the ultrasound and CT appearances often show only splenomegaly and, disappointingly, they have a low sensitivity with a high false-negative rate for the disease.

VASCULAR DISORDERS

The spleen is as liable to infarcts as other organs and tissues. Wedge-shaped defects may be seen on ultrasound and CT. They are usually an incidental finding, but are more common in patients with hypersplenism.

Splenomegaly occurs in portal hypertension (*see* Fig. 4.7) and other causes of increased back pressure on the portal venous system, such as portal vein thrombosis (**Fig. 4.35**). Calcification of the splenic artery is common in the elderly, and atheromatous aneurysms may also occur.

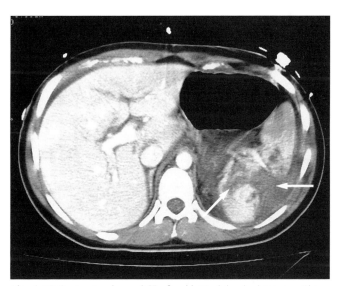

Fig. 4.33 *Contrast-enhanced CT after blunt abdominal trauma. There is extensive laceration of the spleen (arrows), and blood in the peritoneal cavity and tracking around the portal vein.*

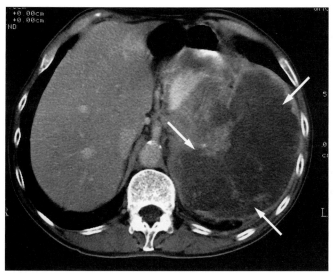

Fig. 4.34 *CT showing splenic metastases from a primary colon cancer. The spleen is entirely replaced by hypodense metastases (arrows).*

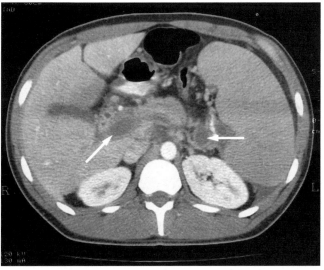

Fig. 4.35 *Contrast-enhanced CT in a patient with thrombosis of the portal and splenic veins (arrows), showing splenomegaly.*

Part 5. Invasive and interventional procedures in the hepatobiliary system

TRANSJUGULAR INTRAHEPATIC PORTOSYSTEMIC SHUNT

The *Transjugular Intrahepatic PortoSystemic Shunt* procedure (TIPSS) is designed to create a shunt to reduce portal venous pressure and hence reduce the risk of bleeding from varices. It is often undertaken before liver transplantation (**Fig. 4.36**). A catheter is introduced into the internal jugular vein and passed through the right atrium into the hepatic veins. Under ultrasound or fluoroscopy control, or using both, a special cutting needle creates a false channel in the liver between the hepatic venous system and the portal venous system. When the channel is established, a metallic stent is inserted, the portal venous pressure decreases, and the risk of variceal bleeding is reduced. Hepatic encephalopathy develops in about 25% of patients after the procedure.

ENDOSCOPIC RETROGRADE CHOLANGIOPANCREATOGRAPHY

The technique of ERCP comprises endoscopic cannulation of the ampulla of vater in the second part of the duodenum, followed by injection of contrast medium. It is the best method of showing the anatomy of the bile ducts and pancreatic duct (**Fig. 4.37**), and is performed to identify the cause of obstructive jaundice, and in assessing the pancreatic duct. A complication of the procedure is acute pancreatitis. Endoscopic cannulation of the common bile duct can also be a prelude to sphincterotomy, basket stone extraction, and stent insertion.

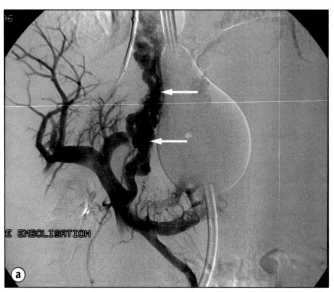

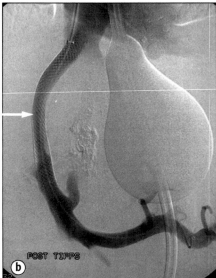

Fig. 4.36 (a) Portal venogram in a patient with oesophageal varices (arrows) and portal hypertension. A sengstaken tube has been inserted to stop variceal bleeding. **(b)** Post-TIPPS. The portal venous system has been decompressed into a hepatic vein by an intrahepatic stent (arrow).

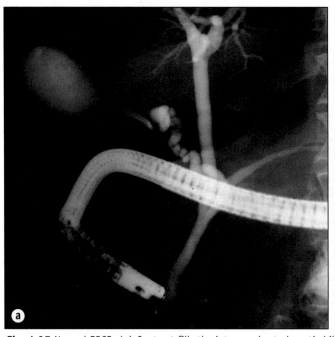

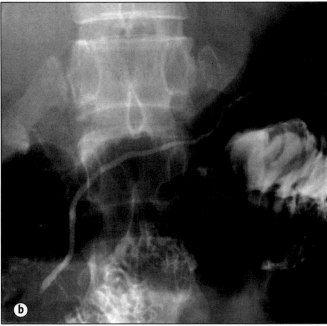

Fig. 4.37 Normal ERCP. **(a)** Contrast fills the intra- and extrahepatic bile ducts, cystic duct, and gall bladder. **(b)** Normal pancreatogram.

PERCUTANEOUS TRANSHEPATIC CHOLANGIOGRAPHY

PTC may be performed to investigate obstructive jaundice or prior to biliary drainage or stenting procedures. A thin needle is introduced into the bile ducts using a lateral approach, often under ultrasound or fluoroscopic control. Contrast medium is then injected to outline the duct system (*see* Fig. 4.24). Complications include biliary peritonitis, subphrenic abscess, and haemorrhage. Contraindications are bleeding and clotting disorders, biliary sepsis, and lack of surgical cover in case of complications.

BILIARY DRAINAGE AND STENTING

Biliary drainage may be undertaken either transhepatically after PTC (**Fig. 4.38**), or endoscopically. The drainage may be internal or external, depending on the cause of the obstruction.

If it is possible to cross an obstructing lesion with a guidewire, then a metallic stent can be inserted to restore biliary patency, without the need for a drainage catheter (**Fig. 4.39**).

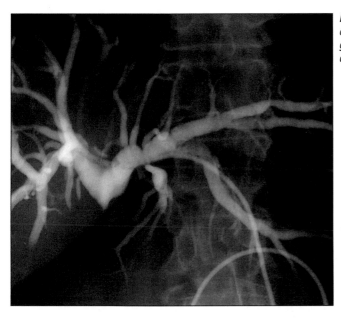

Fig. 4.38 *External biliary drain in a patient with extrinsic compression of the porta hepatis by metastatic lymph nodes. After a PTC, a guidewire and drainage catheter have been manipulated into the dilated bile ducts.*

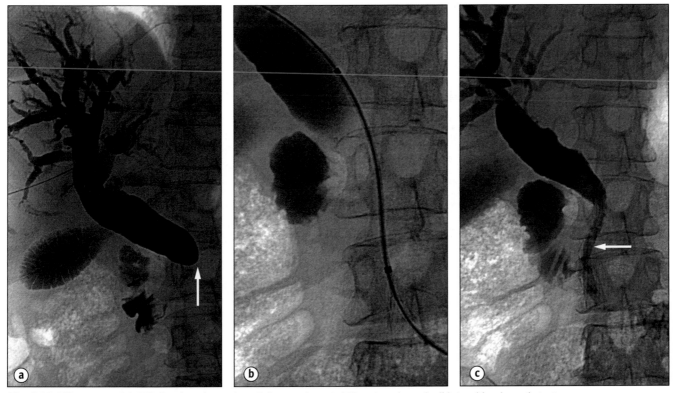

Fig. 4.39 *Biliary stent. (**a**) PTC showing obstruction of the extrahepatic biliary tree (arrow). (**b**) A guide wire and stent delivery system have been placed across the obstructing tumour. (**c**) Stent in situ (arrow) with contrast flowing into the duodenum.*

LIVER BIOPSY

Biopsy of focal (or diffuse) liver lesions may be performed under ultrasound or CT control, depending on many factors, including operator preference. As with any invasive procedure using needles, it is essential to establish that the patient has normal bleeding and clotting parameters before any intervention.

EMBOLIZATION

Embolization of liver tumours and other vascular lesions can be performed as a curative procedure, to reduce vascularity before operation, or to relieve symptoms in the carcinoid syndrome (Fig. 4.40).

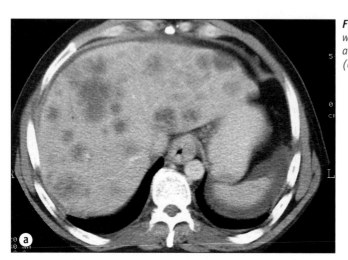

Fig. 4.40 (*a*) *Multiple hepatic metastases seen on CT in a patient with carcinoid syndrome.* (*b*) *Selective hepatic angiography in the late arterial phase, showing the tumour 'blush' of the multiple metastases (arrows).* (*c*) *Image after embolization of hepatic arterial branches.*

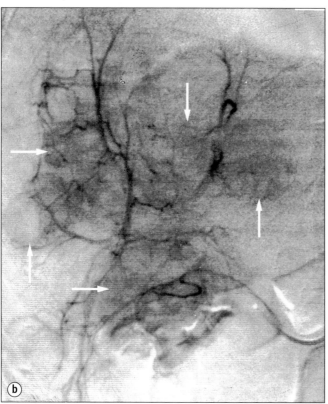

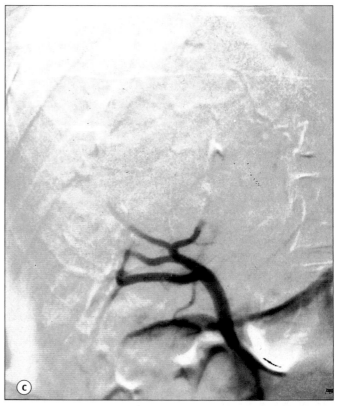

INVESTIGATION OF JAUNDICE

The pathways for the investigation of jaundice are shown in **Fig. 4.41**, with examples in **Figures 4.42** and **4.43**.

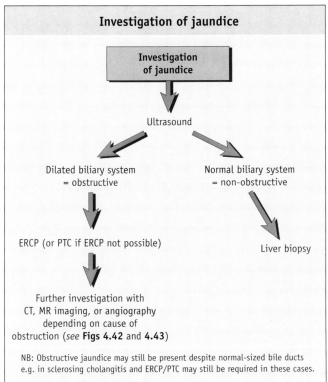

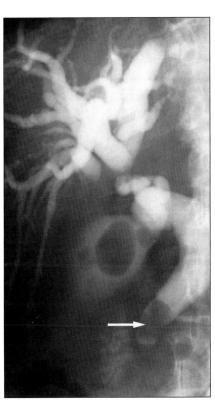

Fig. 4.42 ERCP in a jaundiced patient, showing a large gall stone (arrow) in the distal common bile duct. There is intra- and extrahepatic duct dilatation, and further gall stones are present in the gall bladder.

Fig. 4.41 Investigation of jaundice. ERCP, endoscopic retrograde cholangiopancreatography; PTC, percutaneous transhepatic cholangiography.

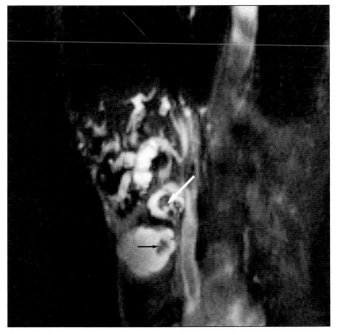

Fig. 4.43 Coronal inversion recovery MR image cholangiogram, demonstrating multiple stones in the dilated common bile duct (arrow), and a further stone in the gall bladder (small arrow).

chapter 5

Urinary Tract and Testes

Part 1. Urinary tract

CONGENITAL, NEONATAL, AND DEVELOPMENTAL ABNORMALITIES

RENAL ABNORMALITIES

Congenital abnormalities of the kidney may result in abnormality of number, position, fusion, or form. These abnormalities may co-exist.

Renal agenesis

Unilateral renal agenesis occurs in 1 in 1000–1500 births. It is associated with other congenital abnormalities of the urogenital tract, for example unicornuate or bicornuate uterus in females, and agenesis of the vas deferens and testicle in males. The remaining, single kidney is hypertrophied.

Bilateral renal agenesis is obviously incompatible with life; it is associated with oligohydramnios and Potter's facies.

An isotope renogram (**Fig. 5.1**) and ultrasound are the best methods of confirming renal agenesis and differentiating this condition from an ectopic or hypoplastic kidney.

Renal ectopy

An ectopic kidney fails to ascend to its normal position, and may lie anywhere along the embryological line of ascent from the pelvis (**Fig. 5.2**) superiorly; occasionally, it may be located in the thorax.

Fused crossed ectopia

Crossed ectopia is said to have occurred when the kidney lies on the side opposite to its ureter; most often it is associated with fusion to the normally located kidney (**Fig. 5.3**). This condition occurs in 1 in 1000 births, and is more common in males than in females. There is an increased incidence of reflux into the ectopic crossed kidney.

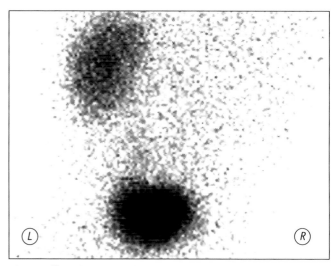

Fig. 5.1 *^{99m}Technetium (Tc) diethylenetriamine pentacetic acid (DTPA) isotope renogram in a child with right renal agenesis. There is no activity on the right side of the abdomen or pelvis. This is a posterior view.*

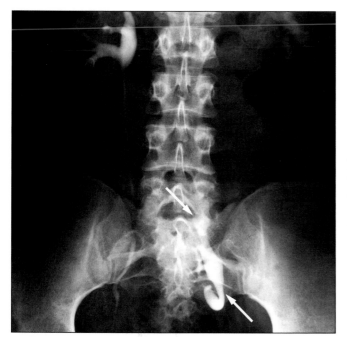

Fig. 5.2 *Intravenous urogram (IVU), showing an ectopic (pelvic) left kidney (arrows).*

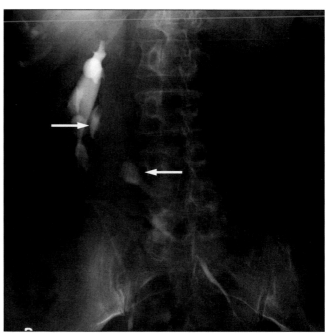

Fig. 5.3 *Fused crossed ectopia. IVU showing the left kidney (arrows) in the right side of the abdomen, fused to the right kidney.*

Horseshoe kidney

The condition known as horseshoe kidney occurs in 1 in 400 births, and is more common in males than in females. The lower poles of the kidneys are joined by an isthmus of renal parenchyma (**Fig. 5.4**) or a fibrous band, and are therefore rotated medially (**Fig. 5.5**); the ureters pass anteriorly. There is an increased incidence of calculi, possibly of Wilm's tumour (in isthmus), and the kidney is more susceptible to injury during abdominal trauma.

Renal dysplasia

Renal dysplasia may affect all or part of one or both kidneys. Dysplastic renal tissue is poorly functioning, with loss of corticomedullary differentiation. The condition includes a spectrum of abnormalities, from a small dysplastic kidney to a large multicystic dysplastic kidney; the latter is one of the possible causes of an abdominal mass in a neonate. There may be associated ureteric atresia.

Inherited cystic diseases of the kidney

Autosomal dominant polycystic kidney disease

The spectrum of severity of autosomal dominant polycystic kidney dis-

ease (ADPKD) varies from asymptomatic to endstage renal disease. ADPKD usually presents in adulthood; it accounts for 10–15% of patients receiving dialysis, and endstage renal disease develops in up to 50% of the patients by the age of 40–60 years. Cysts form within the nephrons, causing progressive loss of renal parenchyma and distortion of the calyceal system (**Fig. 5.6**); enormous renal enlargement may occur.

ADPKD is associated with cysts of the liver, pancreas, spleen, and gonads, intracranial aneurysms, cardiac valvular disease, and colonic diverticula. Complications include haemorrhage into cysts, calculi, and urinary tract infection.

An aggressive form of ADPKD occurs in neonates and results in enlarged kidneys with multiple cysts. It is associated with hepatic cysts and congenital hepatic fibrosis.

Ultrasound is the investigation of choice in diagnosis, and may be used to guide aspiration of a haemorrhagic or infected cyst.

Tuberous sclerosis complex

Tuberous sclerosis is an autosomal dominant phakomatosis. Hamartomas occur in the central nervous system, eyes, skin, heart, liver, adrenals, and kidneys. The renal abnormalities that occur in 50% of cases include cysts, angiomyolipomas, and renal cell cancers.

Von Hippel–Lindau disease

Von Hippel–Lindau disease is an autosomal dominant multisystem disease characterized by haemangioblastomas of the central nervous system, retinal angiomas, phaeochromocytomas, pancreatic cysts and tumours, and epididymal cystadenomas. Renal abnormalities may mimic ADPKD, with multiple bilateral renal cysts. Solid and cystic renal cell cancers occur and are often multiple.

ABNORMALITIES OF THE RENAL PELVIS AND URETER

Vesicoureteric reflux

Reflux of urine from the bladder into the ureters, and sometimes into the pelvicalyceal system, is the most common developmental anomaly of the urinary tract; it occurs as a result of a short intramural course of the lower ureter through the bladder wall. It is important because it is associated with urinary tract infection (UTI) and with 'reflux nephropathy' resulting from progressive renal scarring. Because of these potential long-term consequences, any child with a bacterio-

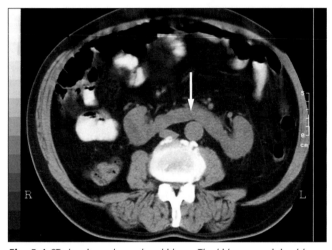

Fig. 5.4 *CT showing a horseshoe kidney. The kidneys are joined by an isthmus of renal parenchyma (arrow).*

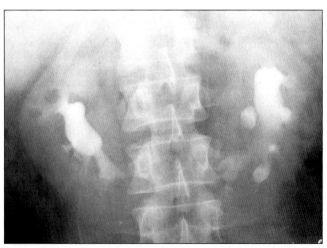

Fig. 5.5 *IVU of a horseshoe kidney, showing medial rotation of the lower poles, which are joined in the midline.*

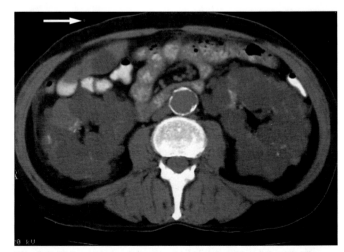

Fig. 5.6 *CT in autosomal dominant polycystic kidney disease. The kidneys are enlarged and almost entirely replaced by multiple cysts. The patient required peritoneal dialysis; the dialysis catheter can be seen outside the anterior abdominal wall (arrow).*

logically proven UTI should be investigated for reflux.

Reflux is graded as follows:

- **Grade I:** ureter only.
- **Grade II:** ureter and upper tract, not dilated.
- **Grade III:** ureter and upper tract, calyces normal.
- **Grade IV:** ureter and upper tract, calyces blunted.
- **Grade V:** gross tortuosity of ureters, with no papillary impressions in calyces.

In the investigation of proven UTI in childhood, ultrasound will show any renal cortical scarring and dilatation of the pelvicalyceal system. Renal cortical scarring and differential renal function can also be demonstrated on isotope renography using ^{99m}Tc dimercaptosuccinic acid (DMSA). Isotope renography using other agents (^{99m}Tc DTPA or ^{99m}TcMAG3) can demonstrate renal function and importantly can show reflux during micturation (**Fig. 5.7**). In patients who give equivocal results in ultrasound and isotope studies, and for whom surgery is being considered, a micturating cystogram is indicated.

Mild grades of vesicoureteric reflux resolve as the child grows and the intramural portion of the lower ureter lengthens. Long-term antibiotic therapy is given to maintain sterile urine and prevent reflux nephropathy (**Fig. 5.8**).

Bifid renal pelvis

Bifid renal pelvis is common, occurring in 10% of the population; it is usually an incidental finding on intravenous urography (IVU). The renal pelvis is divided in two, with one part draining the upper pole and the other the middle and lower poles. The condition has no pathological associations.

Ureteric duplication

Ureteric duplication may be partial or complete and is believed to be caused by the formation of an additional ureteral bud (**Fig. 5.9**). In the complete form, the ureter that enters the bladder nearest the trigone is the 'normal' or orthotopic ureter, and drains the lower moiety of the kidney. The 'ectopic' ureter drains the upper moiety, and enters the bladder at an abnormally low and medial position. Unilateral duplication is much more common than bilateral duplication; ureteric triplication is very rare.

Abnormalities associated with ureteric duplication are stenosis of the ectopic ureteric orifice, leading to obstruction (**Fig. 5.10**), and reflux into the orthotopic ureter.

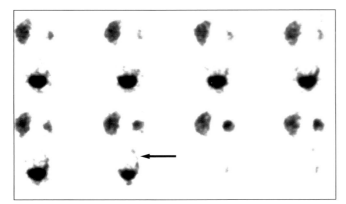

Fig. 5.7 ^{99m}Tc-DTPA isotope renogram with micturating study, showing vesicoureteric reflux. Activity appears in the ureter (arrow) and increases in the kidney as the bladder empties.

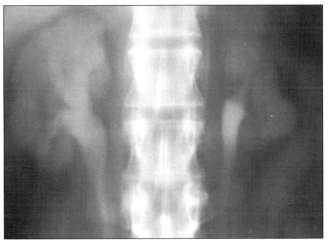

Fig. 5.8 IVU showing chronic reflux nephropathy. There is atrophy of both kidneys, particularly the left, with multiple cortical scars.

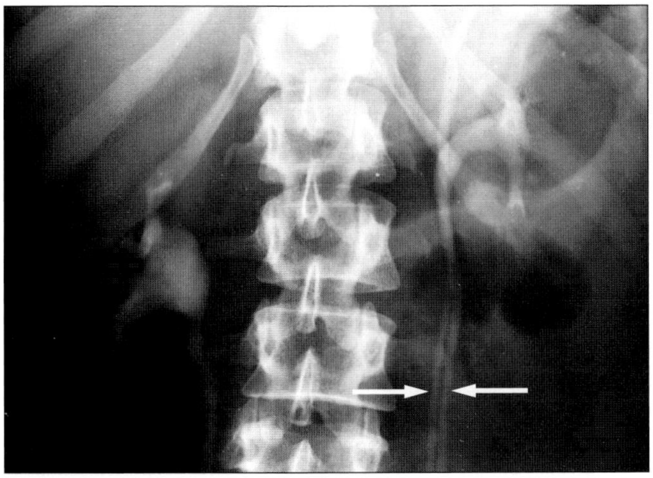

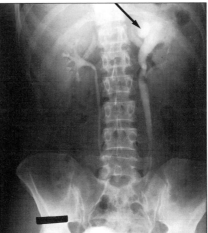

Fig. 5.10 IVU showing a left duplex collecting system and ureters, with obstruction of the upper moiety (arrow).

Fig. 5.9 IVU showing a left duplex collecting system and ureters (arrows).

Ectopic ureter

The term 'ectopic ureter', when not associated with ureteric duplication, refers to a ureteric orifice that inserts below the bladder neck. It is much more common in girls than in boys, and usually presents with incontinence.

Ureteropelvic junction anomalies

Obstruction of the ureteropelvic junction (UPJ) is a common congenital abnormality of the urinary tract; it is the most common cause

of an abdominal mass in a neonate, and can be diagnosed antenatally with ultrasound. In 10% of affected individuals, it is bilateral. It can present later in life with flank pain, urinary tract infection, or an abdominal mass (Fig. 5.11). Most cases are caused by a functional abnormality of the circular muscle at the junction of the renal pelvis and ureter; this results in hydronephrosis and dilated calyces, which can be shown on ultrasound and IVU.

Isotope renography demonstrates obstruction at the UPJ (Fig. 5.12): there is no clearing of isotope after administration of a diuretic.

Ureterocele

Prolapse of the lower ureteric mucosa into the bladder produces a ureterocele, which consists of a tube formed from ureteric and bladder musoca and may occur with normal or ectopic ureters. The IVU appearance is typical and is termed a 'cobra head'; ureteroceles can also be seen on ultrasound (Fig. 5.14). They may be complicated by calculi (Fig. 5.15).

Prune belly syndrome

The rare congenital abnormality known as prune belly syndrome occurs only in males and is caused by a defect of the abdominal musculature (Fig. 5.16), as a result of which the skin wrinkles like a prune. The urinary tract is dilated, with a dilated prostatic urethra, distended bladder, and tortuous ureters. The kidneys may be dysplastic.

ABNORMALITIES OF THE BLADDER AND URETHRA
Exstrophy

Exstrophy of the bladder is caused by deficiency of the lower abdominal wall; there is externalization of the bladder mucosa, which merges with adjacent skin.

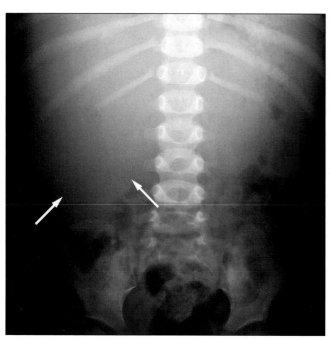

Fig. 5.11 *Plain abdominal radiograph in a child with right ureteropelvic junction obstruction. There is a large right flank mass (arrows) caused by hydronephrosis.*

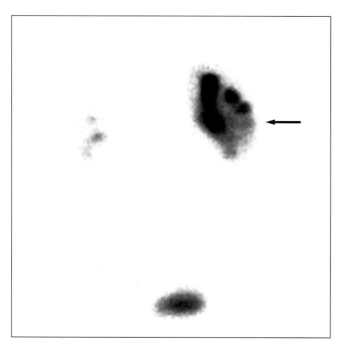

Fig. 5.12 *^{99m}Tc-DTPA isotope renogram in UPJ obstruction, showing isotope accumulating in the hydronephrotic kidney (arrow).*

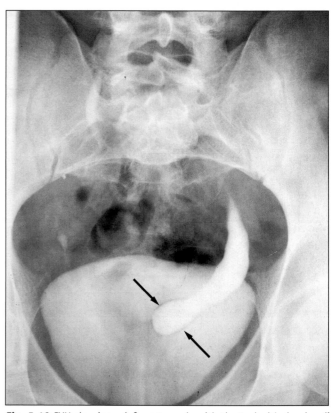

Fig. 5.13 *IVU showing a left ureterocele with the typical 'cobra head' appearance (arrows).*

Epispadias

Epispadias is a condition in which the male urethra is open on the dorsal aspect of the penis. It may occur alone, or with associated bladder exstrophy; in either case, there is usually widening of the symphysis pubis (Fig. 5.17). Ureteric obstruction occurs as a result of fibrosis or ureterocele formation, and inguinal and umbilical hernias may occur. Imaging is used to assess the upper urinary tract and for follow up after reconstructive surgery.

Urachal anomalies

Embryologically, the bladder is connected to the umbilicus. Failure of this attachment to obliterate can result in a patent urachus (through which urine discharges from the umbilicus), a urachal cyst (at the bladder end), or an umbilical cyst (at the umbilical end).

Bladder duplication

Duplication of the bladder is rare and may be complete, with two urethral orifices, or incomplete, with a bladder septum.

Posterior urethral valves

Posterior urethral valves are mucosal folds that persist embryologically as a result of abnormal migration of the Wolfian duct orifices.

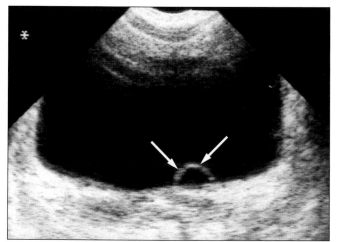

Fig. 5.14 Ultrasound image showing a left ureterocele (arrows) through a full bladder.

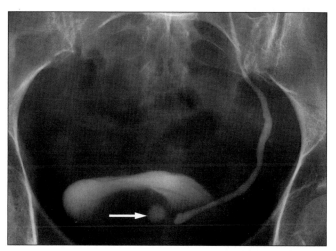

Fig. 5.15 IVU in a patient with a left ureterocele in which a calculus has formed (arrow).

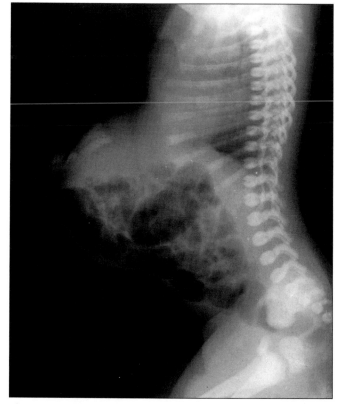

Fig. 5.16 Lateral abdominal and thoracic radiograph in a neonate with prune belly syndrome.

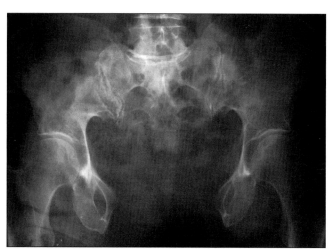

Fig. 5.17 Pelvic radiograph in an adult with bladder exstrophy, showing gross widening of the symphysis pubis.

They are present only in males and occur in the bulbomembranous urethra. If there is complete obstruction of bladder outflow, renal failure and intrauterine death can result. Postnatally, there may be abdominal distension, palpable kidneys, a distended bladder, and poor urinary output. Less severe cases present later with urinary tract infection or chronic renal failure.

Posterior urethral valves and urethral dilatation are best demonstrated with a micturating cystourethrogram (**Fig. 5.18**).

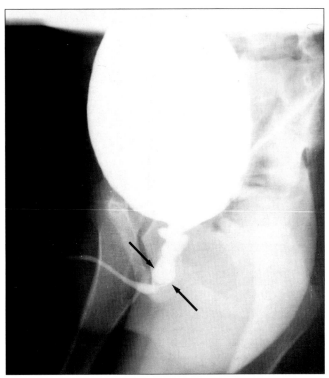

Fig. 5.18 *Micturating cystourethrogram in a boy with posterior urethral valves. There is obstruction of the posterior urethra (arrows), and gross distension of the urinary bladder.*

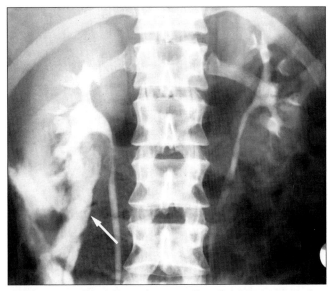

Fig. 5.19 *IVU after right renal trauma. There is laceration through the renal cortex into the collecting system, with extravasation of contrast (arrow).*

TRAUMA

RENAL INJURY

Renal injuries may be classified as follows:
- **Mild:** 75–85% of cases. Contusion, minor cortical lacerations, no disruption of the collecting system.
- **Major:** 10–15% of cases. Cortical lacerations through the renal capsule or into the collecting system (**Fig. 5.19**). The patient's condition is usually unstable, with a flank mass, frank haematuria, and peri- or paranephric haematoma.
- **Catastophic:** 5% of cases. This group includes shattered kidney and pedicle injuries, with renal artery avulsion or thrombosis. Arteriography is indicated, with a view to possible revascularization.

Haematoma and laceration

Renal injury may be caused by penetrating or blunt trauma, or may be iatrogenic, usually as a result of interventional procedures to the kidney, such as biopsy or nephrostomy.

Renal avulsion

Patients with complete renal avulsion may not have haematuria.

URETERIC INJURY

The most common causes of ureteric injury are iatrogenic:
- **Surgical:** obstetric and gynaecological procedures, abdomino-perineal resection of rectum.
- **Endoscopic:** retrograde catheterization, basket extraction of calculi.
- **Trauma:** deceleration injuries may result in pelviureteric junction avulsion.
- **Radiotherapy:** ureteric stricture as a result of fibrosis.
- **Obstruction:** ureteric rupture proximal to a calculus obstruction can be seen on IVU (**Fig. 5.20**).

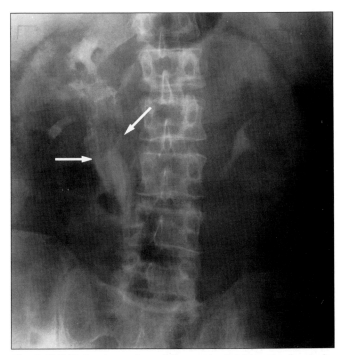

Fig. 5.20 *IVU showing rupture of the proximal right ureter (arrows), secondary to an obstructing calculus.*

BLADDER INJURY

The bladder is not commonly injured. The following types of injury may occur:

- **Trauma:** accounts for 95% of cases. The majority of cases are caused by blunt trauma, particularly with pelvic fractures. The infant bladder is more susceptible because of its relatively more intraperitoneal position. Rupture may be extraperitoneal or intraperitoneal.
- **Runner's bladder:** contusion of the bladder wall against the pubic arch during running results in haematuria.
- **Spontaneous:** may occur in the presence of bladder outflow obstruction, when the bladder wall is weakened by tumour or a diverticulum.

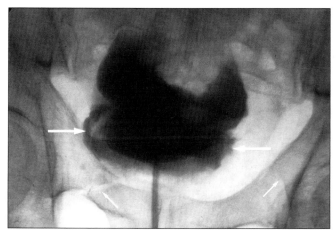

Fig. 5.21 *Cystogram after extraperitoneal bladder rupture. Contrast extravasates from the bladder (arrows); bilateral superior pubic rami fractures can also be seen (small arrows). There were also fractures of both inferior pubic rami.*

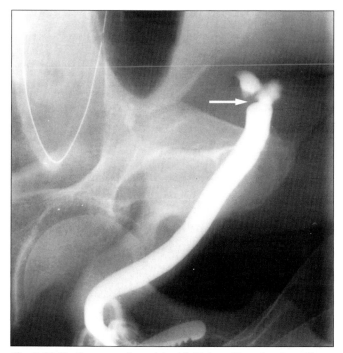

Fig. 5.22 *Urethrogram after a 'straddle' injury. There is a type II posterior urethral injury (arrow).*

The best method of diagnosing bladder rupture is cystography, provided there is not an associated urethral injury (**Fig. 5.21**). IVU is inadequate.

URETHRAL INJURY

Injuries to the anterior urethra are usually caused by instrumentation (catheterization, cystoscopy etc.), or by falling astride, with injury to the bulbous urethra (straddle injury). Injuries to the posterior urethra are more common and virtually always associated with pelvic fracture; they are seen in 12% of those with pelvic fracture. Such injuries occur as a result of shearing of the prostatomembranous urethra during deceleration injuries (**Fig. 5.22**).

Diagnosis is with a retrograde urethrogram. Three types of posterior urethral injuries are recognized on imaging:

- **Type I:** stretching of the prostatic urethra, but no extravasation of contrast.
- **Type II:** contrast extravasates extraperitoneally, but is limited inferiorly by an intact urogenital diaphragm.
- **Type III:** contrast is present above and below the urogenital diaphragm, which is ruptured.

Late complications of urethral injury include stricture, incontinence, and impotence.

INFECTION

URINARY TRACT INFECTION

The vast majority of patients with UTI are managed in the community and never undergo imaging; in most instances there will be no radiological abnormality. Imaging is indicated in children, to look for reflux (*see* pages 98–99), and in adults with recurrent or persisting infection, to look for underlying abnormalities such as obstruction, calculi, tumour, or anatomical variants such as a horseshoe kidney or duplex system.

Acute pyelonephritis

In acute pyelonephritis, ultrasound may show swelling of the kidney, with hypoechoic renal pyramids, but may be normal.

Renal abscess

On ultrasound, a renal abscess is a focal renal mass that is mainly cystic. If the abscess ruptures, peri- or pararenal collections of pus will be apparent on CT (**Fig. 5.23**).

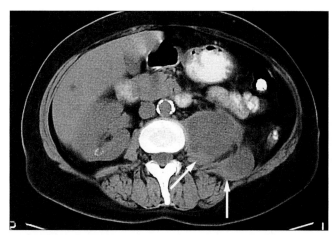

Fig. 5.23 *CT showing an abscess in an atrophic left kidney. The abscess has extended into the adjacent psoas and quadratus lumborum muscles (arrows).*

Cystitis

Ultrasound in cystitis may show diffuse thickening of the bladder mucosa, with cellular debris in the urine; however, ultrasound may be normal.

Prostatitis

Prostatitis can be persisting and difficult to treat. There is no imaging abnormality.

Urethritis

A long-term complication of urethritis in males is a urethral stricture, which can be demonstrated by a retrograde urethrogram (**Fig. 5.24**).

INFECTIONS WITH SPECIFIC RADIOLOGICAL APPEARANCES
Tuberculosis

Tuberculosis (TB) can affect any part of the urinary tract. Initially,

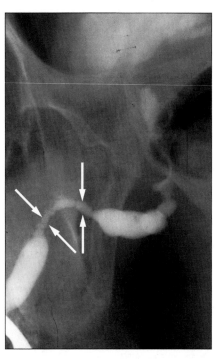

Fig. 5.24 Urethrogram demonstrating a stricture (arrows) that has occurred as a result of chronic urethritis.

there is blood-borne spread to the kidney; subsequently, the renal tubules and collecting system are sequentially involved.

Renal TB is characterized by papillary destruction on IVU; there is renal calcification in 30% of cases. Caseous pyonephrosis may involve the whole kidney (**Fig. 5.25**), and the condition may progress to tuberculous autonephrectomy.

TB of the ureter typically shows calcification that appears beaded. Fibrotic strictures may cause obstruction, and are often multiple.

TB of the bladder rarely causes calcification. The bladder is small, with a fixed, trabeculated wall.

Urinary schistosomiasis (Bilharzia)

Although urinary schistosomiasis is uncommon in Britain, it is a major cause of ill-health in Africa, Asia, the Middle East, and Southern Mediterranean countries, where it is acquired from water infected with *Schistosoma haematobium*. The organism enters by penetration of the skin, progresses through the lymphatics to the venous system, and deposits ova in the bladder and lower ureter.

Bladder. Ova in the submucosa of the bladder produce calcification (**Fig. 5.26**); granulomas and mucosal oedema appear as filling defects. Carcinoma of the bladder is a long-term complication.

Ureters. Tramline calcification is characteristic, rather than the beaded calcification seen in TB. The ureters may be dilated because of obstruction by strictures or calculi, secondary to reflux due to fibrosis of the vesicoureteric junction.

Kidney involvement in urinary schistosomiasis is only secondary to bladder and ureteric abnormalities, in contrast to TB, which involves the kidney first.

Xanthogranulomatous pyelonephritis

Xanthogranulomatous pyelonephritis occurs in the presence of renal stones complicated by infection (usually *Proteus*), and takes its name from the yellow colour of the cut surface of the kidney at pathological examination. The condition can be focal or diffuse, with an inflammatory mass containing fat, which may be indistinguishable from tumour; more commonly, there is an obstructed, poorly functioning kidney.

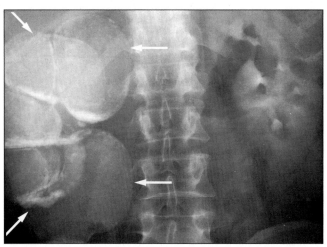

Fig. 5.25 IVU in a patient with right renal TB. There is a caseous pyonephrosis (arrows).

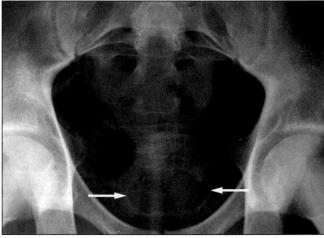

Fig. 5.26 Plain film of the bladder area in bilharzia (urinary schistosomiasis), showing calcification in the submucosa (arrows).

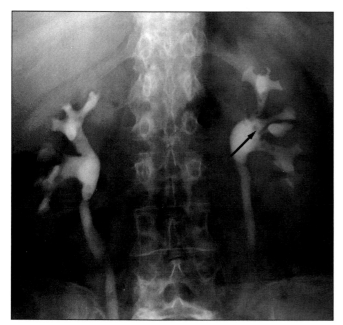

Fig. 5.27 IVU in pyeloureteritis cystica. There are multiple small filling defects in the pelvicalyceal system, most obvious on the left (arrow).

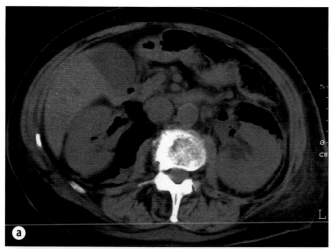

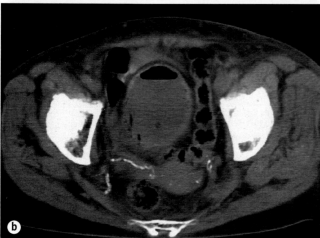

Fig. 5.28 CT showing gas in the renal collecting systems and perinephric tissues (a) and in the urinary bladder (b). This is an example of emphysematous pyelonephritis and cystitis in a patient with diabetes mellitus.

Pyeloureteritis cystica

The condition known as pyeloureteritis cystica is associated with urinary tract infection. There are multiple small cysts involving the mucosa of the renal pelvis and upper ureter; they appear as filling defects on an IVU (Fig. 5.27).

Emphysematous pyelonephritis and cystitis

Emphysematous pyelonephritis and cystitis occurs in patients with diabetes, usually because of infection with *Escherichia coli* or *Candida*; it may be fatal. Gas forms within the renal parenchyma and often extends into the peri- and pararenal spaces (Fig. 5.28). The bladder and ureters may also be involved.

INFLAMMATORY CONDITIONS

Inflammatory change in the urinary tract is part of many other pathologies e.g. infection, calculi or vascular disease. See relevant sections.

Glomerulonephropathies

Patients with glomerulonephritis may present with nephrotic syndrome, acute nephritis, or chronic renal failure. The role of imaging is to exclude obstruction and to guide renal biopsy, which is performed under ultrasound control.

Retroperitoneal fibrosis

Retroperitoneal fibrosis may occur as a consequence of surgery or the use of drugs such as methysergide, but there is an idiopathic form. The condition is characterized by progressive retroperitoneal fibrosis that encases the lower ureters, inferior vena cava (IVC), and aorta, resulting in urinary obstruction and renal failure. IVU shows the typical appearance of focal narrowing of the ureters, with medial deviation around the L4/5 level (Fig. 5.29). An association exists between retroperitoneal fibrosis and the rare condition of pelvic lipomatosis, in which extraperitoneal fat proliferation causes characteristic deformity of the bladder and may compress the sigmoid colon and lower ureters (Fig. 5.30).

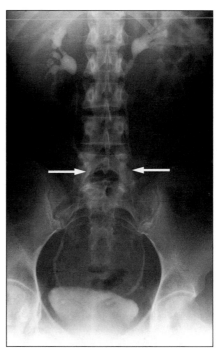

Fig. 5.29 IVU in retroperitoneal fibrosis. There is focal, medial deviation of the right ureter and underfilling of the left ureter at this level (arrows).

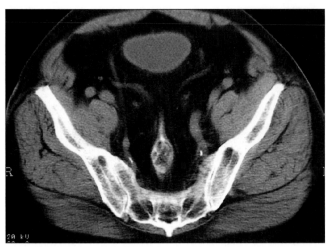

Fig. 5.30 *CT in pelvic lipomatosis. Note the large amount of fat (which appears black) in the pelvis.*

VASCULAR DISORDERS

ARTERIAL ABNORMALITIES
Renal artery stenosis
Reduction in blood flow to the kidney in renal artery stenosis results in release of renin, which activates formation of angiotensin I; this in turn is converted to angiotensin II, which produces hypertension. There are two main causes of the renal artery stenosis:

- **Atheroma:** either of the portion of the abdominal aorta that involves the renal artery origin, or of the renal artery itself (**Fig. 5.31**). Patients with atheroma are usually older than 40 years.
- **Fibromuscular hyperplasia:** involves the renal artery and its branches, giving a 'string of sausages' appearance (**Fig. 5.32**); it is bilateral in 60% of cases. The condition is more common in women, and usually presents before the age of 40 years.

Renal artery stenosis is confirmed by arteriography; MR and CT are emerging as non-invasive methods for imaging the renal arteries, but ultrasound can be difficult due to overlying bowel gas. An isotope renogram will show delayed perfusion of the kidney, with reduced differential function with or without reduced renal size.

Other causes of renovascular disease
Large arteries may be affected by:
- Renal artery thrombosis/embolization.
- Renal artery aneurysm (multiple in 30% of cases, bilateral in 20%).
- Extrinsic compression from an adjacent mass.
- Arteriovenous fistula (after renal biopsy (**Fig. 5.33**), trauma, congenital, or tumour-associated).

Small arteries may be affected by:
- Atheroma.
- Polyarteritis nodosa (has renal involvement in 80% of cases, with small aneurysms of intrarenal arteries (**Fig. 5.34**) and renal infarcts).
- Scleroderma.
- Kawasaki disease.
- Churg-Strauss syndrome.

Renal infarct
Renal infarcts are usually caused by a renal artery embolus, with occlusion of an interlobar artery, resulting in pain and haematuria. IVU shows part or all of the kidney to be non-functioning. In the late stage, there is a focal cortical defect, but a normal collecting system.

Acute tubular necrosis
The term 'acute tubular necrosis' refers to acute renal failure caused by renal ischaemia (shock, trauma, infection, or childbirth) or nephrotoxins. Ultrasound will show enlarged kidneys and is indicated only to exclude obstruction as a cause of renal failure.

Acute cortical necrosis
The causes of acute cortical necrosis are the same as those of acute tubular necrosis, but the majority of cases follow obstetric shock. In the late stages, plain films show renal cortical calcification.

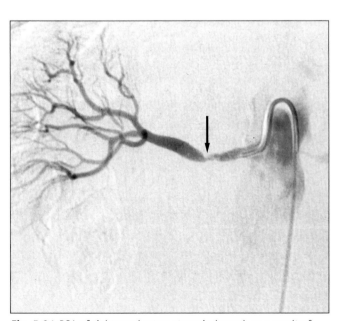

Fig. 5.31 *DSA of right renal artery stenosis (arrow) as a result of atheroma, demonstrating typical poststenotic dilatation.*

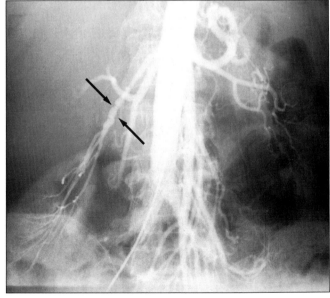

Fig. 5.32 *Aortogram showing fibromuscular hyperplasia of the right renal artery (arrows). The patient has an ectopic right kidney.*

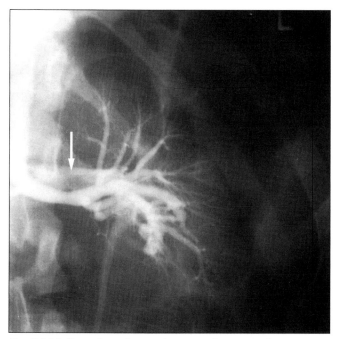

Fig. 5.33 *Left renal arteriogram demonstrating an arteriovenous fistula, with early opacification of the left renal vein (arrow). This occurred as a complication of renal biopsy.*

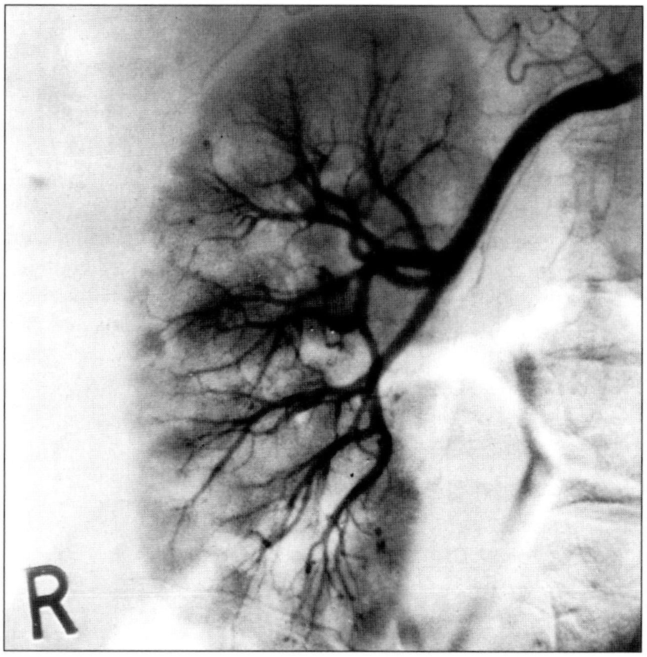

Fig. 5.34 *Right renal DSA in polyarteritis nodosa, showing multiple small aneurysms arising from the arcuate arteries.*

VENOUS ABNORMALITIES
Renal vein thrombosis

If renal vein thrombosis is complete and acute, it causes venous infarction of the kidney, which becomes painful and enlarged. If the condition is chronic, the clinical picture is one of nephrotic syndrome, which in turn is a cause of renal vein thrombosis. The wide variety of possible causes of renal vein thrombosis are shown in **Figure 5.35**.

Causes of renal vein thrombosis	
Diseases causing nephrotic syndrome	Glomerulonephritis Systemic lupus erythematosus Amyloidosis
Tumours	Renal-cell carcinoma (*see* **Fig. 5.36**) Nephroblastoma (Wilm's tumour) Retroperitoneal tumour
Reduced renal vein perfusion	IVC thrombosis Shock (particularly in infants)
Hypercoagulable states	Malignancy Burns

Fig. 5.35 *Causes of renal vein thrombosis.*

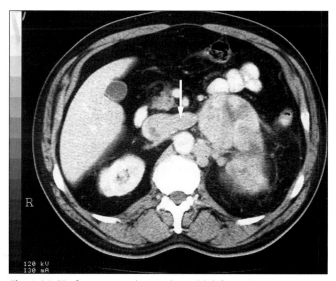

Fig. 5.36 *CT after contrast, in a patient with left renal carcinoma. Tumour thrombus can be seen in the left renal vein (arrow) and IVC.*

NEOPLASTIC DISEASE

TUMOURS OF THE KIDNEY
Renal adenocarcinoma

Renal adenocarcinoma is the most common renal tumour, accounting for 85% of renal malignancies; it is bilateral in 5% of cases. It arises from the proximal convoluted tubular cells. The condition is more common in males than in females and can occur at any age, but peaks in sixth decade of life. Predisposing factors include endstage renal disease, long-term dialysis, and von Hippel–Lindau disease.

Clinically, renal adenocarcinoma may present with haematuria (usually frank) in 50% of patients, flank pain in 30%, a flank mass in 30%, endocrine manifestations (**Fig. 5.37**), or varicocele (caused by tumour extension obstructing the testicular vein).

Stage 1 tumours are confined within the renal capsule. Local spread is initially within Gerota's fascia, and then beyond; direct extension into the renal vein and IVC is a common feature. Lymphatic spread is initially to the renal hilar lymph nodes, and haematological spread is to the liver, lungs, and bone.

Calcification is found on plain films in 10% of patients, but ultrasound is the best first-line investigation and will show a renal mass, which may be partly cystic and is usually of increased vascularity (**Fig. 5.38**). A tissue diagnosis can be obtained by ultrasound-guided biopsy. Ultrasound can also enable assessment of the renal vein, IVC, and right atrium for tumour extension, and is improved by the use of colour flow. On isotope renograms and bone scans, renal-cell carcinomas are demonstrated by a photopenic area, because the tumour is non-functioning (**Fig. 5.39**).

Endocrine presentations of renal adenocarcinoma	
Presentation	**Hormone**
Hypertension	Renin
Erythrocytosis	Erythropoietin
Hypercalcaemia	Parathyroid hormone
Galactorrhoea	Prolactin
Gynaecomastia	Gonadotrophins
Cushing's syndrome	Adrenocorticotrophic hormone

Fig. 5.37 *Endocrine presentations of renal adenocarcinoma.*

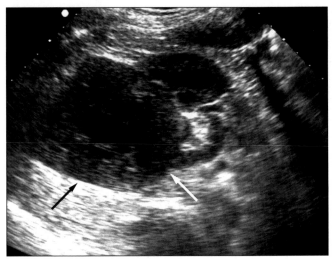

Fig. 5.38 *Transverse ultrasound of the right kidney, which is partly replaced by renal carcinoma (arrows).*

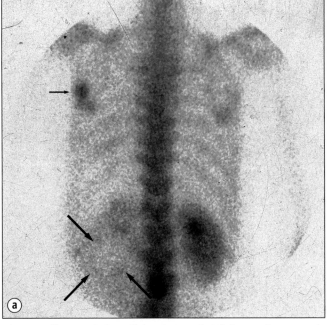

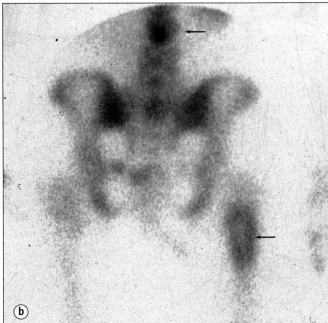

Fig. 5.39 ^{99m}Tc-methylene diphosphonate (MDP) isotope bone scan in a patient with metastatic left renal carcinoma. The istope is excreted by the kidneys, which are normally visible on a bone scan, but here there is a large photopenic area representing the primary tumour (arrows), and bony metastases in the lumbar spine, a left upper rib (**a**) and proximal right femur (**b**) (small arrows).

Staging of renal adenocarcinoma is best performed with contrast-enhanced CT, which will show the extent of the renal mass, lymphadenopathy, and any venous extension of the tumour (**Fig. 5.40**). Embolization of vascular renal-cell carcinomas may be performed before nephrectomy, to reduce the operative risk of haemorrhage (**Fig. 5.41**).

Nephroblastoma (Wilm's tumour)

Wilm's tumour, which arises from a metanephric blastema, is the most common cause of a solid abdominal mass presenting after the neonatal period. It is associated with aniridia, hemihypertrophy, and Beckwith–Wiedemann syndrome. The condition affects young children, 50% before the age of 2 years, and 75% before 5 years; tumours are bilateral in 5–10% of cases. The incidence is equal in the two sexes.

Ultrasound will show a solid renal mass, which is usually large and may have cystic areas that represent necrosis, haemorrhage, or both. Plain film reveals calcification in 5–10% of cases. As with renal-cell carcinoma, spread into the renal vein and IVC can occur; haematogenous metastases to the liver, lung (**Fig. 5.42**), bone, and brain are common.

CT is currently the best method of staging nephroblastoma (**Fig. 5.43**), but the role of MR imaging is increasing.

The following must be differentiated from nephroblastoma:

Mesoblastic nephroma (fetal renal hamartoma). This is the most common neonatal solid abdominal mass, and shows as a well-defined soft-tissue mass on ultrasound. There is no associated calcification.

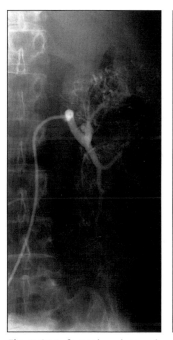

Fig. 5.40 *CT after contrast, of a large right renal carcinoma. There has been spread of tumour beyond the renal capsule (arrow) and there is tumour thrombus in the IVC (small arrow).*

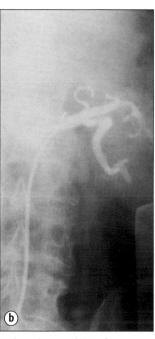

Fig. 5.41 *Left renal angiogram in renal carcinoma.* **(a)** *Before embolization.* **(b)** *After embolization. There has been a significant reduction in tumour vascularity after embolization; this makes nephrectomy easier.*

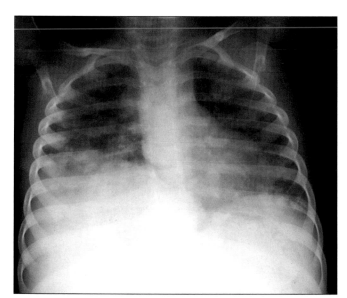

Fig. 5.42 *Chest radiograph in a child with metastatic Wilm's tumour, showing multiple pulmonary metastases.*

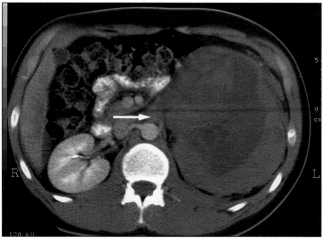

Fig. 5.43 *CT in a child with a left Wilm's tumour. There is a huge left renal mass with preaortic lymphadenopathy (arrow).*

Neuroblastoma (arising from the adrenal gland or lumbar sympathetic chain within the abdomen) can be difficult to distinguish from nephroblastoma, if there is invasion of the upper pole of the kidney. It usually presents before the child is 2 years old (30% before 1 year), as an abdominal mass that may be due to the primary tumour, or hepatomegaly. Metastases occur early, with invasion of adjacent organs, lymph node spread, and haematogenous spread to the liver, bone, brain, lung, orbits, and skin.

Calcification is present on 50% of plain films; however, CT is more sensitive for this feature than plain films, and also defines the extent of retroperitoneal disease. Ultrasound shows a large mass, frequently crossing the midline. The kidney is pushed inferolaterally

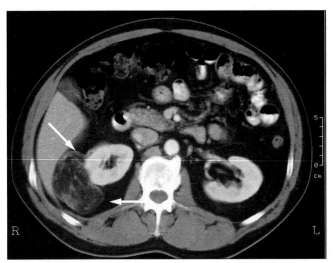

Fig. 5.44 *CT showing a right angiomyolipoma (arrows). This contains fat which is characteristic.*

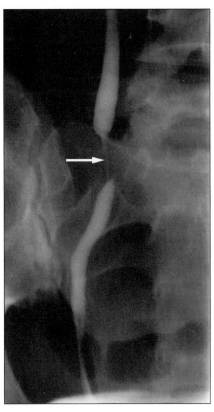

Fig. 5.45 *Retrograde pyelogram of a transitional-cell tumour of the right ureter demonstrating a stricture (arrow).*

in the 60% or more of cases of neuroblastoma that arise in the adrenal gland.

Oncocytoma

Oncocytoma is a specific type of renal adenoma that arises from proximal tubular cells. It is indistinguishable from renal-cell carcinoma on imaging, showing as a solid renal mass, which is usually well defined from surrounding tissue. Biopsy is required to exclude a malignant lesion.

Angiomyolipoma

Angiomyolipoma is a benign, hamartomatous renal mass that is seen usually in middle-aged women. It is associated with tuberous sclerosis, and may then be multiple and bilateral.

On ultrasound an angiomyolipoma is an echogenic mass, and on CT it has a characteristic appearance due to its fat contents (**Fig 5.44**).

Lymphoma

Lymphoma may occur as a discrete soft-tissue mass or diffuse lymphomatous involvement of the kidney. Retroperitoneal lymphadenopathy may result in hydronephrosis. On ultrasound, hypoechoic masses may be seen within or around the kidney. Vascular invasion is rare.

Multiple myeloma

Myeloma may involve the kidneys and can be complicated by amyloidosis.

Metastases to the kidney

Metastatic tumours in the kidney represent haematogenous spread, commonly from primaries in the bronchus, breast, or gastrointestinal tract.

UROTHELIAL TUMOURS

Urothelial tumours can occur wherever there is urothelium, from the renal pelvis to the urethra. The most common site is the bladder, followed by the renal pelvis; ureteric tumours are rare. Ninety per cent of urothelial tumours are malignant (transitional-cell carcinoma); 20% are multifocal at presentation, and 40% of patients will develop further urothelial tumours.

Risk factors predisposing to these tumours include smoking, exposure to aniline dyes and organic chemicals, contact with leather and rubber products, and abuse of phenacetin (tumours of the upper tract).

Painless haematuria occurs in 80% of patients with urothelial tumours and is the most common presenting complaint of bladder transitional cell carcinoma. Renal colic and haematuria (caused by blood clot in the ureter, from a renal pelvis tumour), silent obstruction (ureteric tumours), and urinary frequency (bladder tumours) can also occur.

Cystoscopy is indicated in all patients with frank haematuria (*see* flow diagram, page 121) and will diagnose bladder tumours; however, IVU is indicated before cystoscopy, as a bladder tumour may co-exist with an upper tract tumour (**Fig. 5.45**). Ultrasound with a full bladder will show many bladder tumours (**Fig. 5.46**); some may cause obstruction of the ureteric orifice (**Fig. 5.47**).

CT is used for staging of transitional-cell carcinomas, and can guide biopsy to obtain a tissue diagnosis (**Fig. 5.48**). It is particularly indicated for the staging of poorly differentiated transitional-cell tumours, and if bladder wall invasion is suspected at the time of cystoscopy.

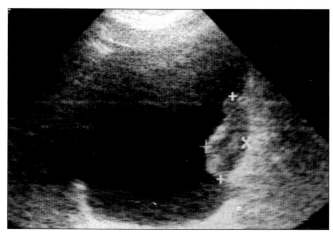

Fig. 5.46 *Ultrasound image through the full bladder, showing a polypoid bladder transitional-cell carcinoma (crosses).*

If ultrasound, IVU and cystoscopy have failed to reveal the cause of haematuria, retrograde ureterography is indicated. This is performed by injecting contrast into a catheter inserted retrogradely into the ureter at the time of cystoscopy. The causes of pelvicalyceal and ureteric filling defects that may be revealed include:

- Normal anatomy (accessory renal papillae and impressions from adjacent arteries).
- Transitional-cell tumour.
- Renal-cell carcinoma.
- Radiolucent calculi (uric acid).
- Blood clot.
- Papillary necrosis.
- Pyeloureteritis cystica.
- Metastases (rare, from melanoma or renal-cell carcinoma).
- Leucoplakia.

OTHER TUMOURS INVOLVING THE URINARY TRACT
Squamous carcinoma of the urinary tract
Squamous carcinoma of the urinary tract is rare. It is associated with chronic irritation of the urinary tract from infection and calculi, and with leucoplakia. Urinary schistosomiasis is a predisposing factor.

Prostatic carcinoma
Prostatic carcinoma is most commonly diagnosed when the curettings from transurethral resection of the prostate are examined pathologically. The role of imaging is evaluation of tumour spread in the pelvis, using CT (**Fig. 5.49**) and MR, and in diagnosing bony metastatic spread on isotope bone scintigraphy (**Fig. 5.50**) or plain films, which show skeletal hot spots or sclerotic areas, respectively.

Pelvic rhabdomyosarcoma
Twenty per cent of paediatric rhabdomyosarcomas occur in the pelvis, originating in the bladder, vagina, or prostate. The age of the patient is usually less than 2 years, and the ratio of males to females is 2:1.

If the tumour grows into a cavity, such as the bladder or vaginal lumen, it gives rise to characteristic grape-like clusters. Cross-sectional imaging is required to assess the extent of the tumour, initially using ultrasound, then CT or, preferably, MR to minimize radiation dose. On imaging alone, it can be impossible to differentiate rhabdomyosarcoma from pelvic teratoma or neuroblastoma.

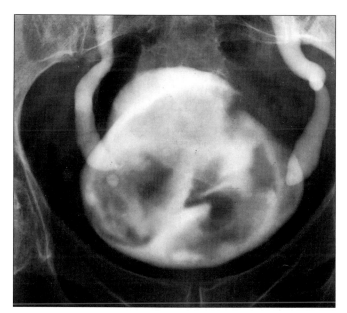

Fig. 5.47 *IVU showing a large bladder carcinoma, which is causing obstruction of both the vesicoureteric orifices.*

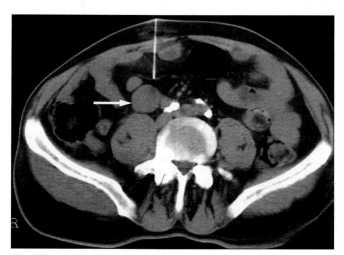

Fig. 5.48 *CT of a transitional-cell carcinoma of the ureter (arrow) that is being biopsied under CT control.*

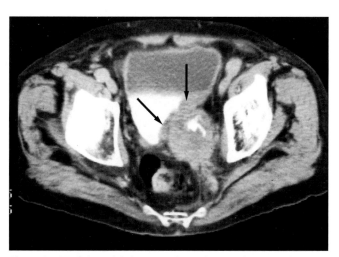

Fig. 5.49 *CT of the pelvis in prostatic carcinoma. The prostatic tumour (arrows) is invading the left posterior bladder wall.*

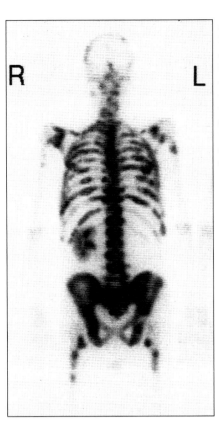

Fig. 5.50 *^{99m}Tc-MDP isotope bone scan in metastatic prostatic carcinoma. There are multiple skeletal metastases in the ribs, skull vault, spine, pelvis, and proximal long bones. The patient has had a previous left nephrectomy.*

for urinary tract calculi and bony metastases from possible prostatic carcinoma. Ultrasound of the urinary tract after the bladder has been emptied is indicated, to assess the residual volume of the bladder, to exclude hydronephrosis and exclude other urinary tract pathology.

Postobstructive atrophy

The normal kidney can withstand complete obstruction for up to 1 week and recover complete function. Obstruction for longer than this causes progressive nephron loss, with thinning of the renal cortex and blunting of the normally cup-shaped calyces.

Reflux nephropathy

Long-standing vesicoureteric reflux will cause upper tract dilatation; if reflux is into the renal collecting system, it will result in loss of renal cortex (*see* Fig. 5.8).

Renal cysts

Simple renal cysts are frequently seen on renal ultrasound as an incidental finding (**Fig. 5.51**); their prevalence increases with age, and they are frequently multiple. They are very thin walled and transonic; any wall thickening or internal echoes should raise the suspicion of haemorrhage or tumour.

Acquired cystic kidney disease (ACKD) is a condition seen in patients with chronic renal failure but without a history of hereditary cystic disease. Multiple small parenchymal cysts are found in patients with endstage renal disease of whatever cause, and their prevalence increases with increasing duration of dialysis. With time, the cysts increase in size and number, and there is an increased risk of haemorrhage into them, and of renal-cell carcinoma. Such tumours occur earlier and with a higher ratio of males to females among those with ACKD, compared with the normal population. The risk of ACKD and renal-cell carcinoma is not removed by successful renal transplantation.

Amyloidosis

The kidneys are involved in 80% of secondary amyloidosis and 30% of primary amyloidosis: amyloid is deposited in the renal interstitium and glomeruli. Initially, the kidneys are enlarged; in the chronic stage they are small. This condition may be complicated by renal vein thrombosis.

DEGENERATIVE CONDITIONS

Benign prostatic hyperplasia

Benign prostatic hyperplasia is common. Patients present with 'prostatism', which is characterized by difficulty in micturition, poor stream, dribbling, nocturia, and frequency. Imaging has a role in the search for evidence of bladder outflow obstruction and the exclusion of other urinary tract pathology before transurethral resection of the prostate.

A plain film of the kidneys, ureters, and pelvis is indicated, to look

Fig. 5.51 *Longitudinal ultrasound image of the left kidney, showing a simple cyst in the lower pole (arrows).*

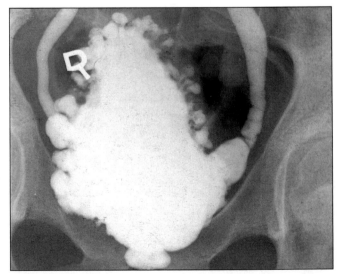

Fig. 5.52 *Cystogram in a patient with spina bifida and a neurogenic bladder. The bladder is extensively trabeculated, and has a vertical orientation, with bilateral vesicoureteric reflux.*

Neurogenic bladder

The innervation of the bladder is complex, and normal voiding requires intact sympathetic (hypogastric, T11–L2), parasympathetic (pelvic, S2–4), and somatic (pudendal, S2–4) nerves. Any abnormality of any of these can result in loss of bladder control.

The most common causes of an upper motor neurone abnormality are spinal cord injury, multiple sclerosis, and cerebrovascular disease. The result of such an abnormality is a hyper-reflexic bladder, with failure of relaxation of the detrusor sphincter. Eventually, this can lead to a trabeculated bladder, which has a vertical orientation (**Fig. 5.52**).

Lower motor neurone lesions are most often caused by a central lumbar disc prolapse or lumbosacral myelomeningocele; they result in an areflexic bladder, with urinary retention.

METABOLIC AND TOXIC CONDITIONS

METABOLIC DISORDERS
Nephrocalcinosis

The term 'nephrocalcinosis' refers to calcification in the renal parenchyma. It has many causes (**Fig. 5.53**).

Causes of nephrocalcinosis	
Focal nephrocalcinosis	Calcification within a focal renal abnormality, e.g. tumour, haematoma, vascular or inflammatory lesion
Cortical nephrocalcinosis	Chronic glomerulonephritis (GN) Post acute cortical necrosis Alport's syndrome (hereditary GN and deafness) } Very rare Oxalosis Rejected renal transplant
Medullary nephrocalcinosis	Hyperparathyroidism Renal tubular acidosis Medullary sponge kidney (see **Fig. 5.54**) } Most common causes Milk alkali syndrome Nephrotoxic drugs

Fig. 5.53 *Causes of nephrocalcinosis.*

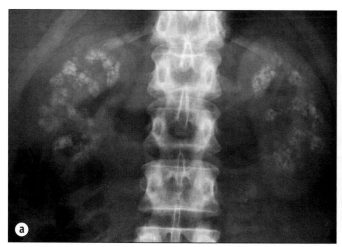 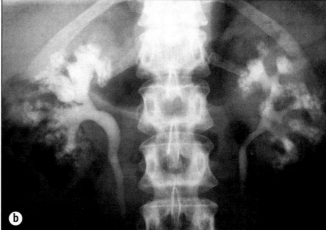

Fig. 5.54 *Control (**a**) and IVU (**b**) films in medullary sponge kidney. In this condition, multiple calculi form in dilated collecting tubules.*

Nephrolithiasis

'Nephrolithiasis' refers to stone formation within the collecting system of the urinary tract. The most common presenting complaint of urinary calculi is renal colic, but at least 85% of patients also have haematuria. Calyceal calculi may sometimes cause pain.

Because 80% of urinary tract stones are radio-opaque, they can be seen on a plain film (**Fig. 5.55**). **Figure 5.56** shows the classification of urinary calculi according to their chemical origins.

Investigation of renal colic

In investigating renal colic, a plain film of the *Kidneys*, *Ureters* and *Bladder* (KUB) should be performed first, to identify any calcification in the line of the urinary tract.

IVU shows whether a radio-opacity on the KUB is within the urinary tract, and identifies the level of the obstruction (**Fig. 5.58**). If an obstructing ureteric calculus is present, a 'standing column' or continuous column of contrast may be seen from the pelvicalyceal system to the obstructing stone (**Fig. 5.59**). A radiolucent obstructing lesion may represent a radiolucent calculus, thrombus, or ureteric tumour.

On ultrasound, both radio-opaque and radiolucent calculi are echogenic, and intrarenal stones can be seen clearly. Ureteric calculi, however, are frequently missed because of overlying bowel gas, although any urinary tract obstruction is seen as hydronephrosis and hydroureter. Calculi obstructing the vesicoureteric junction can be seen with a full bladder.

Bladder calculi

Calculi in the urinary bladder are often large and multiple (**Fig. 5.60**). They are predisposed to by immobility and indwelling catheters.

Diabetic nephropathy

Patients with diabetes mellitus are susceptible to urinary tract infection, particularly with gas-forming organisms (*see* Fig. 5.28), glomerulosclerosis and progressive renal failure, and renal papillary necrosis.

Papillary necrosis

Destruction of the renal papillae causes the calyces to look cup-shaped on an IVU. The causes of this condition include analgesic nephropathy, sickle-cell disease, diabetes mellitus, acute pyelonephritis, TB, and chronic obstruction.

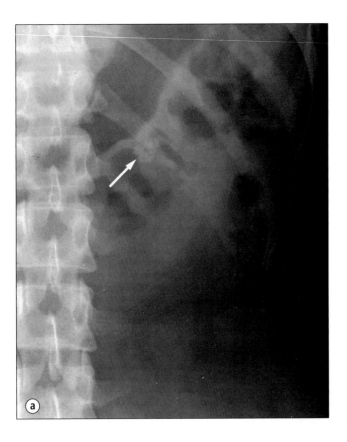

(a)

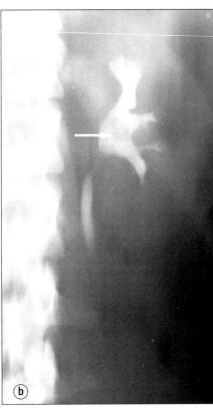

(b)

Fig. 5.55 (a) *Control film showing a spiculated calculus (arrow) projected over the left renal area.* **(b)** *After contrast, the calculus (arrow) is outlined with contrast in the left renal pelvis.*

Classification of urinary calculi

Types of urinary calculi	Predisposing factors
Calcium oxalate and/or calcium phosphate (70–75%)	**Increased calcium absorption from gut** Hypervitaminosis D Milk–alkali syndrome Sarcoidosis Beryllium toxicity Idiopathic **Oxaluria** Primary oxaluria: inborn error of metabolism Secondary oxaluria: small-bowel disease or resection, pyridoxine deficiency **Increased calcium mobilization from bone** Hyperparathyroidism Immobilization Bone metastases Multiple myeloma Hyperthyroidism Cushing's syndrome **Decreased tubular reabsorption** Renal tubular acidosis Fanconi's syndrome Wilson's disease Nephrotoxic drugs
Magnesium ammonium phosphate (struvite) ± calcium salts (15%) account for 70% of all staghorn calculi (*see* **Fig. 5.57**)	**Urinary tract infection** (especially with *Proteus* organisms, which possess urease)
Uric acid (5–10%) Radiolucent on plain films but opaque on CT and echogenic on ultrasound	**Increased uric acid in urine** Idiopathic Gout Lesch–Nyhan syndrome (rare) Acidic urine, e.g. chronic diarrhoea or ileostomy **Increased serum uric acid** Salicylates Thiazides High dietary protein/purine
Xanthine and matrix stones These are rare and radiolucent	

Fig. 5.56 *Classification of urinary calculi.*

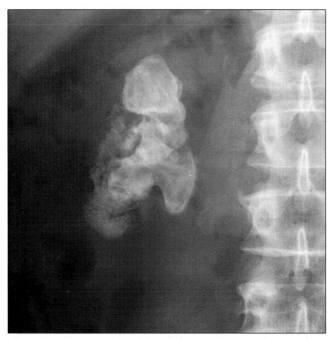

Fig. 5.57 *Plain film of the right renal area, showing a large staghorn calculus filling the right renal pelvis and calyces.*

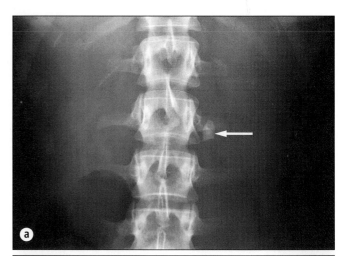

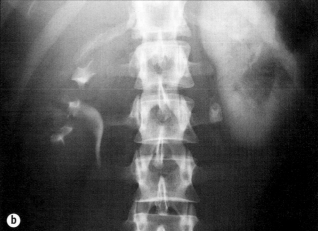

Fig. 5.58 (a) *Control film showing a large radio-opacity projected over the left transverse process of L2 (arrow). (b) After contrast, the dense left nephrogram confirms complete obstruction of the left ureter by the calculus.*

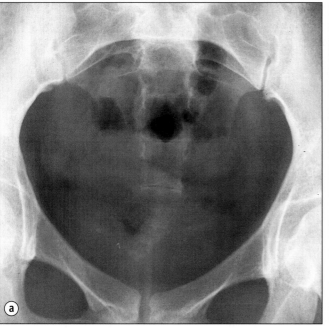

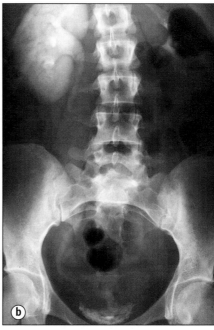

Fig. 5.59 (a) *Control film of the pelvis, showing small bilateral radio-opacities in a patient with right renal colic. (b) After contrast, there is a persistent right nephrogram, with a standing column of contrast in the right ureter confirming an obstructing calculus at the right vesicoureteric orifice.*

TOXIC CONDITIONS
Analgesic nephropathy
It was in 1953 that it was first noted that combinations of aspirin and phenacetin could result in renal papillary necrosis. Several mechanisms are involved, including a direct toxic effect and vascular occlusion. Other non-steroidal anti-inflammatory drugs, such as indomethacin, may also cause the condition. Calcification of the papillae is seen on a plain film (**Fig. 5.61**).

SURGICAL PROCEDURES

RENAL TRANSPLANTATION
Renal transplantation has been possible since the early 1950s. The transplant is usually from a cadaver donor, or occasionally from a living, related donor. After a successful transplant, patients have improved long-term survival and a better quality of life than can be achieved with haemo- or peritoneal dialysis. The procedure is now common; indications include almost anyone with endstage renal disease, the most common causes of which are diabetic nephropathy, chronic glomerulonephritis, and polycystic kidney disease. Contra-indications are active malignancy or infection.

The transplant kidney is placed in an extraperitoneal position within the recipient, usually in the right iliac fossa, with anastomosis of the renal artery to the external iliac artery (end-to-side) or internal iliac artery (end-to-end), and anastomosis of the renal vein to the external iliac vein (end-to-side). The transplant ureter is anastomosed to the recipient bladder, with creation of a submucosal tunnel.

Interventional procedures such as nephrostomy, angioplasty (**Fig. 5.62**), stenting, and dilatation are readily applicable to the transplanted kidney (*see* page 119).

Imaging and complications after renal transplantation
After renal transplantation, patients require long-term immuno-suppressive therapy and are therefore immunocompromised and at risk of a range of malignancies, including skin, rectal, cervical, Kaposi's, and lymphoma. Lymphoproliferative diseases form a spectrum—from diffuse lymphadenopathy to malignant B-cell lymphoma—that is known as post-transplant lymphoproliferative disorder (PTLD).

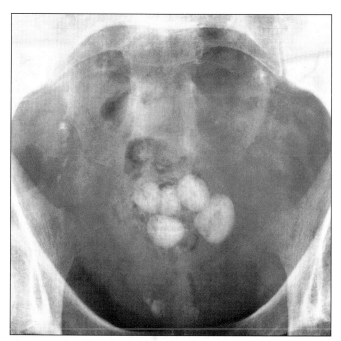

Fig. 5.60 *Plain film of the bladder area, showing multiple radio-opaque bladder calculi.*

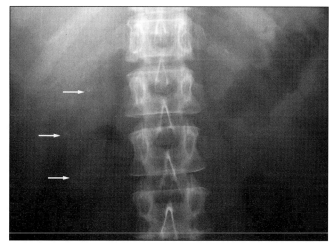

Fig. 5.61 *Plain film of the renal areas in analgesic nephropathy. The kidneys are small, and there is calcification of several right papillae (arrows).*

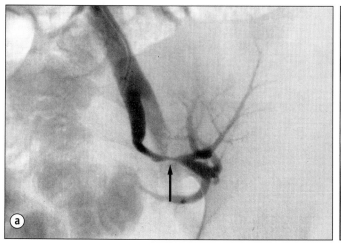
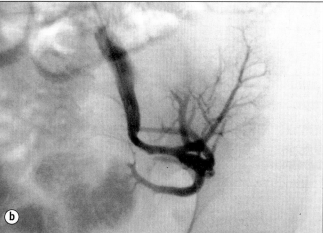

Fig. 5.62 *(a) DSA of a transplant renal artery, showing renal artery stenosis (arrow). (b) After angioplasty, there is a normal-calibre renal artery, with improved transplant perfusion.*

Ultrasound is the imaging modality used most widely for assessing the transplanted kidney, which is easily seen because of its superficial position. Ultrasound will show peri- and intrarenal abnormalities; the blood vessels can be assessed using Doppler and colour flow.

Perinephric fluid collections

Small perinephric collections of fluid are a common ultrasound finding in the immediate postoperative period; they may be caused by haematoma, urinoma, lymphocele, or abscess. Aspiration of the collected fluid may be undertaken under ultrasound control.

Hydronephrosis

Hydronephrosis is often transient, and is caused by postoperative oedema at the ureteric anastomosis. Other causes include stenosis at the ureteric anastomosis, denervation/devascularization of the ureter, calculi, and thrombus (**Fig. 5.63**).

Parencymal complications

Parenchymal complications that may follow renal transplantation include pyelonephritis, infarction, rejection, PTLD, and renal-cell carcinoma.

Vascular complications

Renal artery stenosis accounts for 10% of the vascular complications (*see* Fig. 5.62) after transplantation. Other complications include intrarenal arteriovenous fistula (AVF), extrarenal AVF or pseudo-aneurysm, and renal vein stenosis. Thrombosis of the renal artery or renal vein is rare.

Rejection

Transplant failure may be due to acute rejection, chronic rejection, acute tubular necrosis, or cyclosporine toxicity.

Rejection cannot be diagnosed specifically on ultrasound, but requires renal biopsy; however, ultrasound may be used to identify increased resistive index (>0.8) in the renal arteries, which is a non-specific finding.

A single nuclear medicine study of renal perfusion and function is not usually helpful in diagnosing rejection, but serial studies can show changes in transplant perfusion and excretion that indicate transplant failure.

ILEAL CONDUIT

After a total cystectomy, usually for invasive bladder transitional-cell carcinoma or prostatic carcinoma, a new bladder is created from a loop of ileum, with implantation of the ureters to this. An ileostomy is then created to allow urine to drain into a collecting bag (**Fig. 5.64**).

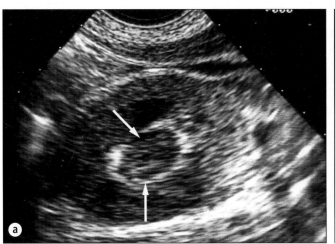 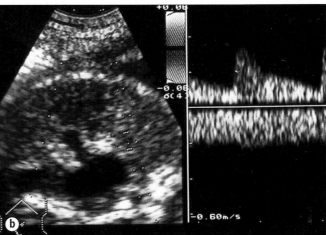

Fig. 5.63 *Ultrasound images of a renal transplant, showing obstruction of the collecting system as a result of thrombus (arrows). On (**a**) transverse and (**b**) longitudinal images with a normal Doppler tracing (right) from an intrarenal artery.*

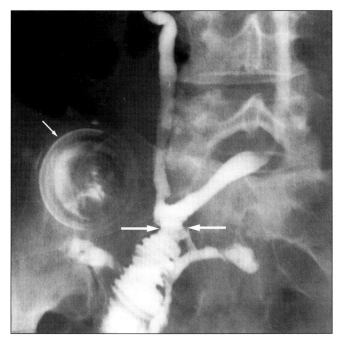

Fig. 5.64 Ileal conduit after total cystectomy. The ureters have been anastomosed to a loop of ileum (arrows), which drains through an ileostomy (small arrow). There is free reflux of contrast from the ileal conduit into the ureters.

INTERVENTIONAL URORADIOLOGY

VASCULAR PROCEDURES
Renal artery angioplasty
Renal artery stenosis may be dilated by angioplasty, with or without stenting, producing resolution of renovascular hypertension and renal failure (**Fig. 5.65**).

Tumour embolization
Preoperative embolization of vascular renal tumours enables safer surgical excision, with reduced operative blood loss (*see* Fig. 5.41).

AVF embolization
Embolization of renal AVFs (which are frequently a complication of renal biopsy or intervention, *see* Fig. 5.33) can be performed to abolish haematuria.

UROLOGICAL PROCEDURES
Nephrostomy
Percutaneous nephrostomy is performed for relief of worsening urinary obstruction. The calyceal system is punctured under ultrasound or radiographic control and a guidewire is inserted. Dilators are used to enlarge the tract from the skin into the collecting system, and finally a nephrostomy catheter with retaining pigtail is introduced. Nephrostomy may be for temporary or long-term relief of obstruction, or may be the initial stage of a more complex intervention such as percutaneous nephrolithotomy or endopyelotomy.

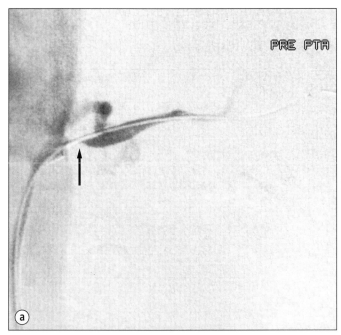

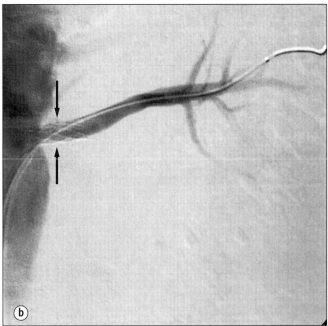

Fig. 5.65 (a) Left renal DSA, showing proximal renal artery stenosis (arrow). A guidewire has been placed across the stenosis. *(b)* After angioplasty and insertion of a stent (arrows), the renal artery is of normal calibre.

Percutaneous nephrolithotomy

Calculi in the collecting system or upper ureter may be removed through a ureteroscope inserted into the calyceal system through a dilated nephrostomy tract (**Fig. 5.66**). This procedure requires general anaesthesia.

Endopyelotomy

Endopyelotomy is used to treat UPJ stenosis or obstruction; it requires a nephrostomy and cystoscopic placement of a ureteric guidewire. The UPJ is incised from within the collecting system.

Ureteric dilatation and stenting

Ureteric strictures may be dilated with a balloon catheter. Long-standing benign strictures, malignant strictures, and those occurring after radiotherapy usually require stenting with a double J-stent. This has pigtail-shaped ends, which are positioned in the renal pelvis and bladder (**Fig. 5.67**).

HAEMATURIA

The sequence of procedures that should be followed in the investigation of frank haematuria is summarized in the flow diagram (**Fig. 5.68**).

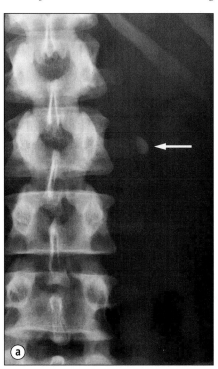
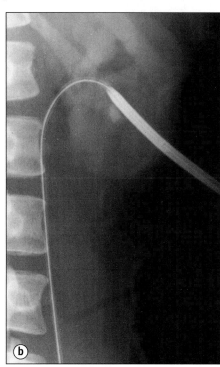
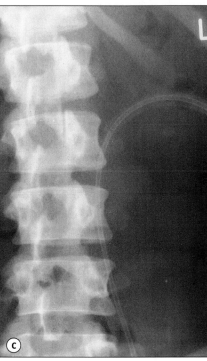

Fig. 5.66 PERC. *(a) Plain film of the left renal area, showing a calculus projected over the lower pole of the left kidney (arrow). (b) After puncture of the collecting system, guidewire is inserted down the left ureter, and the calculus removed through a nephroscope. (c) After percutaneous nephrolithotomy, the calculus is no longer seen. A nephrostomy drainage catheter is left in situ.*

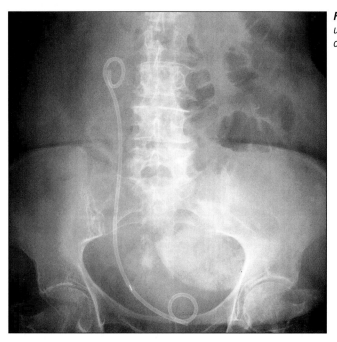

Fig. 5.67 Double J-stent in the right ureter in a patient who has a ureteric stricture as a result of radiotherapy. There is also small bowel obstruction.

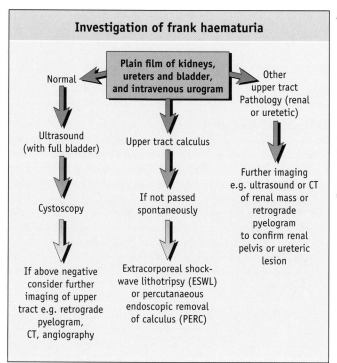

Investigation of frank haematuria

Plain film of kidneys, ureters and bladder, and intravenous urogram

Normal → Ultrasound (with full bladder) → Cystoscopy → If above negative consider further imaging of upper tract e.g. retrograde pyelogram, CT, angiography

Upper tract calculus → If not passed spontaneously → Extracorporeal shock-wave lithotripsy (ESWL) or percutanaeous endoscopic removal of calculus (PERC)

Other upper tract Pathology (renal or uretetic) → Further imaging e.g. ultrasound or CT of renal mass or retrograde pyelogram to confirm renal pelvis or ureteric lesion

Fig. 5.68 Investigation of frank haematuria.

Part 2: Scrotum and testes

Ultrasound is the best method of imaging the scrotal contents, because of their superficial nature and its avoidance of ionizing radiation.

CONGENITAL AND NEONATAL ABNORMALITIES

Undescended testes

Undescended testes are common in preterm male infants. In the majority, the testis completes its descent into the scrotum in weeks or months; fewer than 3% of males have persistent undescended testis, usually unilateral. The testis involved may lie in the abdomen, pelvis, or inguinal canal.

The condition may be complicated by malignant change, torsion, or infertility.

Ultrasound is the method of choice for identifying an undescended testis in the inguinal canal (**Fig. 5.69**). CT or MR imaging are required to hunt for an intra-abdominal or pelvic testis.

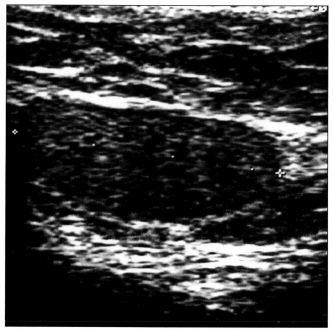

Fig. 5.69 Ultrasound image showing an undescended testis (crosses) in the inguinal canal.

TRAUMA

Direct trauma to the scrotum may cause haemorrhagic epididymitis, a scrotal haematoma, or testicular rupture. The last of these requires urgent surgical exploration, and ultrasound is indicated if rupture is suspected clinically.

INFECTION AND INFLAMMATORY CONDITIONS

Acute epididymitis

Acute epididymitis is common. In young males it is often caused by sexually transmitted pathogens, and in older men it is associated with lower urinary tract infection. Ultrasound shows swelling and hypoechogenicity of the epididymis (**Fig. 5.70**), often with a small associated hydrocele. If severe, the condition may progress to abscess formation or epididymo-orchitis.

Acute orchitis

The most common identifiable pathogen in cases of acute orchitis is the mumps virus. The testis is swollen and hypoechoic. On examination, it is important to look for flow in the testicular vessels, to differentiate the condition from testicular torsion, which can have a similar clinical presentation.

Chronic epididymo-orchitis/periorchitis

In chronic epididymo-orchitis/periorchitis, persisting low-grade or recurrent infection results in thickening of the tunica albuginea and increased echogenicity of the epididymis, with or without areas of calcification. The testis may atrophy.

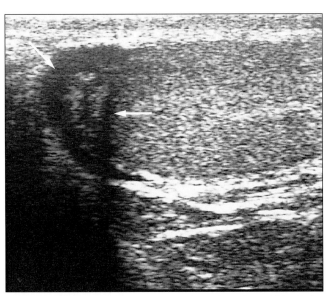

Fig. 5.70 Ultrasound image of acute epididymitis; the epididymis is hypoechoic and swollen (arrows).

Tuberculous epididymitis

Tuberculous spread from the proximal urinary tract is the usual cause of tuberculous epididymitis. The condition can result in abscess and sinus formation, with extensive scrotal calcification.

VASCULAR DISORDERS

Testicular torsion

Torsion of the testis occurs in young males, and testes with a horizontal rather than vertical orientation are at greater risk. Torsion occurs around the spermatic cord, occluding the testicular vessels. This condition is a surgical emergency that must be corrected within 4 hours if the testis is to be salvaged.

Ultrasound shows a swollen, hypoechoic testis, with swelling and sometimes haemorrhage of the epididymis. Reduced or absent flow on Doppler and colour flow is seen on imaging of the testicular artery. Torsion can also be shown as an ovoid photopenic defect on a ^{99m}Tc-pertechnetate nuclear medicine scan, because of the absence of testicular perfusion.

Varicocele

A varicocele is essentially a varicose vein in the scrotum, caused by tortuosity and dilatation of the pampiniform venous plexus. Primary varicocele is most common on the left because of the venous anatomy, with the left testicular vein draining into the left renal vein. Varicoceles may arise secondary to renal or IVC obstruction by renal-cell carcinoma. The condition can result in pain, reduced fertility, and testicular atrophy, but many are asymptomatic (*see page 124*).

Ultrasound of a varicocele shows multiple dilated venous channels in the scrotum (**Fig. 5.71**).

NEOPLASTIC DISEASE

The classification of testicular tumours is shown in **Figure 5.72**. Germ-cell tumours comprise 95% of all testicular tumours.

Seminoma

Seminoma is the most common testicular tumour and usually occurs in men aged between 30 and 45 years. Seminoma is typically a hypoechoic, well-defined, uniform intratesticular mass on ultrasound. These tumours are radiosensitive, and have a good prognosis.

Non-seminomatous germ-cell tumours

Non-seminomatous germ-cell tumours are more aggressive than seminomas, and metastasize early. Lymphatic spread occurs first, with lymphadenopathy around the left renal hilum and aorta from left-sided tumours, and around the IVC from right-sided tumours. Haematogenous spread to the liver and lungs occurs later.

On ultrasound, these tumours have a less uniform appearance than seminomas, with areas of increased and decreased echogenicity (**Fig. 5.73**). The main role of imaging is in staging and in monitoring response to therapy. CT of the abdomen is the best imaging method of staging (**Fig. 5.74**) and looking for early relapse. Tumour markers are also monitored during follow-up to detect early relapse.

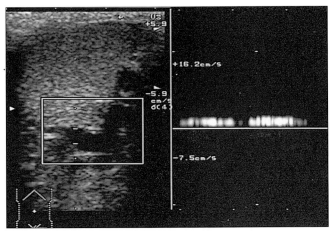

Fig. 5.71 *Ultrasound image of a left varicocele, showing multiple dilated venous channels around the testicle. The Doppler tracing on the right shows normal venous flow.*

Classification of testicular tumours	
Germ-cell	Seminoma Non-seminomatous germ-cell tumours
Gonadal stroma	Leydig-cell tumours Sertoli-cell tumours
Metastases	Any tumour, but especially renal-cell carcinoma and prostatic carcinoma
Lymphoma	Primary testicular or with systemic lymphoma

Fig. 5.72 *Classification of testicular tumours.*

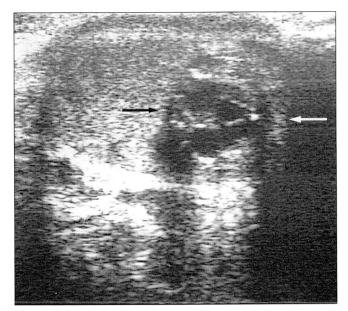

Fig. 5.73 *Non-seminomatous germ-cell tumour of the testis (teratoma). There is an irregular mass, with solid and cystic areas replacing the normal testicular tissue (arrows).*

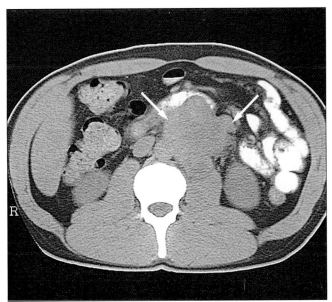

Fig. 5.74 *CT of the abdomen in non-seminomatous germ-cell tumour of the testis, demonstrating abdominal lymph-node metastases (arrows).*

INTERVENTIONAL RADIOLOGY IN SCROTUM AND PENIS

Varicocele embolization

The indications for embolization of a varicocele are subfertility, pain, and testicular atrophy in adolescents. Occlusion of the testicular vein and collaterals may restore fertility in 30–60% of patients and abolish pain. The procedure is most commonly performed using steel coils inserted through an angiographic catheter into the testicular vein or veins (**Fig. 5.75**). Embolization is most successful when coils are placed as far distally as possible—that is, close to the inguinal ligament.

Impotence

Impotence may be vascular in aetiology, because of either reduced arterial supply or venous leakage from the corpora cavernosa. Angioplasty of the internal iliac artery has been used to treat the arterial disease, and it is possible to restore erectile function in some patients by venous embolization to prevent venous leaks.

Priapism

Embolization of the internal pudendal artery has been successful in some cases of spontaneous priapism.

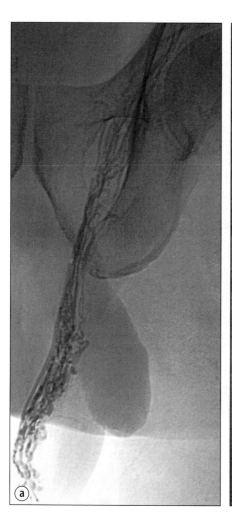
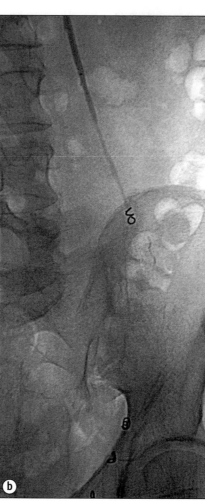

Fig. 5.75 (a) *Left testicular venogram, showing a left varicocele. (b) After embolization with steel coils, there has been occlusion of the testicular vein.*

chapter 6

Obstetrics and Gynaecology

Ultrasound is the principal imaging investigation used in both obstetrics and gynaecology. Its main advantage is the avoidance of ionizing radiation during pregnancy or during imaging of the reproductive organs of women of child-bearing age. Every effort should be made to avoid radiation, and when the diagnosis is not apparent on ultrasound, MR imaging may be indicated. During early pregnancy and in gynaecological imaging, resolution is best with transvaginal ultrasound, as the transducer is closer to the organs being imaged and a higher frequency of ultrasound can be used.

Transabdominal scanning requires a full bladder in non-pregnant patients and in early pregnancy, to displace loops of bowel (which contain gas) out of the pelvis and to act as an 'acoustic window'. A full bladder is also required for some indications in later pregnancy, such as evaluation of placenta praevia. This may be uncomfortable for the patient.

Part 1. Obstetrics

NORMAL PREGNANCY

In some centres, ultrasound is performed routinely in the first trimester of pregnancy, to confirm the following:
- The pregnancy is intrauterine.
- The embryo is viable.
- The number of embryos—singleton or multiple.
- The gestational dates—that is, to confirm the date estimated from the date of the last menstrual period.

Bleeding during the first trimester is common, occurring in 20–50% of women; it is usually limited to slight 'spotting', and is believed to be caused by implantation of the choriodecidua into the endometrium. However, a further 20–30% of those with bleeding will progress to abortion, therefore ultrasound is often indicated to assess whether the pregnancy is viable or not.

NORMAL FIRST TRIMESTER
On transvaginal ultrasound in a normal first trimester, a gestation sac should be visible within thickened, decidualized endometrium by 5 weeks after the first day of the last menstrual period. Within the sac, a second smaller sac—the developing yolk sac—may be visible. This stage corresponds with a beta human chorionic gonadotrophin (β-hCG) level of 500–800 mIU, compared with levels of 1800–3000 mIU that are attained by the time (approximately 6 weeks) a gestation sac can be visualized with transabdominal ultrasound.

Pulsation of the fetal heart can be identified from 5.5 weeks gestation on transvaginal ultrasound (**Fig. 6.1**) and 6.5 weeks on transabdominal ultrasound. After 7 weeks, fetal movement can be seen. By the end of the 8th week, the head and body of the embryo can be identified transabdominally.

During the first trimester, once the embryo is visible, crown–rump length—the longest demonstrable length of the embryo or fetus, excluding yolk sac or limbs (**Fig. 6.2**)—is used to assess gestational age. It is accurate to within 3 days from 7 to 10 weeks, and to within 5 days from 10 to 14 weeks. After 10 weeks, fetal movement and variable curvature increase the error.

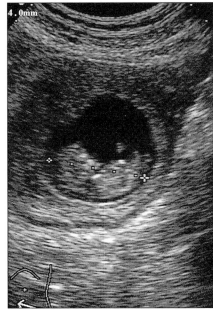

Fig. 6.2
Transabdominal ultrasound of an 8-week gestation, showing the crown–rump length (crosses).

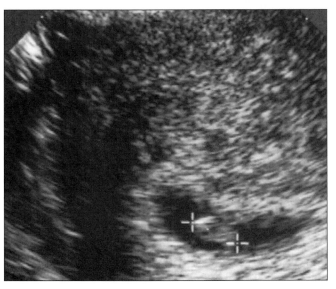

Fig. 6.1 *Early pregnancy on transvaginal ultrasound. The embryo (crosses) can be seen within the gestation sac.*

SECOND TRIMESTER

Many centres have now stopped performing routine scans in the first trimester in favour of scans in the second trimester, when a more detailed examination of fetal anatomy can be made.

After 14 weeks, the bi-parietal diameter of the fetal skull is used to assess gestation: an axial image of the brain is obtained through the thalamus and cavum septum pellucidum, and the distance from the outer table of the more superficial parietal bone to the inner table of the opposite parietal bone is measured (**Fig. 6.3**). The bi-parietal diameter can be measured from 12 weeks and can be used in conjunction with the crown–rump length from 12–14 weeks. Also measurable from 12 weeks is the femoral length (**Fig. 6.4**); at this stage, the epiphyses have not ossified, and the femoral shaft is measured from its proximal to its distal end.

Assessment of fetal age becomes less accurate as pregnancy progresses, and is best achieved with a combination of parameters. In addition to bi-parietal diameter and femoral length, the abdominal circumference can be measured. This is done on an axial image of the upper abdomen, including the liver and umbilical vein (**Fig. 6.5**).

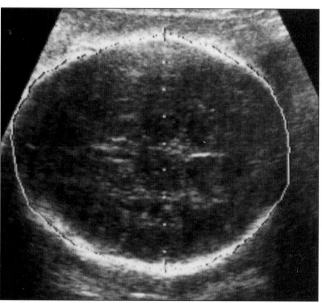

Fig. 6.3 *Axial scan through the fetal skull. The bi-parietal diameter is measured as the distance from the outer table of the more superficial parietal bone to the inner table of the distant parietal bone. The occipitofrontal circumference has also been measured in this fetus.*

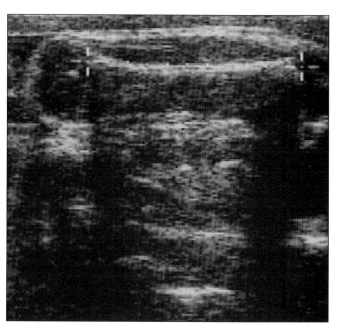

Fig. 6.4 *Ultrasound image of the fetal thigh showing measurement of the femoral length (crosses).*

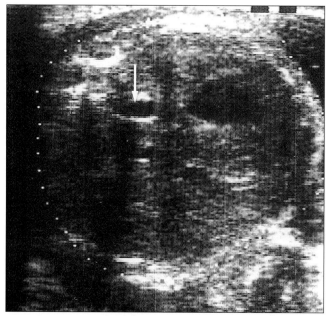

Fig. 6.5 *Axial scan through the fetal abdomen at the level of the umbilical vein (arrow) showing measurement of the abdominal circumference.*

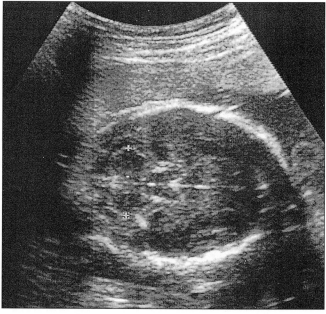

Fig. 6.6 *Transverse scan through the fetal brain, showing measurement of the cerebellum (crosses).*

THIRD TRIMESTER

Assessment of fetal age is inaccurate in the third trimester, but the above parameters can be measured on serial scans to assess fetal growth if, for example, the mother has pre-eclampsia or the uterus is 'small for dates'. From these measurements, an estimate of fetal weight can be made.

As the fetus develops, many anatomical structures can be seen on ultrasound (**Figs 6.6–6.9**). The importance of recognizing these structures lies in the diagnosis of fetal abnormalities in which the normal structures are absent or abnormal.

TWIN PREGNANCY

Twin or greater multiple-gestation pregnancy carries a greater risk than a singleton pregnancy, with perinatal mortality up to 10 times greater, particularly with monozygotic twins. The main cause of this is prematurity, with its associated complications. Twins are also at greater risk of congenital abnormalities, intrauterine growth retardation, and twin–twin transfusion (with monozygotic twins). Maternal complications are also more likely; they include hypertension, anaemia, and postpartum haemorrhage, while labour may be complicated by malposition of the fetus.

The aim of antenatal ultrasound in multiple-gestation pregnancy is initially to diagnose the number of gestation sacs (**Fig. 6.10**) and determine zygosity. The membranes and placenta may vary from dichorionic, diamniotic with two placentae to monochorionic, monoamniotic with a shared placenta. The importance of assessing the membranes and placenta is that there is a greater incidence of congenital abnormalities and perinatal mortality in twins sharing the same placenta and chorionic cavity. In the rare case of monoamniotic cavity, a careful examination of the fetuses should be made, to exclude conjoined twins.

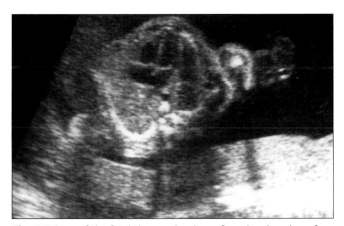

Fig. 6.7 *Scan of the fetal thorax, showing a four-chamber view of the heart; both ventricles and both atria can be seen clearly.*

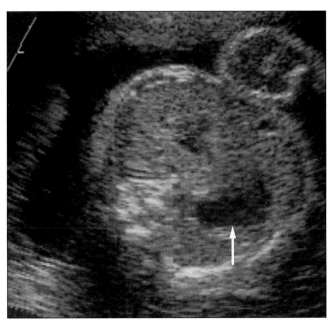

Fig. 6.8 *Normal fluid-filled stomach (arrow), indicating that the oesophagus is patent and the fetus is able to swallow amniotic fluid.*

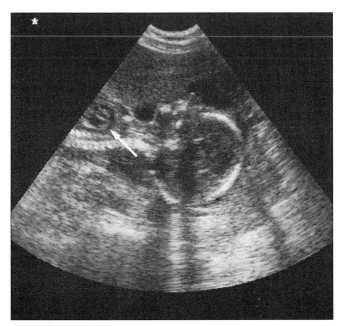

Fig. 6.9 *Coronal scan through the fetal face and aortic arch (arrow).*

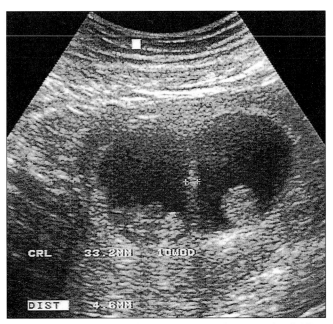

Fig. 6.10 *Twin pregnancy: there are two gestation sacs. The dividing membranes (crosses) are fairly thick, indicating that this is likely to be a dichorionic gestation.*

In the third trimester, ultrasound to assess fetal growth is important, as this is when twin growth may slow, compared with that of a singleton fetus.

Twin–twin transfusion syndrome is said to have occurred when there is shunting of blood from one fetus to the other through arteriovenous anastomoses in the placenta. This occurs to a significant extent only with monozygotic twins, it can result in growth disparity, with one twin that is larger and may have hydrops, and a smaller, growth-retarded twin.

ABNORMAL PREGNANCY

BLEEDING IN EARLY PREGNANCY

Bleeding in early pregnancy is common, and in most cases is minor and without pain. However, in 20% of cases the pregnancy does not continue. Ultrasound is indicated, to look for the following abnormalities.

Ectopic pregnancy

Implantation of the conceptus outside the endometrial cavity constitutes an ectopic pregnancy. The majority occur in the Fallopian tube, with only 5% occurring in the peritoneal cavity, ovary, or cervix. The risk of tubal pregnancy is increased in women with a history of salpingitis or tubal surgery, but women with an intrauterine contraceptive device (IUCD) or who have undergone infertility treatment also have an increased risk of ectopic pregnancy.

Undiagnosed ectopic pregnancy can lead to maternal bleeding and death if tubal rupture occurs. Ectopic pregnancy should be suspected in any woman with amenorrhoea and lower abdominal pain, with or without vaginal bleeding; the important investigations are a pregnancy test (β-hCG level) and transvaginal ultrasound.

On transvaginal ultrasound, it is important to exclude a viable intrauterine pregnancy. In an ectopic pregnancy, ultrasound will show a thickened endometrium, possibly with some blood in the endometrial lumen. An adnexal mass is the typical finding, and may vary from 1 to 3 cm in diameter. The embryo is not usually identifiable, and there may be a further cystic structure in the ovary—a corpus luteum cyst.

Unruptured ectopic pregnancies may bleed through the fimbriated end of the Fallopian tube. Fluid can be seen in the peritoneal cavity in both ruptured and unruptured ectopic pregnancies.

Anembryonic pregnancy (blighted ovum)

In anembryonic pregnancies, the embryo either fails to develop or develops abnormally, usually as a result of a chromosomal abnormality. A gestation sac and decidual reaction are seen, but without a recognizable embryo (**Fig. 6.11**).

Missed abortion

The gestation sac and embryo can be seen in missed abortion, but there is no fetal heart movement, and often the size of the embryo is smaller than would be expected for the menstrual dates (**Fig. 6.12**).

Incomplete abortion

In cases of incomplete abortion, the patient has usually passed some solid tissue with vaginal bleeding. Ultrasound is indicated, to exclude any retained intrauterine products of conception that could later become infected if not evacuated (**Fig. 6.13**). If a gestation sac is seen it is irregular, and there is no fetal heart activity.

Complete abortion

When there has been heavy bleeding and expulsion of the entire gestation sac, ultrasound is not indicated unless there is clinical concern that the abortion is incomplete.

Retrochorionic haemorrhage

Bleeding beneath the chorion may threaten the pregnancy (**Fig. 6.14**); there is fetal loss in approximately 20% of such cases.

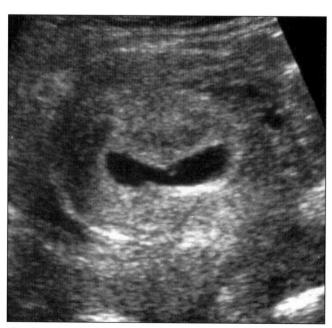

Fig. 6.11 *Anembryonic pregnancy (blighted ovum): there is a gestation sac, but no identifiable embryo.*

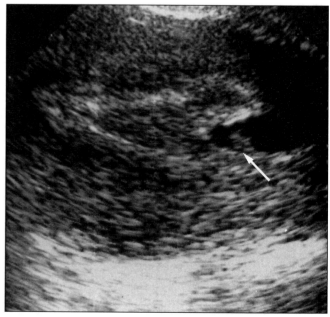

Fig. 6.12 *In this missed abortion, the endometrium is thickened, and a small embryo (arrow) can be seen within an irregular, partly collapsed gestation sac.*

FETAL ABNORMALITIES

Detailed scanning in the second trimester should include assessment of the fetal brain, spine, face, heart, aorta, stomach, kidneys, bladder and limbs, and size of the fetus in relation to the gestational dates. The volume of amniotic fluid, umbilical cord vessels, and placenta are examined. Any single abnormality of the above prompts a careful hunt for any associated anomalies; for example, with oligohydramnios the fetal urinary tract is scrutinized carefully.

BRAIN AND SPINE ABNORMALITIES
Ventriculomegaly

Enlargement of the ventricular system in ventriculomegaly can indicate a variety of underlying pathologies (**Fig. 6.15**).

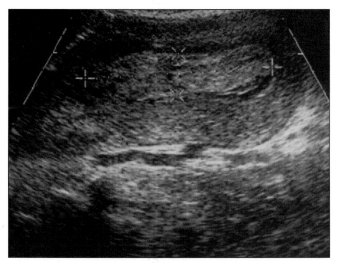

Fig. 6.13 *Incomplete abortion. Note the echogenic retained products of conception (crosses) within the uterine lumen.*

Causes of fetal ventriculomegaly	
Ultrasonic abnormality	**Underlying pathology**
Lemon-shaped skull with square-shaped, dilated frontal horns of lateral ventricles, effacement of cisterna magna, and cerebellar hypoplasia	Spina bifida (the spinal abnormality of a meningocele or myelomeningocele can also be seen)
Posterior fossa cyst (± ventriculomegaly)	Dandy–Walker malformation
Lateral and third ventricles dilated	Aqueduct stenosis Communicating hydrocephalus

Fig. 6.15 *Causes of fetal ventriculomegaly.*

Severe malformations of the brain can be diagnosed on ultrasound; they include anencephaly (absence of the skull vault and cerebral hemispheres) (**Fig. 6.16**), holoprosencephaly (malformation of the forebrain, with a single large ventricle), and porencephaly (multiple cystic collections within the brain).

Other abnormalities that may be diagnosed antenatally are encephalocele (protrusion of part of the brain through a skull vault defect), microcephaly (small head, usually associated with other abnormalities), agenesis of the corpus callosum, and choroid plexus abnormalities (cysts and papillomas that may be associated with trisomies 13 and 21 and fetal mortality).

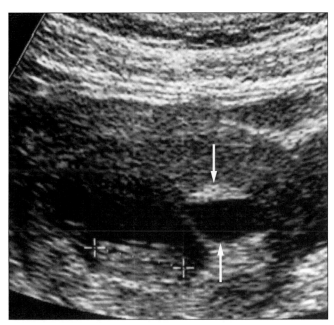

Fig. 6.14 *Retrochorionic haemorrhage. A collection of blood (arrows) can be seen beneath the chorion, separate from the gestation sac.*

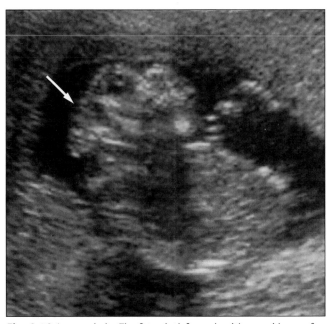

Fig. 6.16 *Anencephaly. The fetus is deformed, with no evidence of a normal skull vault (arrow).*

CARDIOVASCULAR ABNORMALITIES

The chambers of the fetal heart can be identified from 14 weeks, but fetal cardiac anatomy is not well demonstrated until 20–24 weeks. A transverse scan of the fetal thorax gives a four-chamber view of the heart, and many abnormalities can be demonstrated on this view (**Figs 6.17** and **6.18**). More detailed examination involves assessment of the aorta and pulmonary trunk, and colour and Doppler assessment of direction and velocity of flow.

The following abnormalities can be diagnosed antenatally.

Cardiovascular abnormalities	
Structural abnormalities	Atrial and ventricular septal defects Pulmonary and aortic stenosis Fallot's tetralogy Transposition of the great arteries Double-outlet right ventricle Hypoplastic left-heart syndrome (see Fig. 6.18) Coarctation of the aorta Univentricular heart Pulmonary atresia
Cardiomyopathies	Infants of diabetic mothers Secondary to outflow obstruction Infections
Fetal arrhythmias	Tachyarrhythmias Atrioventricular block (mothers with connective-tissue disease and fetal structural cardiac anomalies)

Fig. 6.17 *Cardiovascular abnormalities.*

Causes of non-immune hydrops	
Fetal	Congenital heart disease Arrhythmias Hydrocephalus Vein of Galen aneurysm Pulmonary abnormalities Urinary tract abnormalities Chromosomal abnormalities Intrauterine infection Cystic hygroma Twin–twin transfusion
Placental/cord	Cord knots Umbilical vein thrombosis Chorioangioma
Maternal	Diabetes mellitus Pre-eclampsia/eclampsia Severe anaemia

Fig. 6.19 *Causes of non-immune hydrops.*

Hydrops fetalis

The term 'hydrops fetalis' means an 'oedematous fetus'; this may be found in association with a wide variety of conditions. It is categorized broadly as isoimmune and non-immune, the latter being seen much more commonly now.

Isoimmune hydrops is caused by a severe haemolytic anaemia in the fetus as a result of isoimmunization against an erythrocyte antigen. It has declined in incidence because of the widespread use of Rhesus immunoglobulin immunization.

Non-immune hydrops can occur as a result of fetal, placental, or maternal abnormalities; the most common causes are congenital heart disease and arrhythmias (**Fig. 6.19**).

The ultrasound signs of hydrops are skin thickening and oedema, ascites (**Fig. 6.20**), and pleural and pericardial effusions.

URINARY TRACT ABNORMALITIES

At detailed antenatal ultrasound examinations during the second trimester, the fetal kidneys and bladder should be visible and the amniotic fluid volume should be assessed.

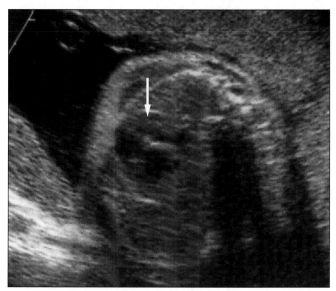

Fig. 6.18 *Four-chamber view of the heart, showing the very small left ventricle (arrow) in a fetus with hypoplastic left-heart syndrome.*

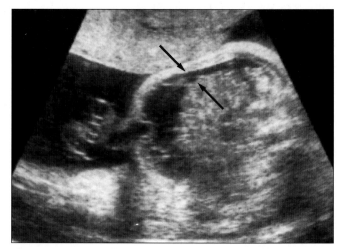

Fig. 6.20 *Fetal ascites in a hydropic fetus, demonstrating fluid within the fetal abdominal cavity (arrows).*

Fetal renal pyelectasis

Fetal renal pyelectasis is the most common fetal abnormality seen on antenatal ultrasound; it is diagnosed when the anteroposterior diameter of the renal pelvis is ≥5 mm (Fig. 6.21). If pyelectasis or renal pelvic dilatation is seen antenatally, then postnatal ultrasound is indicated, to look for the underlying cause and direct further investigation.

Fetal pyelectasis may resolve spontaneously. The most common underlying abnormality is ureteropelvic junction obstruction. Other causes include reflux, ureteral valves or strictures, obstruction at the vesicoureteric junction, ureterocele, and posterior urethral valves (see Chapter 5).

Potter's syndrome

The constellation of abnormalities described by Potter in 1946 consists of bilateral renal agenesis, pulmonary hypoplasia, and facial and limb abnormalities.

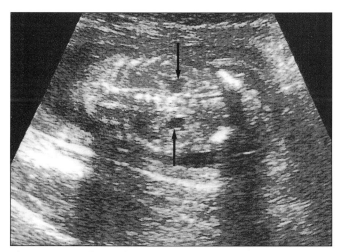

Fig. 6.21 Coronal scan through the posterior aspect of the fetal abdomen, showing the bilateral dilated renal collecting systems (arrows) that are characteristic of fetal renal pyelectasis.

Oligohydramnios (a severe reduction in amniotic fluid volume) (Fig. 6.22) is characteristic of Potter's syndrome. Normally, fetal production of urine contributes to the amniotic fluid volume. In the absence of urine production, severe oligohydramnios occurs, resulting in the facial and limb abnormalities and intrauterine growth retardation, and it is now recognized that the features of the syndrome are the result of bilateral renal agenesis. However, any other abnormality that results in severe oligohydramnios will cause the features typical of Potter's syndrome.

Multicystic dysplastic kidney

Multicystic dysplastic kidney is a common cause of an abdominal mass in a neonate; it can be diagnosed antenatally. The kidney is enlarged and contains multiple cysts, with little functioning renal tissue. There may be oligohydramnios if the contralateral kidney is abnormal, or polyhydramnios, which is believed to be caused by pressure on the gastrointestinal tract. This abnormality must be distinguished from fetal renal pyelectasis.

Mesoblastic nephroma

Mesoblastic nephroma is a fetal hamartoma. Postnatally, it must be distinguished from nephroblastoma (Wilms' tumour); it is very rare for the latter to be diagnosed antenatally.

RESPIRATORY AND NECK ABNORMALITIES
Diaphragmatic hernia

Diaphragmatic hernias can be diagnosed when fluid-filled loops of bowel are seen in the fetal chest (Fig. 6.23).

Cystic adenomatoid malformation of the lung

The condition known as cystic adenomatoid malformation of the lung usually affects the upper lobes or middle lobe. Multiple cysts are seen in the thorax (and should be distinguished from the fluid-filled loops of bowel that are associated with a diaphragmatic hernia). This abnormal lung compresses normal lung and may compress the oesophagus (causing polyhydramnios) or the heart (causing hydrops).

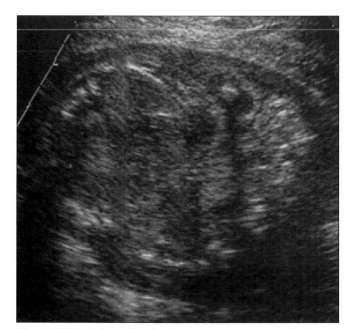

Fig. 6.22 Oligohydramnios: there is scarcely any amniotic fluid, and the fetus is lying in an abnormally flexed position.

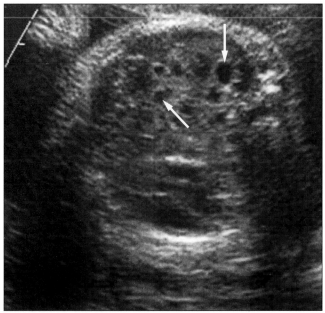

Fig. 6.23 Axial scan in diaphragmatic hernia, showing typical loops of bowel within the fetal thorax (arrows) .

Cystic hygroma

A cystic hygroma is an abnormality of the lymphatics and may occur as an isolated finding or be part of a chromosomal abnormality. It usually involves the back of the fetal neck (**Fig. 6.24**), and can be very variable in size. In severe cases, the fetus is engulfed in cystic collections.

Teratoma of the neck

Teratomas of the neck are benign, bilateral tumours. It is important that they are diagnosed antenatally, as they may obstruct labour.

GASTROINTESTINAL TRACT ABNORMALITIES
Oesophageal atresia

Oesophageal atresia is associated with tracheo-oesophageal fistula in the majority of cases. The ultrasound signs are polyhydramnios and absence of the normal fluid-filled stomach, as the fetus is unable to swallow amniotic fluid; fluid should normally be visible in the stomach from 15 weeks of gestation.

Duodenal atresia

The ultrasound signs of duodenal atresia are polyhydramnios and a 'double bubble', representing the distended fluid-filled stomach and proximal duodenum (*see* Fig. 3.2). It is important to look for other abnormalities, as duodenal atresia is associated with trisomy 21, other gastrointestinal atresias, congenital heart disease, renal and vertebral anomalies, and biliary atresia.

Lower gastrointestinal abnormalities

Anorectal malformations, Hirschprung's disease, and meconium plug syndrome can all give similar antenatal apprearances, with a dilated colon. However, this is a non-specific sign that can also be seen in normal fetuses.

Abdominal wall defects

Herniation of abdominal contents through a defect in the anterior abdominal wall can occur in gastroschisis and omphalocele. In gastroschisis, small bowel herniates through a full-thickness defect that is paraumbilical: on ultrasound, loops of small bowel are seen free in the amniotic fluid (**Fig. 6.25**), with the umbilical cord inserting at the normal site. With omphalocele, on the other hand, the abdominal wall defect is at the site of the umbilicus, and the cord inserts into a membrane covering the herniated abdominal contents.

The importance of distinguishing between these two conditions is that gastroschisis is usually an isolated defect, whereas omphalocele is associated with other congenital abnormalities.

ABNORMALITIES OF THE PLACENTA, CORD AND MEMBRANES

PLACENTAL ABNORMALITIES

The placenta develops from a maternal component, the decidua basalis or basal plate, which is supplied with blood from the spiral arterioles, and a fetal component, the chorionic plate, which consists of chorionic villi that are bathed in maternal blood in the intervillous space. It may have accessory (succenturiate) lobes, and can have a variety of shapes, positions, and configurations. The following are clinically significant.

Placenta praevia

In placenta praevia, the placenta lies over the internal os (**Fig. 6.26**). Massive haemorrhage can occur during labour if this is not diagnosed antenatally.

Succenturiate lobe

If the placenta has an accessory or succenturiate lobe, this may be retained *in utero* and cause postpartum haemorrhage; alternatively, vessels connecting this lobe to the main placenta may cross the internal os (vasa praevia) and cause fetal blood loss in labour.

Circumvallate placenta

The chorionic plate in circumvallate placenta is smaller than the basal plate, and the fetal membranes form a folded ring around the fetal surface of the placenta. This condition is associated with haemorrhage, premature labour, and perinatal mortality.

Placental infarcts

Placental infarcts can occur in normal pregnancy, but they occur to a greater extent when there is pre-eclampsia or maternal essential hypertension.

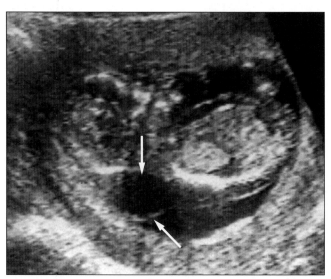

Fig. 6.24 *Cystic hygroma, showing an extensive, fluid-filled collection that is most obvious on the posterior aspect of the fetal neck (arrows).*

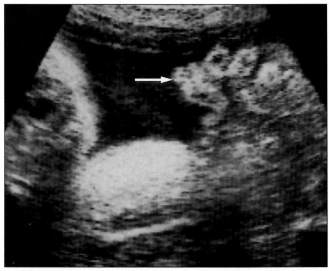

Fig. 6.25 *A defect in the anterior abdominal wall in gastroschisis results in the presence of loops of bowel in the amniotic cavity (arrow).*

Retroplacental haemorrhage

Retroplacental haemorrhage can occur with a normally sited placenta, placenta praevia, a low-lying placenta, or circumvallate placenta. It may present with external bleeding, or may be seen as a haematoma beneath or at the margin of the placenta (Fig. 6.27).

Gestational trophoblastic disease

The group of gestational trophoblastic diseases arise from abnormal fertilization or abnormal development of the blastocyst. The abnormal tissues arise from trophoblastic cells and can therefore invade tissues and produce hCG; this feature is exploited to monitor disease progression and response to treatment.

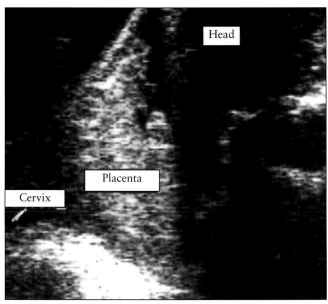

Fig. 6.26 Longitudinal scan through the lower uterine segment with a full maternal bladder, demonstraing placenta praevia, with the placenta covering the internal os.

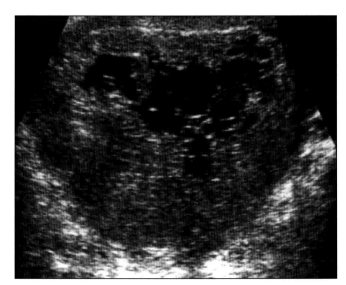

Fig. 6.28 Hydatidiform mole. Note the multiple cystic spaces within the uterus, which have a typical 'cluster of grapes' appearance. There was no evidence of a normal gestation sac or embryo.

Hydatidiform mole

Hydatidiform mole is characterized by swollen, oedematous chorionic villi that have the appearance of clusters of grapes (Fig. 6.28). With a complete mole, there is no fetus; with a partial mole, there may be some normal villi and an abnormal fetus. A hydatidiform mole may co-exist with a normal fetus in a twin pregnancy.

Invasive mole

When the condition known as invasive mole occurs, there is invasion of trophoblastic tissue into the myometrium, with some villus formation.

Choriocarcinoma

No discernible villi are present in choriocarcinoma. This is a highly malignant disease that metastasizes beyond the uterus to the lungs, liver, brain, and other organs.

CORD ABNORMALITIES

The normal umbilical cord contains one umbilical vein and two umbilical arteries (Fig. 6.29); it usually inserts in a position central or eccentric to the placenta. Doppler ultrasound can be used to assess blood flow in the fetoplacental circulation, and to monitor fetal well-being.

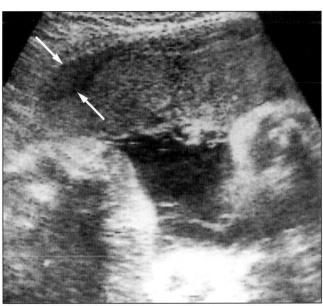

Fig. 6.27 Retroplacental haemorrhage. Echogenic fluid is seen lying between the uterine wall and the placenta (arrows).

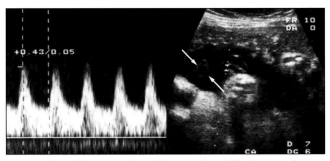

Fig. 6.29 Doppler tracing through a normal umbilical artery. The normal umbilical cord (arrows, right) contains the umbilical vein and two smaller umbilical arteries.

Cord position

The cord may loop around parts of the fetus, or form knots and lead to perinatal mortality. Cord prolapse during labour may occur if the cord lies between the presenting part and the lower uterine segment; this can cause fetal death.

Cord insertion

The cord may insert at the margin of the placenta or, rarely, to the membranes, at a distance from the edge of the placenta (velamentous insertion). Vessels in a velamentous insertion are more likely to tear during labour.

MEMBRANES

The amniotic membranes envelope the embryo and cord, and enlarge progressively until, by 12–14 weeks of gestation, the surrounding chorionic cavity is obliterated. Before this time, ultrasound can show the thin amniotic membrane.

'Amniotic bands' are believed to arise as a result of rupture of the amniotic membrane, with the formation of fibrous bands that may trap parts of the fetus and cause malformations (**Fig. 6.30**).

MATERNAL ABNORMALITIES

DIABETES MELLITUS

Infants of diabetic mothers have a greater incidence of many abnormalities compared with those of non-diabetic women. Congenital abnormalities include neural tube defects and cardiac abnormalities. Macrosomia, defined as birth weight >4 kg or >90th centile for the gestational age, is typically manifest as enlargement of the viscera and an increase in adipose tissue; conversely, women with diabetic vascular disease may instead show evidence of intrauterine growth retardation, as a result of reduced placental blood flow. There is an increased risk of intrauterine fetal death, and also of postnatal respiratory distress.

Antenatal ultrasound examination in diabetic women should assess gestational age and fetal size and growth, and seek evidence of congenital abnormalities.

PRE-ECLAMPSIA

Pre-eclampsia is specific to pregnancy and the immediate postpartum period. The mother becomes hypertensive, and may develop proteinuria and peripheral oedema. The umbilical Doppler waveform may be abnormal, and there is a risk of intrauterine growth retardation and perinatal mortality.

PELVIC PATHOLOGY

Pelvic pain during pregnancy may be caused by a variety of abnormalities. The most common cause is a corpus luteum cyst. This is usually a transonic cyst within an ovary. Most are asymptomatic and regress normally after 16 weeks; occasionally, they may be large, or may bleed (**Fig. 6.31**). Other cystic pelvic lesions include theca lutein cysts, ovarian tumours, and dermoid cysts.

Solid pelvic abnormalities include fibroids (which may increase or decrease in size during pregnancy), and solid ovarian tumours.

UPPER ABDOMINAL PAIN

Pregnant women develop physiological dilatation of the urinary tract, usually on the right side, from as early as 10 weeks of gestation. However, urinary tract pathology, such as calculi or infection, may also occur. Ultrasound is the investigation of first choice in women with abdominal pain during pregnancy, to look for urinary tract pathology and also for gall-bladder disease.

DEEP VEIN THROMBOSIS AND PULMONARY EMBOLI

Pregnancy carries an increased risk of deep venous thrombosis and pulmonary embolism. Doppler ultrasound of the lower limb veins is indicated to look for deep venous thrombosis, and a limited isotope perfusion study for pulmonary embolism.

CEPHALOPELVIC DISPROPORTION AND PELVIMETRY

When a woman has a pelvic deformity (e.g. previous fracture), or there has been failure to progress in a previous labour, it may be desirable to measure the internal pelvic dimensions, to assess any cephalopelvic disproportion and attempt to predict whether vaginal delivery is feasible. This was previously performed radiographically, but is now possible with MR imaging (**Fig. 6.32**).

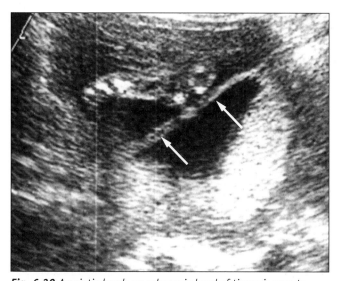

Fig. 6.30 Amniotic band: an echogenic band of tissue is seen to cross the amniotic cavity (arrows).

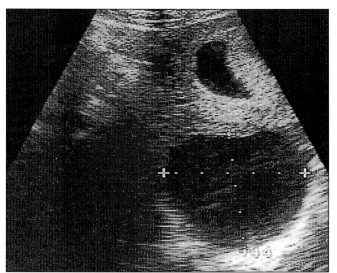

Fig. 6.31 This woman presented with right iliac fossa pain in early pregnancy. There is a cystic structure adjacent to the uterus (crosses), representing haemorrhage into a corpus luteum cyst.

INTERVENTIONAL PROCEDURES

With increasing sophistication of ultrasound equipment in recent years, the ability to guide needle placement carefully into a specific structure has improved dramatically, making possible the interventions described here. As with all intervention, the procedures carry a risk (abortion, infection, fetal injury), and this must be carefully balanced against the benefit of making an antenatal diagnosis.

CHORIONIC VILLUS SAMPLING

Chorionic villi reflect fetal genotype and can be analysed to look for chromosomal abnormalities. Villus sampling is performed at between 9 and 12 weeks of gestation, using either a transabdominal or a transcervical route (**Fig. 6.33**). Indications for this procedure include maternal age >35 years (therefore increased risk of Down's syndrome), previous child with a chromosomal abnormality, or parents who are carriers of chromosomal abnormalities.

AMNIOCENTESIS

Aspiration of amniotic fluid by amniocentesis is usually performed at between 16 and 18 weeks of gestation (**Fig. 6.34**). The desquamated fetal cells obtained from the fluid are cultured for chromosomal and genetic analysis, which takes 3 weeks. The pregnancy is therefore at a more advanced stage by the time the information from the investigation (which may result in termination being advised) is available. Indications for the procedure include possible chromosomal abnormalities, neural tube defects, metabolic abnormalities, and isoimmunization. Later in pregnancy, amniocentesis may be indicated to assess fetal maturity or infection.

FETAL BLOOD SAMPLING

Aspiration of blood directly from the umbilical cord vessels under ultrasound control is indicated to diagnose fetal haematological diseases such as haemolysis in isoimmunization, haemoglobinopathies, and coagulopathies. Other indications include congenital infection and rapid karyotyping late in pregnancy.

FETAL INTERVENTION *IN UTERO*

It is now possible to transfuse a fetus *in utero*. The indication for this is isoimmunization, with fetal anaemia, at a gestation less than 34 weeks. Blood is transfused into the umbilical vein under ultrasound control.

Other indications for possible *in utero* intervention include fetal urinary tract obstruction and hydrocephalus.

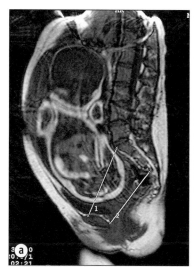
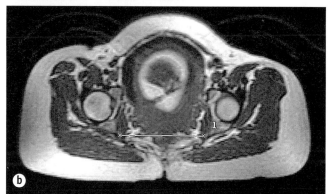

Fig. 6.32 *MR pelvimetry.* *(a)* *T1-weighted sagittal image, showing measurement of the sagittal inlet and outlet diameters.* *(b)* *T1-weighted axial image, showing measurement of the interspinous distance. This is an example of normal anatomy; while it does not predict a normal labour, there is no evidence of cephalopelvic disproportion.*

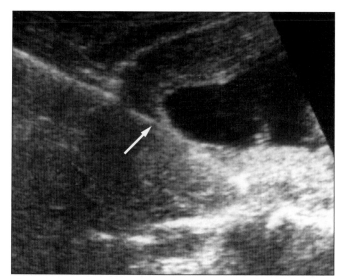

Fig. 6.33 *Placement of the needle tip (arrow) in chorionic villus sampling.*

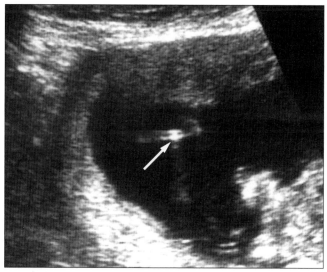

Fig. 6.34 *Amniocentesis. The needle tip (arrow) is within the amniotic cavity.*

Part 2. Gynaecology

CONGENITAL ABNORMALITIES

Congenital abnormalities of the femal reproductive tract may be obvious at birth or may present in later life, at the onset of menarche or with infertility. They are frequently associated with abnormalities of the urinary tract.

UTERINE ABNORMALITIES

Uterine aplasia is very rare; hypoplasia is a cause of infertility. The normal uterus, cervix, and vagina are formed by fusion of paired Müllerian duct structures. Failure of this fusion can result in a spectrum of abnormalities from uterus didelphys (duplication of uterus, cervix, and vagina) to arcuate uterus (prominent fundal concavity); bi-cornuate uterus is an intermediate form (**Fig. 6.35**). These abnormalities are demonstrated by hysterosalpingography, in which contrast is injected into the cervical lumen.

VAGINAL ABNORMALITIES

Vaginal aplasia is associated with severe abnormality of the uterus; urinary tract abnormalities are a common association.

Vaginal atresia and imperforate hymen occur at the junction of the lower third with the upper two-thirds of the vagina—the site of the junction of the urogenital sinus with the Müllerian duct system. They may present in infancy, with an abdominal mass caused by a distended, fluid-filled vagina (hydrometrocolpos); there is usually urinary tract obstruction. However, presentation is usually delayed until after menarche, with amenorrhoea and an abdominal mass as a result of haematometrocolpos (**Fig. 6.36**). These abnormalities are best seen on ultrasound.

ABNORMALITIES OF THE UROGENITAL SINUS AND CLOACA

With persistence of the urogenital sinus, the urethra and vagina share a common orifice. In female pseudohermaphrodites, as a result of androgen production, there may also be clitoromegaly.

Persistence of the cloaca, in which the rectum, vagina, and urethra have a common orifice, occurs at an earlier stage embryologically, with failure of descent of the urorectal septum.

TRAUMA

Most trauma to the female reproductive tract is iatrogenic. Hysterectomy may result in pelvic haematoma because of haemorrhage from the vaginal vault into the extraperitoneal space. Ureteric injury caused by laceration, denervation, or devascularization is a well-recognized risk of hysterectomy. Caesarean section can cause similar complications.

Uterine perforation can occur during diagnostic or therapeutic curettage of the uterus, or during insertion of an intrauterine contraceptive device (IUCD). Asherman's disease is a long-term complication of repeated or excessive endometrial currettage, with adhesions forming within the uterine cavity. These are seen as multiple irregular filling defects at hysterosalpingography.

INFECTION AND INFLAMMATORY CONDITIONS

The following abnormalities, although listed separately, frequently co-exist, and are clinically termed pelvic inflammatory disease. The organisms involved most commonly are *Chlamydia* and gonococci.

OVARIAN DISORDERS

Infection rarely involves the ovary alone, and there is usually associated disease of the Fallopian tube. Ultrasound shows an adnexal mass with a fluid centre, thick septae, and gas bubbles (**Fig. 6.37**). Rupture into the peritoneal cavity may occur.

TUBAL DISORDERS

Acute salpingitis presents with lower abdominal pain, and may mimic appendicitis. Ultrasound shows a thickened Fallopian tube, which may be filled with pus (pyosalpinx), and intraperitoneal fluid in the pouch of Douglas. In the chronic phase, as a result of adhesions at the fimbriated end, a distended tube filled with clear fluid (hydrosalpinx) can be seen on ultrasound or hysterosalpingography (**Fig. 6.38**). This is a cause of infertility.

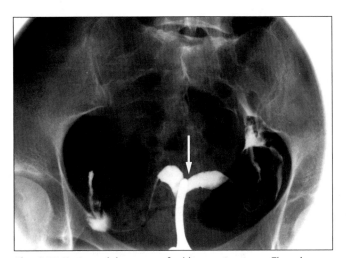

Fig. 6.35 *Hysterosalpingogram of a bi-cornuate uterus. There is a thick septum extending from the uterine fundus to divide the uterine cavity (arrow).*

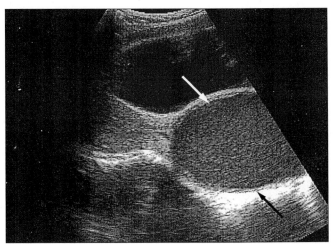

Fig. 6.36 *Longitudinal ultrasound of haematometrocolpos. The vagina is distended with echogenic blood (arrows).*

UTERINE DISORDERS

Endometritis is seen on ultrasound as a thickened, echogenic endometrium with a surrounding hypoechoic rim. A condition in which the uterus is distended with pus is known as pyometra. Uterine infection with *Clostridium* can occur after abortion, and may spread rapidly into the myometrium and surrounding structures; gas bubbles may then be seen on a plain film.

VAGINAL DISORDERS

Vaginal infection is common, and imaging is rarely indicated. In young girls, infection can occur secondary to a foreign body. The foreign body can be demonstrated on ultrasound or plain films if it is not obvious on clinical examination.

TUBERCULOSIS

In the female genital tract, tuberculosis primarily involves the Fallopian tubes, leading to strictures and occlusion. Plain films show calcification, and hysterosalpingography demonstrates irregular beading of the tubes. This is another cause of infertility.

ENDOMETRIOSIS

Although not strictly an inflammatory condition, endometriosis is considered here as its presentation can be similar to that of chronic pelvic inflammatory disease. It is characterized by the presence of endometrial tissue outside the uterus, usually in the pelvic peritoneum or ovary. Bleeding from this ectopic endometrium during menstruation results in haemorrhagic cysts ('chocolate cysts'), with subsequent fibrosis and pelvic adhesions. The condition is associated with infertility.

Adenomyosis is a related condition that can co-exist with endometriosis, and in which endometrial tissue extends into the myometrium.

MR imaging is the best method of demonstrating endometriosis (**Fig. 6.39**) and adenomyosis, showing cysts containing blood products in the former, and focal abnormalities in the myometrium in the latter.

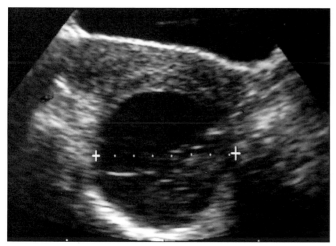

Fig. 6.37 *Tubo-ovarian abscess, showing an adnexal cystic structure containing echogenic debris, representing pus and thick septae.*

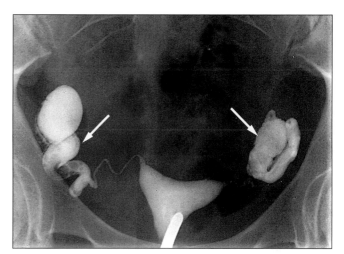

Fig. 6.38 *Hysterosalpingogram showing bilateral hydrosalpinx. The fimbriated ends of the Fallopian tubes (arrows) are distended and obstructed, with no free spill of contrast into the peritoneal cavity.*

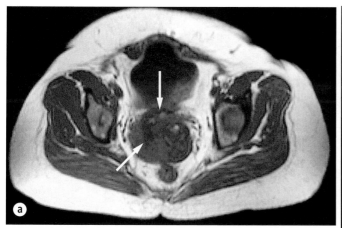

Fig. 6.39 *Axial T1-weighted (**a**) and sagittal T2-weighted (**b**) MRI of the pelvis in endometriosis. Note the multiloculated 'chocolate' cyst containing fluid of different signal intensities; this is typical of blood of varying ages (arrows).*

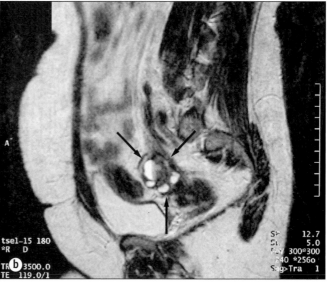

NEOPLASTIC DISEASE

OVARIAN TUMOURS
Ovarian carcinoma

Ovarian carcinoma is an important cause of death from malignant disease in the female population. The mortality is high because the disease is usually insidious in onset and presents late; the tumour has spread beyond the ovary in 75% of cases at diagnosis. The most common clinical presentation is abdominal swelling as a result of the primary tumour and ascites.

There is a genetic predisposition to ovarian carcinoma in some women, a proportion of whom are also at increased risk of breast cancer. It is believed that the risk of ovarian carcinoma is increased with increasing ovulatory events, and that pregnancy and combined oral contraceptives provide some protection.

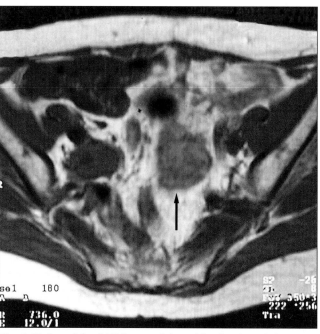

Fig. 6.40 *T1-weighted MR image of the pelvis, showing a left ovarian mass (arrow) that is an early ovarian carcinoma.*

Ultrasound is the initial investigation of choice, and in late presentations will show a large, partly solid, partly cystic mass; these tumours can be very large (>10 cm) at diagnosis, which may make it impossible to identify the ovary of origin. Ultrasound readily demonstrates any ascites, and sometimes shows peritoneal masses; however, although spread to para-aortic lymph nodes and the liver may be shown by ultrasound, they are more accurately assessed with MR imaging (**Fig. 6.40**) or CT (**Fig. 6.41**). The use of transvaginal ultrasound is undergoing assessment as a screening method for ovarian cancer in postmenopausal women.

Ovarian cystadenomas
Ovarian cystadenomas may be serous or mucinous; on ultrasound they are predominantly cystic, with internal septae (**Fig. 6.42**). However, it is not possible to exclude malignancy in an ovarian lesion that contains solid components on ultrasound, therefore excision is usually indicated.

Ovarian fibroma
Ovarian fibromas are benign, solid ovarian tumours that may show calcification on plain films. They are associated with Meig's syndrome, which comprises:
- A benign solid ovarian tumour.
- Ascites.
- Pleural effusion.
- Spontaneous resolution of the ascites and pleural effusion on removal of the ovarian tumour.

Other benign ovarian tumours that can present in the same way are granulosa-cell tumours, thecal-cell tumours, and Brenner's tumours.

Ovarian germ-cell tumours
Dermoid cyst
Dermoid cysts are benign cystic teratomas that can contain a variety of ectodermal tissues including hair, skin, teeth (**Fig. 6.43**), and fat. Ultrasound shows a complex cystic mass with acoustic shadowing; the different components can be readily identified on CT or MR imaging (**Fig. 6.44**).

Malignant teratoma
Malignant teratomas are rare ovarian germ-cell tumours; they are usually solid on ultrasound.

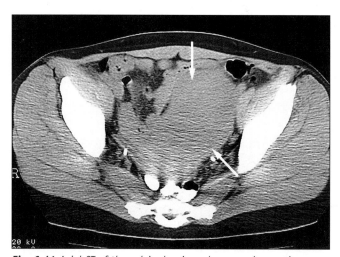

Fig. 6.41 *Axial CT of the pelvis showing a large ovarian carcinoma (arrows).*

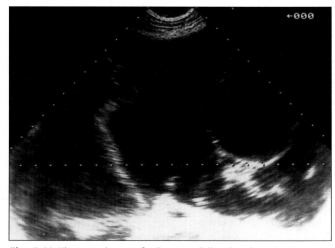

Fig. 6.42 *Ultrasound scan of a large, multiloculated ovarian cystadenoma. It is not possible on imaging to differentiate this from a cyst adenocarcinoma.*

Ovarian metastases

Ovarian metastases are rare, but may occur bilaterally. They are usually derived from a gastric primary, in which case they are termed Krukenberg tumours.

UTERINE TUMOURS
Endometrial carcinoma

Endometrial carcinoma usually presents with postmenopausal bleeding. The investigation of choice is transvaginal ultrasound. Normal postmenopausal endometrium (in the absence of hormone replacement therapy) should be uniformly thin (≤4 mm) and smooth; any increase in thickness or irregularity is an indication for endometrial biopsy. Extension of tumour into the myometrium is best seen on MR imaging (**Fig. 6.45**).

Fibroids

Fibroids are benign tumours of the myometrium and are common. They may be asymptomatic, or may give rise to dysmenorrhoea and menorrhagia. Rarely, they undergo malignant change.

Ultrasound shows well-defined, rounded lesions, often several centimetres in diameter, that may lie in a subserosal, intramural, or submucosal position. They are usually bright, with a typical whorled appearance (**Fig. 6.46**). Central degeneration is seen as a hypoechoic area, and calcification is common, giving rise to acoustic shadowing. Occasionally, fibroids are pedunculated, and can be confused with an ovarian mass. Pedunculated fibroids may undergo torsion.

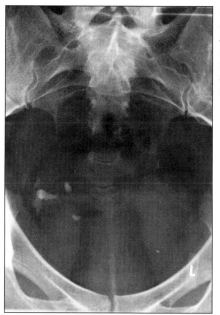

Fig. 6.43 *Pelvic radiograph, showing several teeth in the right iliac fossa, typical of a dermoid cyst (benign ovarian teratoma).*

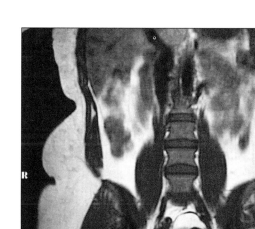

Fig. 6.44 *Coronal T1-weighted MR image of the pelvis, showing a left ovarian dermoid (arrows). The cyst contains tissues of various signal intensity, with characteristic fat returning a high signal.*

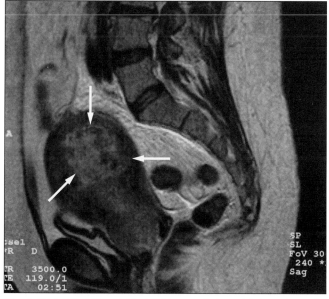

Fig. 6.45 *Sagittal T2-weighted MR image of the pelvis in endometrial carcinoma. There is a large mass involving the fundal endometrium and invading the myometrium (arrows).*

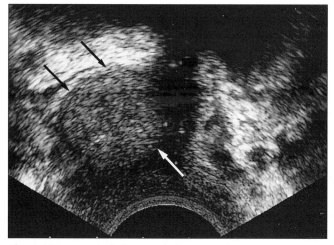

Fig. 6.46 *Transvaginal ultrasound of a uterine fibroid, demonstrating a well-circumscribed soft-tissue mass that has a typical whorled appearance (arrows).*

CERVICAL TUMOURS
Cervical carcinoma

Cervical carcinoma is the second most common female malignancy, after breast cancer, but has a lower mortality than ovarian cancer. Imaging does not have a major role in diagnosing this cancer, which is found as the result of an abnormal cervical smear, visual inspection at colposcopy, and presence of cervical neoplasia on biopsy. Imaging is important, however, in staging cervical cancer; staging is preferably performed with MR imaging (**Fig. 6.47**) or with CT (**Fig. 6.48**), to look for parametrial invasion, pelvic lymphadenopathy, urinary tract obstruction, and distant metastases.

VULVAL AND VAGINAL TUMOURS

Because of the superficial nature of vulval and vaginal tumours, imaging is usually not required in assessment of local tumour extent, but metastases from vulval carcinoma occur in the inguinal and pelvic lymph nodes and can be seen on CT and MR imaging. Vaginal fibromyoma is a rare benign tumour that causes bladder outflow obstruction.

VASCULAR DISORDERS

OVARIAN TORSION

An enlarged ovary, for example one containing a cyst or tumour, may undergo torsion, thus occluding its blood supply. Ultrasound shows an enlarged ovary containing haemorrhage, with peritoneal fluid, and Doppler examination demonstrates absence of blood-flow within the ovary.

UTERINE ARTERIOVENOUS SHUNTS

Uterine arteriovenous shunts may occur with congenital arteriovenous malformations, or may be acquired as a result of Caesarean section, other uterine surgery, or retained placenta. Ultrasound with colour Doppler will show enlarged vessels, with arteriovenous shunting.

PELVIC CONGESTION SYNDROME

Varicose veins in the broad ligament are frequently seen on pelvic ultrasound. In some women, they may be due to retrograde flow in the ovarian vein (analogous to a varicocele in males), and may cause pelvic pain. Embolization has been reported to produce resolution of the symptoms of this pelvic congestion syndrome (*see* Interventional procedures, page 141).

MISCELLANEOUS CONDITIONS

NON-NEOPLASTIC OVARIAN CYSTS

The most common ultrasound finding in the ovary is a physiological or follicular cyst. Normal follicles appear as transonic cysts up to 2.5 cm in diameter; above this size they are termed follicular cysts. They may be associated with pelvic pain, but the vast majority of cases resolve spontaneously, which can be confirmed with repeat ultrasound.

Luteal cysts are those which persist after ovulation and have a slightly thicker wall than follicular cysts. Haemorrhage may occur into a luteal cyst, and can mimic a solid mass on ultrasound. Follow-up ultrasound can be used to show resolution of the haemorrhage.

Polycystic ovarian syndrome

Polycystic ovarian syndrome comprises a spectrum of abnormalities including obesity, hirsutism, amenorrhoea, and abnormal levels of gonadotrophins. Ultrasound can demonstrate multiple, simple, peripherally orientated cysts in one or both ovaries (**Fig. 6.49**); these are best seen on transvaginal scanning.

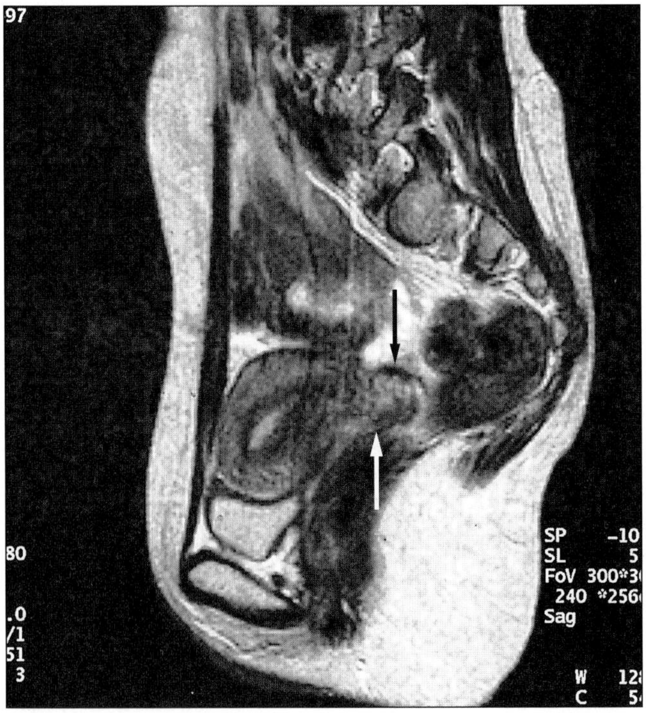

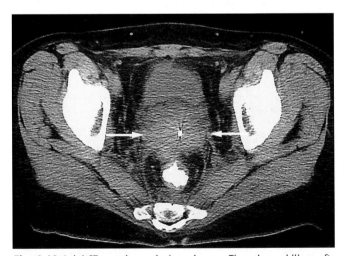

Fig. 6.48 *Axial CT scan in cervical carcinoma. There is a midline soft-tissue mass (arrows), with early parametrial invasion.*

Fig. 6.47 *Sagittal T2-weighted MR image of the pelvis in cervical carcinoma. There is high signal within the cervix (arrows), with loss of definition of the normal cervical canal.*

FISTULAE

Fistulae can occur between the uterus or vagina and any of the surrounding pelvic viscera: for example, a uterovesical fistula is between the uterus and urinary bladder. Fistulae may occur secondary to surgery, radiotherapy, tumour invasion, or inflammatory bowel disease (particularly Crohn's disease, *see* Fig 3.31). A fistula can be demonstrated by carefully injecting contrast into the relevant cavity (fistulogram), or by intravenous urogram or barium enema if the fistula involves the urinary tract or colon respectively.

INTRAUTERINE CONTRACEPTIVE DEVICE

A correctly positioned IUCD should lie in the cavity of the uterine fundus and body, with the threads projecting through the cervical canal (**Fig. 6.50**). If the threads can no longer be felt, then ultrasound is appropriate to locate the device. The IUCD may be found to lie in a normal position, but with the threads drawn up into the cervical canal; in such a case, a gestation sac should be looked for, as pregnancy and resulting uterine enlargement is another reason why the threads may have been drawn up into the cervical canal. Alternatively, the IUCD may have migrated into the myometrium or even into the peritoneal cavity, in which case it can be seen on a plain film.

POSTOPERATIVE APPEARANCES AND INTERVENTIONAL PROCEDURES

TUBAL LIGATION

Clips applied to the tubes at laparoscopic sterilization have a typical appearance on plain films (**Fig. 6.51**).

TUBAL RECANNALIZATION

Occlusion of the Fallopian tubes as a result of pelvic inflammatory disease or endometriosis can cause infertility. It is now possible, in a proportion of women, to recannalize the Fallopian tubes under hysterosalpingography or ultrasound control. The cornual end of the tube is cannulated and a catheter is advanced until free spill of contrast into the peritoneal cavity occurs.

OVARIAN VEIN EMBOLIZATION

Women with retrograde flow in the ovarian vein, pelvic varicosities, and no other cause for their pelvic pain, may benefit from embolization of the ovarian vein, using stainless steel coils. This procedure is analogous to embolization of a varicocele (*see* page 124).

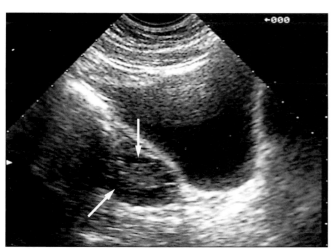

Fig. 6.49 *Transabdominal ultrasound image of a polycystic ovary, showing multiple small follicles (arrows) around the periphery of the ovary. The contralateral ovary had a similar appearance.*

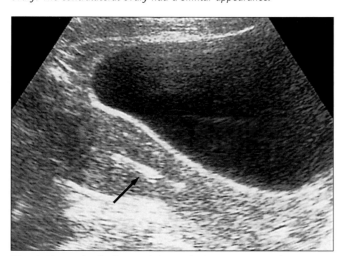

Fig. 6.50 *Longitudinal transabdominal ultrasound scan of the uterus, showing an IUCD in the uterine lumen (arrow).*

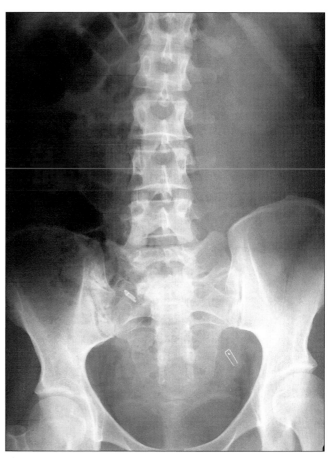

Fig. 6.51 *Abdominal radiograph showing tubal clips after sterilization. The right Fallopian tube is displaced superiorly because of an ovarian mass.*

141

chapter 7

Musculoskeletal System

The imaging of the skeletal system relies heavily on standard 'bone' radiographs. Soft tissue, cartilage and joint pathology is poorly shown on plain films and requires other imaging methods including MR, CT and radionuclide scanning as well as diagnostic interventional procedures such as arthrography. Much joint pathology is only recognized by MR which has become the standard investigation in certain areas, particularly the knee and shoulder joints.

CONGENITAL ABNORMALITIES

There are many complex congenital and hereditary bone diseases that, because of their rarity, are outside the scope of this text. The summary that follows covers the main important disorders that may be encountered in clinical practice. The full classification of bone dysplasias can be simplified into those disorders affecting bone formation (e.g. polydactyly), bone growth (e.g. dwarfism), bone modelling (e.g. osteopetrosis), bone fusion (e.g. Madelung's deformity), and cartilaginous or osseous maldevelopment (e.g. the chondrodysplasias).

CLEIDOCRANIAL DYSOSTOSIS
Absence of the clavicles, combined with craniofacial abnormalities, occurs in this condition (**Fig. 7.1**).

POLYDACTYLY/SYNDACTYLY
Multiple digits or parts of digits (polydactyly or syndactyly) may be isolated findings (**Fig. 7.2**), or part of a widespread disorder, for example in trisomy 13.

DWARFISM
Achondroplasia
Achondroplasia is an autosomal dominant anomaly that affects cartilage growth and development (**Fig. 7.3**). The individual is a short-limbed dwarf with a relatively normal-sized trunk, large head, frontal bossing, and a depressed nasal bridge.

Thanatophoric dwarf
Thanatophorism is a severe form of dwarfism in which babies are either stillborn or die in infancy. Diagnosis can be made *in utero*. The appearances are a severe form of achondroplasia, with very short limbs and marked reduction in vertebral ossification.

Asphyxiating thoracic dystrophy
The rare condition of asphyxiating thoracic dystrophy results, in most cases, in early death during infancy. The thorax is elongated, with horizontally placed ribs associated with abnormalities of pelvic modelling.

Morquio–Brailsford syndrome
The Morquio–Brailsford syndrome forms part of the group of mucopolysaccharidoses that result in short-trunk dwarfism as a result of one form of spondyloepiphyseal dysplasia.

OSTEOGENESIS IMPERFECTA
This hereditary disorder causes a primary defect in the bone matrix. It varies from the common, relatively mild form to the severe

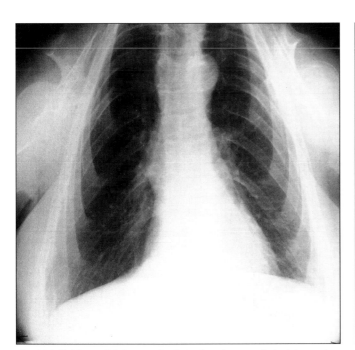

Fig. 7.1 Cleidocranial dysostosis. Note the absence of clavicles and the abnormal conical shape to the chest, with developmental abnormalities of the scapulae.

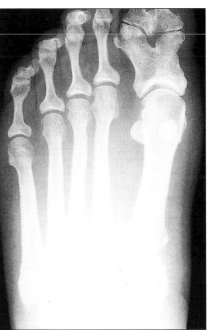

Fig. 7.2 Bifid left great toe was an isolated congenital abnormality in this patient.

progressive form with fetal fractures, blue sclerae, and multiple wormian bones in a thin calvarium (skull vault) (**Fig. 7.4**). One of the important aspects of this disease is the need to make the correct diagnosis, as patients may be misdiagnosed as victims of abuse or non-accidental injury.

NEUROFIBROMATOSIS

Neurofibromatosis is an autosomal dominant disorder. In at least 50% of cases there are skeletal changes including pseudoarthroses,

bowing deformities, and kyphoscoliosis, with scalloping of the posterior vertebral bodies (**Fig. 7.5**).

MUCOPOLYSACCHARIDOSES

The mucopolysaccharidoses are a collection of hereditary disorders secondary to specific enzyme deficiencies.

Morquio–Brailsford syndrome

(*see* Dwarfism, page 143.)

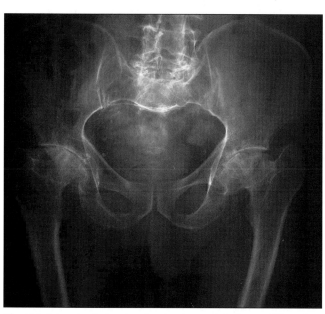

Fig. 7.3 *Achondroplasia, showing developmental abnormalities of the hips, and premature osteoarthritis.*

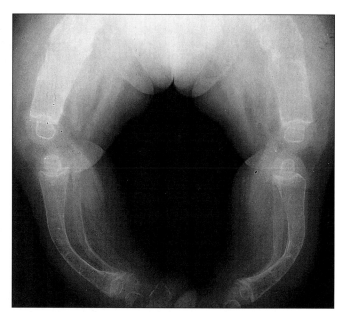

Fig. 7.4 *Osteogenesis imperfecta. There is an abnormal bony pattern, with generalized demineralization and growth deformity.*

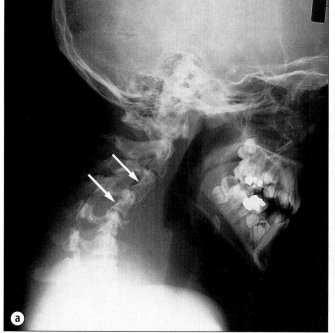

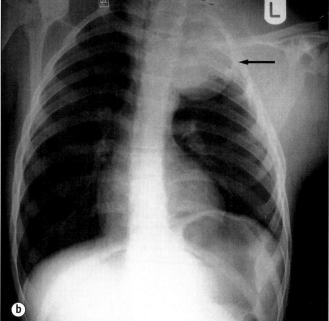

Fig. 7.5 *Neurofibromatosis. (**a**) Lateral cervical spine film, showing abnormal developmental of the cervical spine, with typical posterior scalloping of the vertebral bodies (arrows). (**b**) Chest radiograph, demonstrating a large neurofibroma at the left apex (arrow).*

Hurler syndrome or gargoylism

An abnormal, hook-shaped vertebral body (**Fig. 7.6**) is the characteristic finding in Hurler syndrome or gargoylism, which is usually fatal within the first 10 years of life.

SCLEROTIC BONY LESIONS
Osteopetrosis

Osteopetrosis, or marble bone disease, results in excessive cortical bone and widespread sclerosis (**Fig. 7.7**). There are modelling deformities of the long bones.

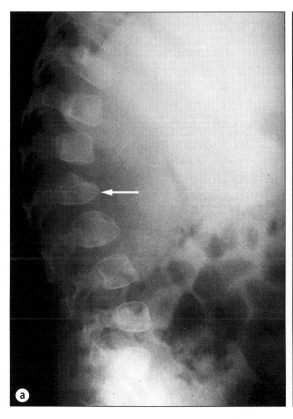

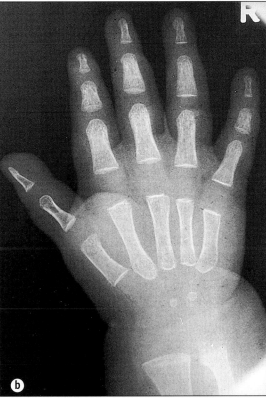

Fig. 7.6 Hurler syndrome is characterized by this lateral lumbar spine abnormality of a hook-shaped vertebra (**a**) at the dorsolumbar junction (arrow). An abnormal bony trabecular pattern throughout the bones of the hand can also be seen (**b**).

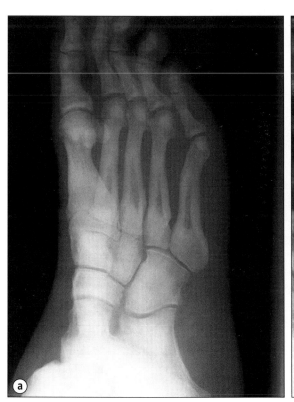

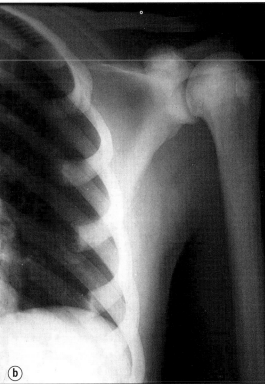

Fig. 7.7 Osteopetrosis, showing a generalized increase in sclerosis throughout the bones (**a**), with increased thickening of the cortex and reduction in the size of the bony medulla. A metaphyseal modelling abnormality is also demonstrated in the upper humerus (**b**).

Osteopoikilosis

Areas of sclerotic bone often seen around large joints are characteristic of the asymptomatic disorder known as osteopoikilosis, which is often diagnosed incidentally (**Fig. 7.8**).

Madelung's deformity

Madelung's deformity is characterized by premature fusion of the distal radius, with subsequent developmental abnormalities of the ulna and wrist (**Fig. 7.9**).

HIP DYSPLASIAS
Congenital dislocation of the hip

Congenital dislocation of the hip is a common anomaly that is more frequent in girls than in boys, and affects both hips in 25% of cases.

There is acetabular dysplasia, shown by an increased acetabular angle, delayed maturation of the femoral capital epiphysis, and lateral subluxation of the hip (**Fig. 7.10**). Recognition of the condition is important, as correct treatment will prevent the secondary complication of a disorganized hip and premature osteoarthritis.

Perthes' disease

Osteonecrosis of the proximal femoral capital epiphysis in Perthes' disease may occur around the age of 6 years, is much more common in boys than in girls, and may be bilateral (**Fig. 7.11**). The ischaemic necrosis may result from repeated minor trauma to the blood supply, but the cause has yet to be fully identified. The result is deformity of the femoral head, with premature osteoarthritis.

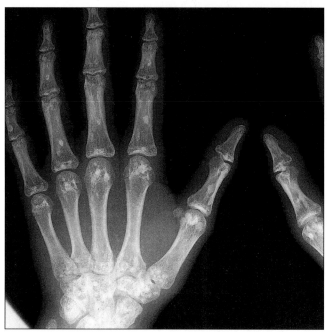

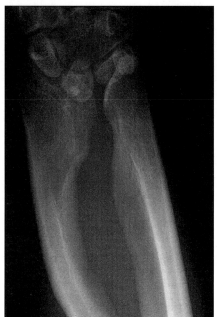

Fig. 7.9 Madelung's deformity is characterized by abnormal modelling of the distal radius and ulna, associated with anomalies of the proximal carpal bones.

Fig. 7.8 Osteopoikilosis. The widespread sclerotic, punctate areas of bone adjacent to joints are characteristic of this condition.

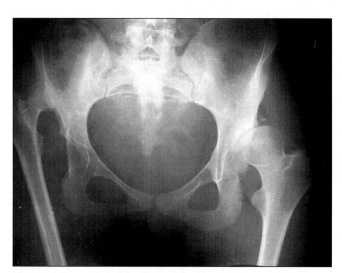

Fig. 7.10 Congenital dislocation of the hip. There is total dislocation of the right hip, with partial subluxation of the left hip, and abnormal acetabular formation.

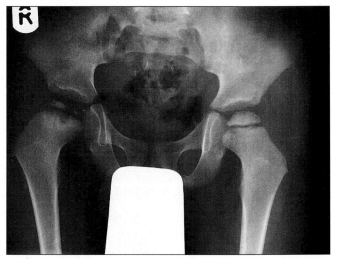

Fig. 7.11 Perthes' disease. Necrosis of the proximal femoral capital epiphysis may be seen on the right, with abnormality of the epiphyseal plate and associated metaphysis. Note also the increased joint space.

Slipped upper femoral epiphysis

Slipped upper femoral epiphysis is a condition that afflicts adolescents, and is more common in boys. It is caused by posterior slip of the femoral capital epiphysis (**Fig. 7.12**); 30% of cases are bilateral. The aetiology is believed to be related to growth spurts.

MYOSITIS OSSIFICANS PROGRESSIVA

Myositis ossificans progressiva is a rare, autosomal dominant disorder that manifests itself by the formation of bone throughout the muscle planes, ligaments, and soft tissues. The disease progresses from the upper thoracic spine, downwards and outwards, resulting in extensive formation of bone around the thorax. The patient dies of respiratory failure before reaching adulthood (**Fig. 7.13**). There is no effective treatment for this condition.

SPINA BIFIDA

Spina bifida is a variable developmental abnormality resulting from failure of fusion of the posterior elements of the vertebral column (**Fig. 7.14**).

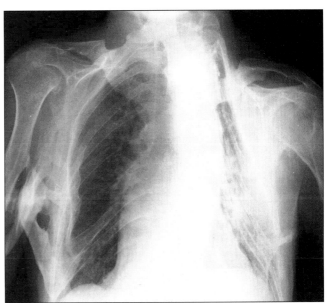

Fig. 7.12 *Left slipped upper femoral epiphysis (SUFE) (arrows). The abnormal angulation of the femoral head in relation to the femoral neck indicates a posterior slip.*

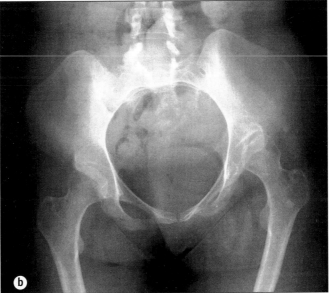

Fig. 7.13 *Myositis ossificans progressiva. New bone formation is evident in the right side of the chest, with deformity of the left side of the chest resulting from fixation of the thoracic cage by extraosseous bone.*

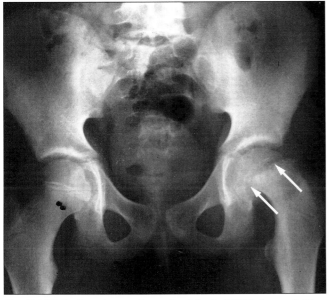

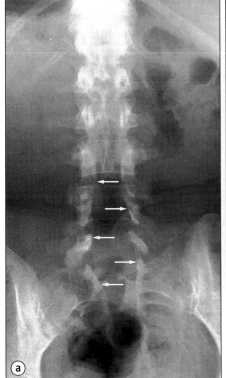

Fig. 7.14 (a and b) *Spina bifida extending from L3 through to S3 (arrows). There is widening of the interpedicular distance below L4. The neurological abnormality of paraplegia has resulted in the abnormal development of the pelvis and lower limbs.*

TRAUMA

GENERAL POINTS
Definitions: types of fracture

Comminuted: multiple pieces of bone are found at the fracture site.

Open (compound): a penetrating fracture, in which the bone is exposed to the air.

Closed (simple): the fracture is contained within the soft tissues.

Greenstick: only one side of the cortex is involved in the fracture; this type is common in children.

Varus deformity: the proximal bone points laterally, with the distal fragment pointing medially (bow-legged).

Valgus deformity: the proximal bone points medially, and distal fragment points laterally (knock-kneed).

Salter–Harris classification: refers to a fracture of the long bones of children, in which the fracture involves the metaphysis, the epiphysis, and the epiphyseal line or growth plate. Types I and II are shown in **Figure 7.15**. Premature fusion is a common complication of such fractures.

Assessment

If a fracture of a limb bone is confirmed, the joints either side of the fracture should be radiographed, as accompanying damage is not uncommon, particularly when dealing with the paired bones—that is, the radius and ulna, the tibia and fibula. Fracture assessment includes the site and extent of the fracture, its alignment, involvement of the surrounding soft tissues and joints, and the presence of any special features such as pathological fracture. It is important to obtain two views of a fracture or dislocation at 90° to each other; otherwise, missed diagnoses and misinterpretations may result.

Complications of a fracture
Mal-union

Failure to position a fracture correctly can result in abnormal alignment or mal-union, which may be unacceptable clinically.

Delayed union

Most fractures heal in weeks or months, but, depending on the site of fracture and the age of the patient, and any systemic condition that may co-exist, union may be significantly delayed.

Non-union

Non-union may be the result of poor alignment of the original fracture, with considerable separation between the bone ends; a reactive sclerosis, with poor joining qualities; ischaemic necrosis; or infection.

Diffuse osteoporosis

Diffuse osteoporosis, which may be severe, results from bone immobilization by plaster casts. A severe form, Sudeck's atrophy, is accompanied by pain, soft-tissue swelling, and skin changes.

Soft-tissue damage

Extensive soft-tissue damage accompanying a fracture may result in traumatic myositis ossificans. If blood-vessel damage occurs, for example to the brachial artery in a supracondylar humeral fracture, distal ischaemic (Volkmann) contracture may result.

Ischaemic necrosis

Certain fracture sites are associated with the condition ischaemic necrosis, which prevents satisfactory healing and leads to further complications, depending on the site involved. Common sites affected are the femoral head after subcapital fracture, the humeral head, and the scaphoid. The changes in the ischaemic bone, which may later collapse and fragment, can be detected on MR imaging; this is now the investigation of choice when dealing with this specific complication.

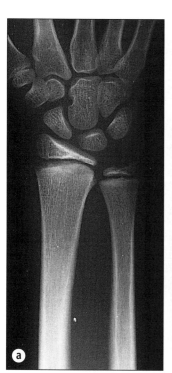 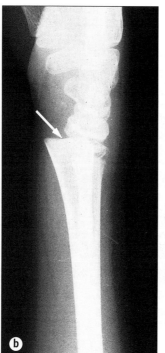 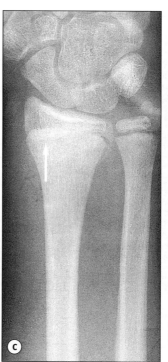 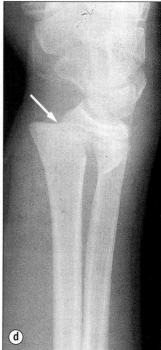

Fig. 7.15 Salter–Harris epiphyseal fractures (arrows). (**a** and **b**) Type I. (**c** and **d**) Type II.

TRAUMA TO THE AXIAL SKELETON
Cervical spine

One of the most important features in spinal injuries relates to the stability of the vertebral column and its relationship to the spinal cord. An unstable fracture involves the loss of integrity of the spinal ligaments, indicated radiologically by vertebral displacement, widening of the apophyseal joints, disruption of the posterior vertebral line, and changes to the interpedicular distance and interspinous spaces.

The types of cervical spine fracture caused by trauma result from the direction and force of injuries received; these may be flexion, extension, compression, shearing, rotation, or distraction. Severe compression or transection of the upper cervical cord is fatal unless assisted ventilation is commenced immediately. However, the phrenic nerve supplying the diaphragm has its origin from the C3, C4, and C5 spinal nerves; thus damage to the spinal cord below C5, although often accompanied by tetraplegia, has the potential for unassisted respiration.

Specific cervical spine injuries

Odontoid peg fractures may result from flexion or, less commonly, extension injury. They may be stable or unstable, depending on the associated posterior column fractures or ligamentous injuries (**Fig. 7.16**).

Jefferson's fracture, produced as a result of direct trauma to the top of the skull vault, causes unstable compression fractures of the anterior and posterior arches of C1 (atlas); the force of the occiput displaces apart the lateral masses of the atlas.

Hangman's fracture occurs when hyperextension and distraction result in bilateral fractures through the pedicles of the axis (C2), with anterior dislocation of the vertebral body, and tearing of the spinal cord. This injury mechanism is also common in road traffic accidents, in which there is sudden hyperextension as a result of acute deceleration (**Fig. 7.17**).

Teardrop fracture is the most severe, unstable injury to the cervical spine, involving fracture of the posterior vertebral elements, ligamentous disruption, and associated damage to the spinal cord (**Fig. 7.18**).

Simple compression vertebral body fractures result from flexion and compression injuries, their importance lying in the presence or absence of displacement of bone into the spinal canal, causing possible cord compression.

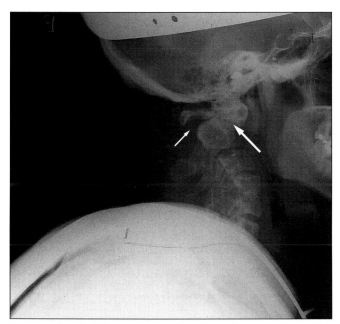

Fig. 7.16 *Ununited fracture of the odontoid peg (large arrow) resulting in gross atlantoaxial subluxation and a compromised cord (small arrow).*

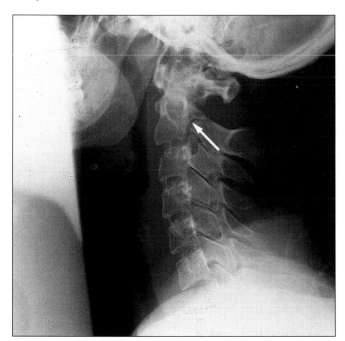

Fig. 7.17 *Hangman's fracture, showing bilateral fractures through the pedicles of C2 (arrow), with only minor anterior dislocation of the body.*

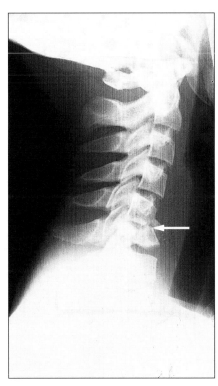

Fig. 7.18 *Teardrop fracture involving C5 and C6 (arrow), with angulation of the cervical spine and compromise of the spinal canal.*

Thoracolumbar fractures

Most thoracolumbar fractures are compression, burst, or distraction injuries, sometimes associated with dislocation. The classification of fractures to this area of the spine is based on the three-column description: the anterior column is the anterior two-thirds of the vertebral body and the annulus fibrosus; the middle column relates to the posterior vertebral body and annulus, together with the posterior longitudinal ligament; and the posterior column comprises the posterior neural arch, supraspinous and interspinous ligaments, facet joints, and ligaments. One-column fractures are stable, three-column fractures are unstable, and two-column fractures are variable, depending on the severity and type of injury.

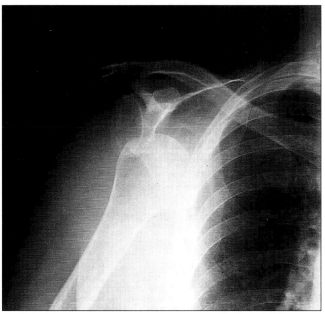

Fig. 7.19 *Anterior dislocation of the shoulder. The humerus lies inferior and anterior to the glenoid.*

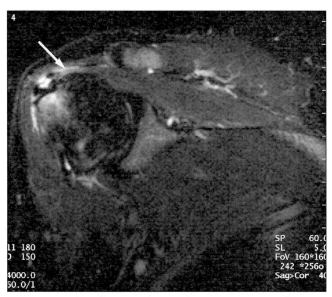

Fig. 7.20 *Coronal oblique MR image of the shoulder using short tau inversion recovery sequence demonstrating a complete tear of the supraspinatous tendon (arrow) shown by the increased signal across the tendon.*

APPENDICULAR FRACTURES, DISLOCATIONS, AND LIGAMENTOUS DAMAGE
Upper limb and shoulder girdle

Shoulder dislocation

The most common position for dislocation of the humeral head is anterior to the glenoid (**Fig. 7.19**). A compression fracture to the posterior aspect of the humeral head may occur at the time of dislocation, producing the Hill–Sacks lesion. Posterior dislocation is rare, but may be missed if only a single anteroposterior view of the shoulder is obtained.

Rotator cuff damage

A tear to the rotator cuff usually involves the supraspinatous tendon; it is best shown by MR imaging (**Fig. 7.20**) or MR arthrography. Calcification in the supraspinatus tendon can be shown on plain film radiography (**Fig. 7.21**).

Neck of humerus

Fractures involving the neck of the humerus may interrupt the blood supply to the humeral head, resulting in osteonecrosis and significant deformity.

Supracondylar fracture of the humerus

Supracondylar fracture of the humerus is an important fracture, seen often in children, because of its association with brachial artery damage and subsequent ischaemic fibrosis of the forearm and hand (Volkmann's contracture).

Dislocation of the elbow

The nature of an elbow dislocation depends on whether the dislocation is related to the ulna, the radius, or both. Posterior dislocations of the radius and ulna account for more than 90% of elbow dislocations (**Fig. 7.22**).

Fracture of the radial head

Radial head fractures may be undisplaced, comminuted, or impacted; occasionally, they are associated with dislocation.

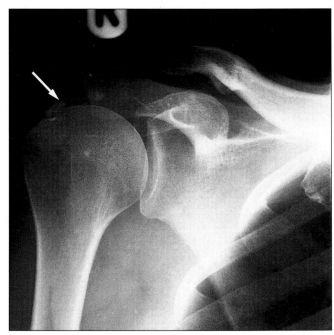

Fig. 7.21 *Calcification in the supraspinatus tendon (arrow).*

Paired-bone fracture–dislocations

The forearm is the site of paired-bone fracture–dislocations. The Monteggia fracture–dislocation is a fracture of the ulna combined with radial head dislocation (**Fig. 7.23**). A Galeazzi lesion is a radial fracture with dislocation of the distal ulna at the wrist.

Colles' fracture

Injury through the distal aspects of the radius and ulna, with dorsal angulation of the distal fragments, constitute a Colles' fracture (**Fig. 7.24**). This very common fracture is often the result of a fall on the outstretched hand. If the distal fragment shows ventral angulation—a much more rare feature—it is known as either a Smith fracture or a reverse Colles' fracture.

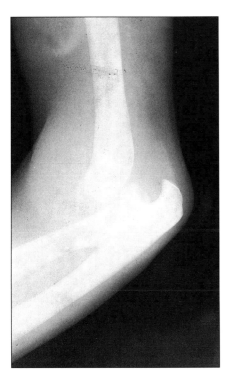

Fig. 7.22 *Posterior dislocation of the radius and ulna at the elbow joint.*

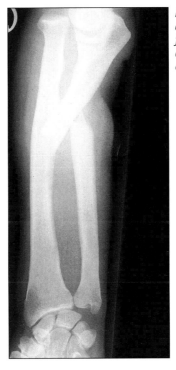

Fig. 7.23 *Monteggia fracture dislocation, with overlapping fracture of the ulna and dislocation of the radius at the elbow joint.*

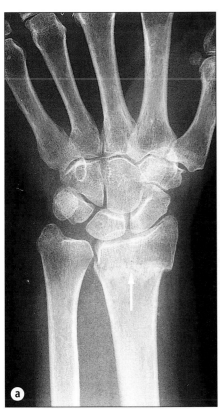

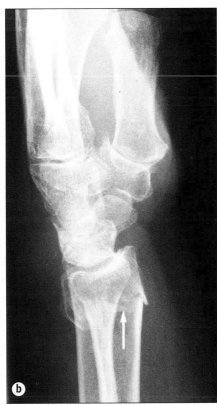

Fig. 7.24 *(**a** and **b**) Colles' fracture through the distal radius (arrows).*

Wrist fractures and dislocations

Scaphoid fracture through the waist of the scaphoid (**Fig. 7.25**), suspected clinically by tenderness in the anatomical snuff box, may be a difficult lesion to show initially in some patients; a repeat radiograph is advisable after 7–10 days if clinical suspicion is high. Failure to immobilize a scaphoid fracture may lead to ischaemic necrosis of the distal fragment and the development of premature osteoarthritis.

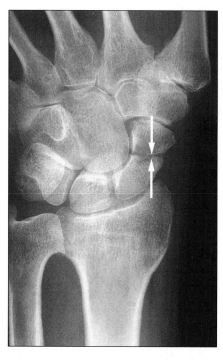

Fig. 7.25 Fracture through the waist of the scaphoid (arrows).

Scapholunate dissociation results from injury to the scapholunate ligament, showing as an increased gap between the two bones on an anteroposterior view of the wrist.

Lunate dislocations comprise isolated dislocation of the lunate itself, the rest of the carpus remaining in a normal position; they are best shown on a lateral view (**Fig. 7.26**). In perilunate dislocation, the lunate is in the correct position, but the rest of the carpus is dislocated.

Trans-scaphoid perilunate dislocation. The most common fracture to be associated with a perilunate dislocation is one through the scaphoid.

Boxer's fracture—of the distal shafts of the fourth and fifth metacarpals—frequently results from the delivery of a punch (**Fig. 7.27**).

Bennett's fracture is an intra-articular fracture of the proximal end of the first metacarpal.

Lower limb and pelvic girdle
Traumatic dislocation of the hip
Three types of dislocation of the hip occur: the common posterior form, the uncommon anterior form, and the central or medial form, which is always associated with a central acetabular fracture.

Pelvic trauma
Fractures of the pelvis are important because of the association of damage to the urinary tracts, the nerves, and blood vessels. Acetabular fractures may involve the anterior and posterior columns, the acetabular roof, or the central portion. Obturator ring fractures are often paired; if involved in substantial injury, with derangement to the shape of the pelvis (**Fig. 7.28**), they may be associated with sacral compression fractures or sacroiliac joint diastasis. Plain films combined with CT give the best assessment of fracture positions and possible complications.

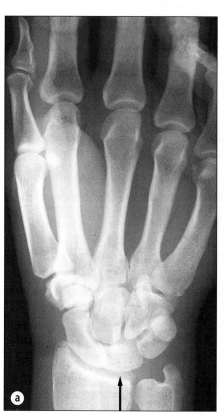

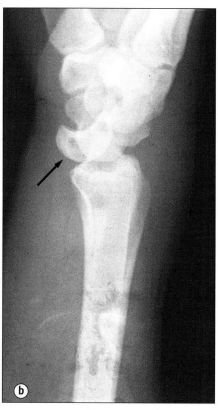

*Fig. 7.26 (**a** and **b**) Lunate dislocation (arrows).*

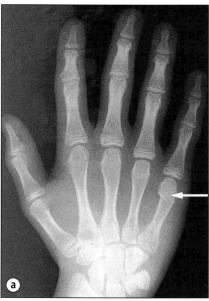

Fig. 7.27 (**a** and **b**) Boxer's fracture of the distal shaft of the fifth metacarpal (arrows) following a punch.

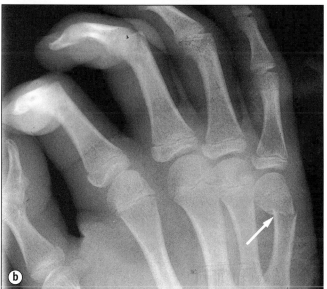

Femoral head/neck fractures

Intracapsular fractures may be capital, subcapital, or transcervical; extracapsular fractures are intertrochanteric or subtrochanteric (**Fig. 7.29**). Most complications occur after the intracapsular fractures, mainly as a result of avascular necrosis. Femoral neck fractures may be undisplaced, impacted, or both, and may be difficult to diagnose on a single film. They will be shown by CT, MR imaging, or radionuclide bone scanning.

The knee

Ligamentous damage involving the cruciate ligaments and fibrocartilage damage to the menisci of the knee are best shown by MR imaging (**Fig. 7.30**). Fractures around the knee joint result from significant trauma; if they involve the joint surfaces, they may produce a lipohaemarthrosis (**Fig. 7.31**). Patellar fractures may be longitudinal or transverse, depending on the type of injury; the former should not be confused with a congenital bipartite patella, which is of no significance.

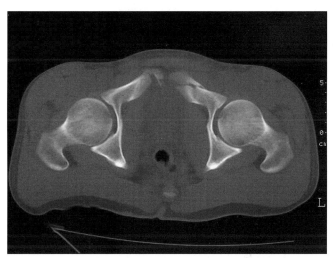

Fig. 7.28 CT scan through the pelvis in a young patient following a road traffic accident showing paired anterior obturator ring fractures with compromise of the proximal urethra.

Fig. 7.29 Fractured neck of femur (arrows).

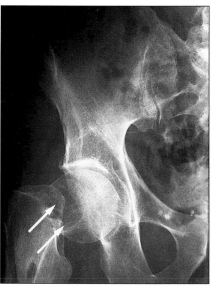

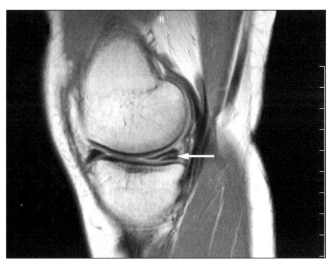

Fig. 7.30 Lateral MR image of a tear in the posterior aspect of the medial meniscus (arrow).

Osgood–Schlatter disease is caused by traumatic avulsion of the anterior tibial tubercle, and has associated pain and soft-tissue swelling (**Fig. 7.32**). Osteochondritis dissecans commonly affects the knee and is the result of chronic damage to a portion of the femoral condyles, with separation of a subchondral fragment of bone together with its overlying cartilage (**Fig. 7.33**).

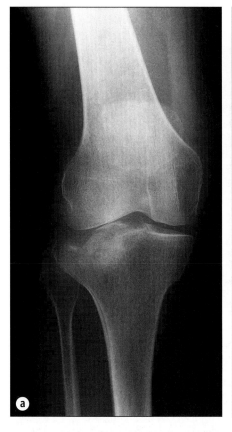
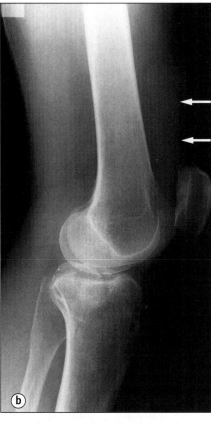

Fig. 7.31 (**a** and **b**) *Fracture of the lateral tibial plateau, with depression and a lipohaemarthrosis (arrows).*

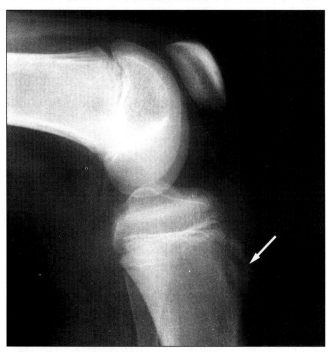

Fig. 7.32 *Lateral view of a knee in an adolescent male demonstrating irregularity and separation of the anterior tibial tubercle (arrow) with an overlying soft-tissue mass. Diagnosis: Osgood–Schlatter's disease.*

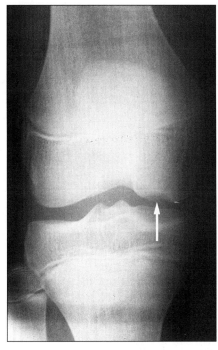

Fig. 7.33 *Osteochondritis dissecans lesion affecting the medial femoral condyle (arrow).*

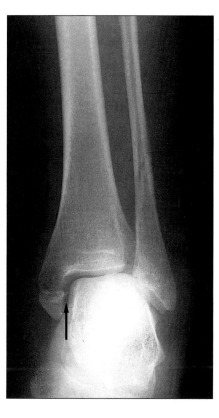

Fig. 7.34 Bi-malleolar fracture, showing some increase in the joint space and lateral subluxation of the talus in relation to the tibia (arrow).

The Pellegrini–Steida lesion comprises traumatic calcification and ossification within the medial collateral ligament.

The ankle

Fractures around the ankle are classified as uni-malleolar, bi-malleolar, or tri-malleolar, and are often associated with complex ligamentous damage, resulting in an unstable ankle joint or frank dislocation (**Fig. 7.34**). These fractures are sometimes referred to as first-, second-, and third-degree Pott's fractures.

The foot

Calcaneal fractures often occur as a result of a fall, and are seen in inexperienced parachutists, cat burglars (who fall off drain pipes!) and other 'jumpers'. Landing on the heel causes the posterior aspect of the calcaneum to wedge-fracture the anterior aspect. This fracture is best shown by CT (**Fig. 7.35**), on which associated joint involvement may be assessed.

Fracture dislocations at the tarsometatarsal joints use the Lisfranc classification, and are the most common dislocations in the foot. The important clinical aspects of this dorsal dislocation, which often results from a fall downstairs, are recognition and appropriate reduction, to reduce the complication of post-traumatic osteoarthritis.

Spondylolysis and spondylolisthesis

A defect in the pars interarticularis of one of the lumbar vertebrae is defined as a spondylolysis (**Fig. 7.36**); if forward slip of the vertebral body occurs as a result of the defect, spondylolisthesis is present (**Fig. 7.37**). Spondylolisthesis may also result from facet (apophyseal) joint degenerative disease alone.

Disc herniation

An intervertebral disc consists of an outer annulus fibrosus and an inner, softer, nucleus pulposus. Herniation posteriorly or postero-laterally of the nucleus pulposus through a damaged or degenerate annulus may result in nerve root compression. MR is now the imaging modality of choice in this common condition.

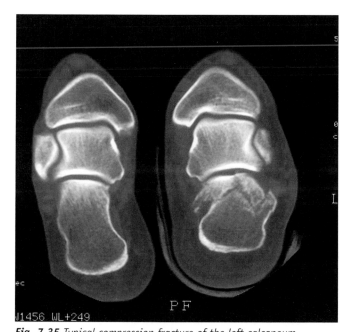

Fig. 7.35 Typical compression fracture of the left calcaneum resulting in reduced anteroposterior diameter, the inverted Y-shaped fracture with involvement of the calcaneo-talar joint surface.

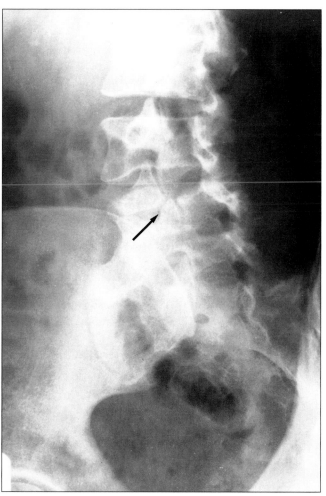

Fig. 7.36 Spondylolysis: a pars interarticularis defect of L5 (arrow).

Non-accidental injury

There are radiological signs of trauma that, when present in children, suggest non-accidental injury. Metaphyseal shear lesions, sub-periosteal haematomas, epiphyseal separation, rib fractures, and cranial vault fractures may all occur, in addition to damage to the abdominal organs. The differential diagnosis of non-accidental injury includes children with scurvy, osteogenesis imperfecta, the rare juvenile osteoporosis, and infantile cortical hyperostosis.

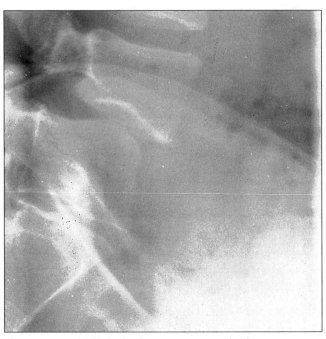

Fig. 7.37 *Spondylolisthesis of L4 on L5 as a result of pars interarticularis defects.*

INFECTION

OSTEOMYELITIS

The earliest signs of osteomyelitic acute bone infection appear about 10 days after the invasion, and comprise a lytic, destructive lesion that progresses to sclerosis, periosteal new bone formation, and further destruction (**Fig. 7.38**). A Brodie's abscess, usually in the metaphysis of the distal femur or proximal tibia, is a subacute infection of insidious onset that shows a lytic area surrounded by reactive sclerosis. Chronic osteomyelitis results from failure of satisfactory treatment of acute or subacute infection, and is manifested by sequestra, sinus tracts, extensive sclerosis, and periosteal reaction (**Fig. 7.39**).

Tuberculous infection may affect the bones or joints, and is characterized by osteoporosis, progressive destruction, and little evidence of sclerosis.

Madura foot is an infective disorder seen in India, Africa, and Central and South America. Fungus infection or 'mycetoma' is the principal infection, which begins as a cellulitis and progresses to involve bone, with osteomyelitis and widespread sequestra formation (**Fig. 7.40**).

INFECTIVE ARTHRITIS

Any joint can be infected by pyogenic organisms, commonly *Staphylococcus aureus*, and signs depend on the site and extent of involvement. In the early stage of the disease, there is soft-tissue swelling and juxta-articular osteoporosis, followed by joint-space narrowing, and progressive destruction if the condition remains untreated (**Fig. 7.41**).

Tuberculous arthritis often affects large joints such as the hip or knee, but may be seen in the wrist and other joints; initially, it has radiographic appearances similar to those seen in pyogenic arthritis. Later, there are bony erosions and joint-space destruction. In the spine, pyogenic and tuberculous infections may occur, with disc-space narrowing, vertebral body and apophyseal joint involvement, and paraspinal masses, which are common to both types of infection (**Figs 7.42** and **7.43**).

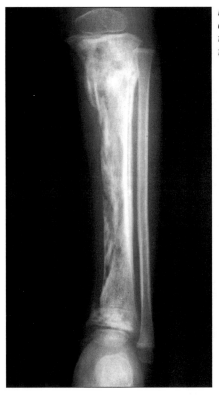

Fig. 7.38 *Extensive osteomyelitis involving the whole of the tibia in a young child.*

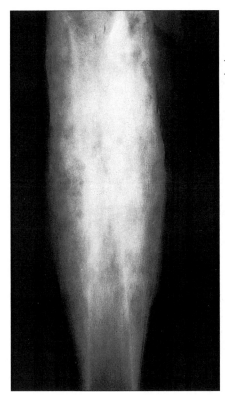

Fig. 7.39 *Chronic salmonella osteomyelitis, causing florid new bone formation in the shaft of the femur.*

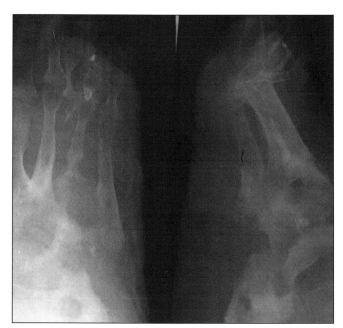

Fig. 7.40 Madura foot, showing gross destructive lesions affecting primarily the tarsus, and evidence of healing via sclerosis.

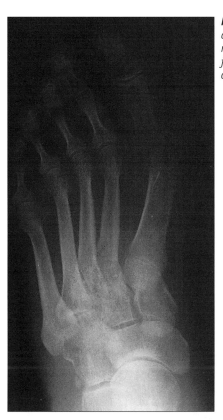

Fig. 7.41 Infective arthritis of the first metatarsophalangeal joint in a patient with diabetes.

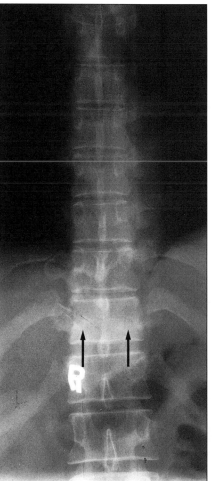

Fig. 7.42 Destruction of both pedicles of T11 (arrows) in a patient with tuberculosis.

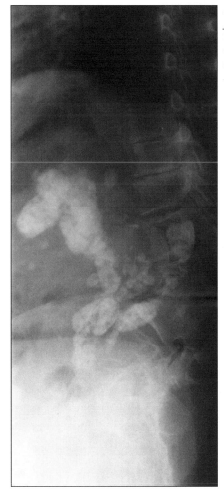

Fig. 7.43 Gibbous formation affecting the lumbar spine, with extensive nodal calcification, after spinal tuberculosis.

INFLAMMATORY CONDITIONS

RHEUMATOID ARTHRITIS

Rheumatoid arthritis is a multisystem disorder characterized in its joint involvement by synovial swelling, erosions, cartilage loss, osteoporosis, and eventual destruction of the joint (arthritis mutilans) (Figs 7.44 and 7.45). It is usually symmetrical, but there is great variability in the degree and site of involvement, and in disease activity.

The earliest radiological signs are synovial swelling and juxta-articular osteoporosis. Later, small erosions develop at the side of the joint—commonly, this is the metacarpophalangeal or metatarsophalangeal joint, the distal interphalangeal joints being involved only rarely. In the cervical region of the spine, erosions commonly affect the synovial apophyseal joints and the odontoid peg, the latter being a particularly important cause of atlantoaxial instability in these patients.

A Baker's cyst is a large popliteal cyst complicating rheumatoid disease. It may rupture and be misdiagnosed as thrombophlebitis.

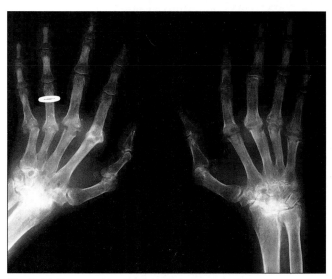

Fig. 7.44 *Rheumatoid arthritis, with implants in the metacarpophalangeal joints. There is extensive erosive arthropathy, with loss of joint space, particularly affecting both carpi.*

JUVENILE RHEUMATOID ARTHRITIS

Rheumatoid arthritis affecting the immature skeleton may cause severe structural abnormalities, with premature fusion and ankylosis; it may be associated with early degenerative joint disease (Figs 7.46 and 7.47).

SERONEGATIVE ARTHROPATHIES
Ankylosing spondylitis

Ankylosing spondylitis is an inflammatory arthritis affecting primarily the spine and sacroiliac joints, but also involving other large joints—particularly the shoulders, hips, and knees. On a lateral view of the spine, there is squaring of the vertebral bodies and the development of syndesmophytes, with subsequent ossification of the anterior longitudinal ligament and fusion of the apophyseal joints, all resulting in a rigid 'bamboo' spine (Fig. 7.48).

Psoriasis

Typically, psoriasis affects the distal interphalangeal joints of the hands and feet, but it can be present in other joints, particularly the sacroiliacs.

Reiter's syndrome

Reiter's syndrome is more common in males than in females. It comprises arthritis, urethritis, and conjunctivitis. The arthritis usually affects the lower limbs, spine, or both; periosteal reaction is occasionally encountered.

MISCELLANEOUS ARTHRITIDES
Scleroderma

Involvement of the distal phalanges, with loss, destruction, and calcification of the soft tissue, are the characteristic findings of scleroderma (Fig. 7.49).

Gout

Gout is a metabolic disorder characterized by hyperuricaemia and the deposition of urate crystals in soft tissues and joints. The joint erosions, classically in the first metatarsophalangeal joint, are 'punched out', point away from the joint margin, and are not associated with osteoporosis (Fig. 7.50). Soft-tissue tophi that frequently calcify may be seen in the feet, elbows, ears, or hands.

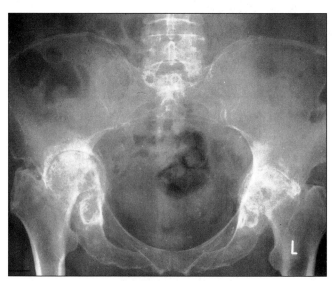

Fig. 7.45 *Protrusio acetabulae caused by rheumatoid disease. Secondary degenerative disease is also present.*

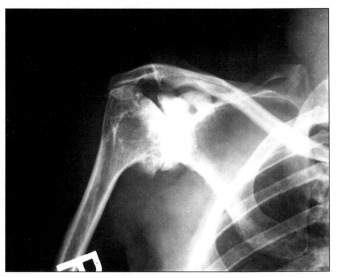

Fig. 7.46 *Premature osteoarthritis in juvenile rheumatoid arthritis.*

Pseudogout or chondrocalcinosis

Deposition of calcium pyrophosphate crystals causes the condition known as pseudogout or chondrocalcinosis. It is shown by calcification in the knee menisci, ligaments, tendons, and joint capsules (**Fig. 7.51**).

Calcium hydroxyapatite crystal deposition

The most common presenting site for calcium hydroxyapatite crystal deposition is in the shoulder, where the condition shows as rotator cuff calcification (*see* **Fig. 7.21**).

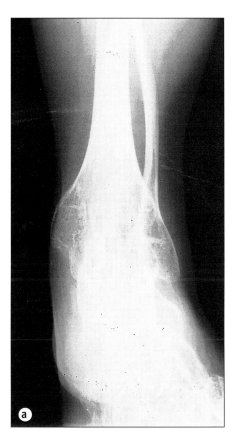

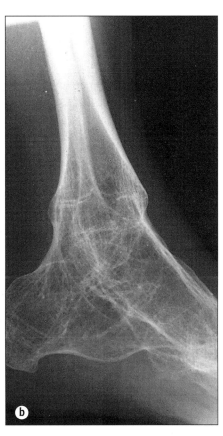

Fig. 7.47 (a and b) Same patient as in Figure 7.46, showing gross ankylosis of the left ankle and foot.

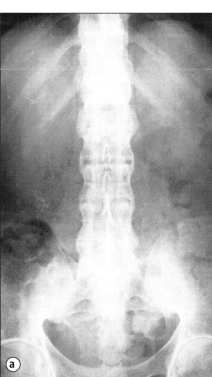

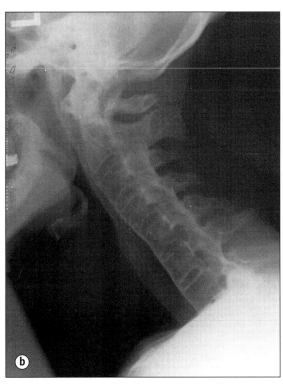

Fig. 7.48 (a and b) Ankylosing spondylitis, with obliteration of both sacroiliac joints and the typical 'bamboo' spine.

Alcaptonuria (ochronosis)

In the condition known as alcaptonuria or ochronosis, absence of the enzyme homogentisic-acid oxidase results in deposition of homogentisic acid, particularly in connective tissue. It is shown by vertebral disc calcification, and marked early degenerative changes of the spine (**Fig. 7.52**).

Charcot's joint (neuropathic arthropathy)

Destruction of articular cartilage, sclerosis, and osteophyte formation in gross degree form a Charcot joint or neuropathic arthropathy (**Fig. 7.53**). Conditions that may be associated with this type of lesion are diabetes mellitus, syringomyelia, absence of pain (sometimes congenital), leprosy, syphilis, and spinal abnormalities such as spina bifida.

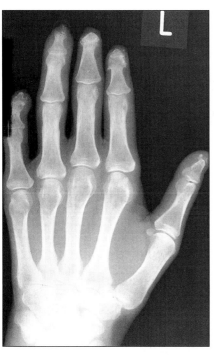

Fig. 7.49 *Scleroderma, demonstrating resorption of the terminal phalanges and calcification in the soft tissues, particularly around the finger tips.*

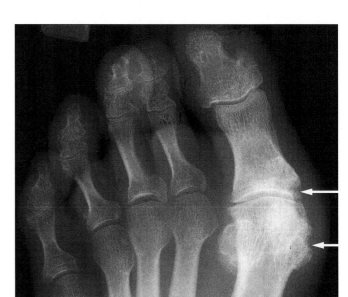

Fig. 7.50 *Gout affecting the first metatarsophalangeal joint, showing classical punched-out erosion and overlying soft-tissue swelling (arrows).*

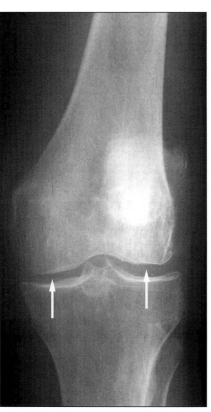

Fig. 7.51 *Chondrocalcinosis. Marginal calcification of the menisci (arrows) with associated degenerative disease.*

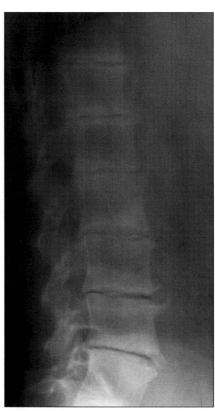

Fig. 7.52 *Ochronosis (alcaptonuria), showing widespread disc degenerative disease, with osteophyte formation and some disc gas.*

NEOPLASTIC DISEASE

The most common bone tumours encountered in clinical practice are metastatic, from a wide variety of primary neoplasms. They may be either lytic or sclerotic. Lytic lesions characteristically metastasize from primary tumours in the breast (**Fig. 7.54**), bronchus, kidney, thyroid, and gastrointestinal tract, whereas sclerotic metastases are principally from prostatic carcinoma (**Fig. 7.55**). Metastases normally involve the axial skeleton or the appendicular skeleton as far as the elbows and knees. Those tumours that disseminate to the distal extremities usually arise from the bronchus or breast (**Fig. 7.56**); lesions that expand may have their origin in the kidney, and must be distinguished from myeloma and other expanding tumour-like conditions. Primary tumours arising in bones and joints relate to the tissue of origin, and may be benign or malignant.

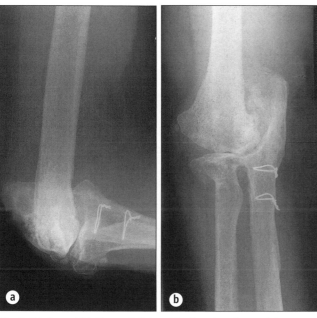

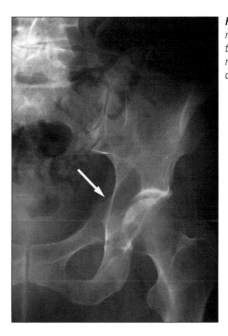

Fig. 7.54 Lytic metastasis affecting the pelvis (arrow), resulting from a breast carcinoma.

Fig. 7.53 (a and *b)* Charcot's joint affecting the elbow, with gross destruction of the joint space.

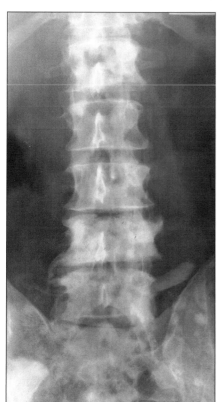

Fig. 7.55 Sclerotic metastases throughout the lumbar spine and pelvis in a patient with carcinoma of the prostate.

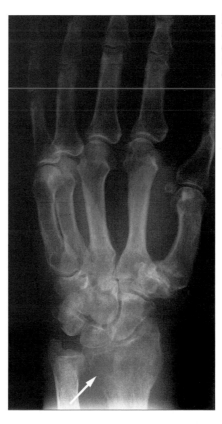

Fig. 7.56 Destructive lesion in the distal end of the radius (arrow) in a patient with carcinoma of the lung.

OSTEOID TUMOURS
Benign tumours
Osteoma
Osteomas are slow-growing, cancellous or cortical (ivory) bone tumours. They often occur in the skull vault or in the frontal or ethmoidal air sinuses, where they may cause blockage of the sinus, resulting in sinusitis, mucocele formation and, occasionally, osteomyelitis.

Osteoid osteoma
Osteoid osteomas occur in the second and third decades of life; they cause pain, and are often found in the femur or tibia. The lesion has a radiolucent centre or nidus, and is surrounded by dense sclerotic bone (**Fig. 7.57**).

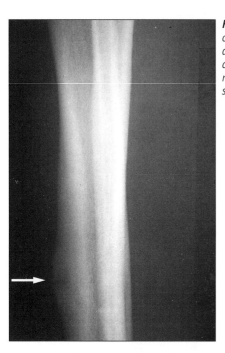

Fig. 7.57 Osteoid osteoma (arrow), demonstrating the characteristic central nidus and bone sclerosis.

Osteoblastoma
Osteoblastoma is a relatively uncommon tumour, found mainly in the vertebral column and pathologically similar to osteoid osteoma.

Malignant osseous lesions
Osteosarcoma
Most osteosarcomas are primary; a few are secondary to Paget's disease, fibrous dysplasia, or radiation damage. Primary osteosarcomas usually occur around the knee or in the upper humerus; they are also found, less commonly, in the pelvis or upper femur. The characteristic features are periosteal reaction, aggressive bone destruction, a soft-tissue mass, and a variable degree of malignant new bone formation (**Fig. 7.58**). MR imaging provides the best definition of the extent and infiltration of the tumour, enabling assessment of involvement of the adjacent vessels and nerves—features that have a direct bearing on treatment.

CARTILAGE TUMOURS
Benign tumours

Enchondroma
Enchondromas are benign cartilage tumours that are found from the second to the fourth decade of life, most often occurring in the fingers and metacarpals. Usually, the lesion is radiolucent and causes expansion of the bone (**Fig. 7.59**). If the lesion develops near the surface of the bone, it is given the name periosteal (juxta-articular) chondroma (**Fig. 7.60**). This tumour has the potential to undergo malignant transformation into a chondrosarcoma if it exists in a long bone or flat bone; lesions in the hand are rarely involved in this complication.

Multiple enchondromas
Multiple enchondromas (Ollier's disease) affect the skeleton extensively. Because there are often many lesions, is not surprising to find malignant change in one of them, given the potential for such change that is recognized in this particular cartilaginous tumour.

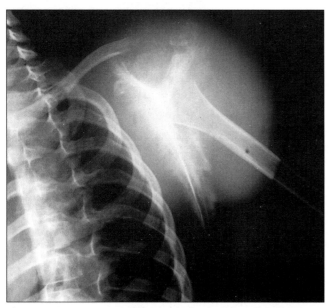

Fig. 7.58 Osteosarcoma of the scapula in a young male Extensive soft-tissue mass with widespread spiculated new bone formation characteristic of a malignant osteoid tumour.

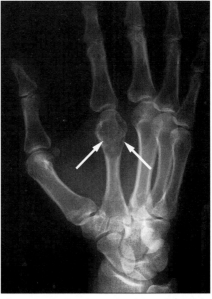

Fig. 7.59 Enchondroma involving the distal aspect of the second metacarpal (arrows).

Osteochondroma

Osteochondroma is a cartilage-capped exostosis arising from metaphyseal areas of long bones, often around the shoulder or knee.

Multiple osteochondromas or exostoses

In common with Ollier's disease, multiple osteochondromas or exostoses are associated with a significant possibility of malignant sarcomatous change in the cartilage cap where they occur (**Fig. 7.61**).

Malignant cartilage lesions

Chondrosarcoma

Chondrosarcomas are malignant cartilage tumours arising in adults older than 30 years, most frequently in the pelvis, femur, or upper humerus. Radiographically, there is an expansile medullary lesion, with endosteal scalloping, calcification, and a soft-tissue mass (**Fig. 7.62**). MR imaging will delineate the tumour more succinctly than plain films.

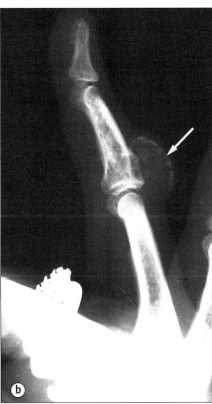
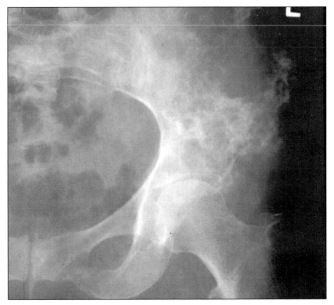

Fig. 7.60 *(a and b) Juxta-articular chondroma (arrows) arising from the cortex of the base of the middle phalanx.*

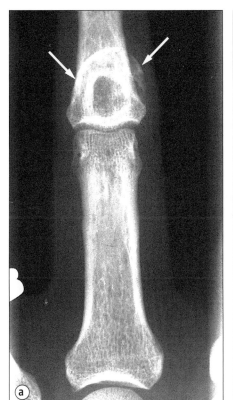

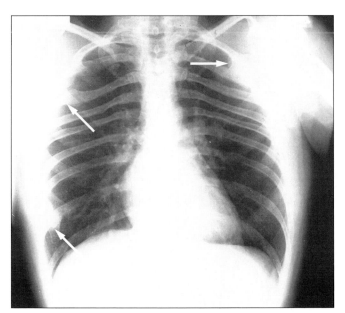

Fig. 7.61 *Multiple exostoses (osteochondromas) affecting the scapulae and ribs (arrows).*

Fig. 7.62 *Chondrosarcoma arising from the left iliac blade. Large lytic destructive lesion with areas of calcification and soft-tissue enlargement.*

TUMOURS OF THE FIBROUS MATRIX OF BONE
Benign lesions

Fibrous cortical defects
Together with non-ossifying fibromas, fibrous cortical defects are the most common fibrous bony lesions, usually seen in the first two decades of life. They are of little significance.

Fibrous dysplasia
Fibrous dysplasia can be classified here, or as a developmental dysplasia. It may be single (monostotic) or multiple (polyostotic). Single lesions usually affect the femoral neck, whereas multiple lesions can be seen in the skull and facial bones, the ribs, pelvis, and both upper and lower limbs (Fig. 7.63). The polyostotic form is more aggressive than the monostotic form, as demonstrated by scalloped medullary expansile lesions, often extending over a considerable portion of the bone and having a ground-glass appearance. Pathological fractures are common. Fibrous dysplasia is associated with endocrine abnormalities in the McCune–Albright syndrome, a condition affecting young girls.

Malignant fibrous lesions
Fibrosarcoma and malignant fibrous histiocytoma
Fibrosarcoma and malignant fibrous histiocytoma both produce lytic bone destruction, often near the ends of long bones. They occur in middle age (Fig. 7.64).

MISCELLANEOUS TUMOURS AND TUMOUR-LIKE LESIONS
Miscellaneous benign conditions

Simple bone cyst
Most simple bone cysts occur in the proximal humerus or femur. Radiographically, the lesion is lucent and well defined, with sclerotic margins; there is no periosteal reaction, unless a pathological fracture has occurred (Fig. 7.65).

Aneurysmal bone cyst
Aneurysmal bone cyst is an expansile cystic lesion in children that affects the metaphyseal region of the long bones, commonly the proximal femur and humerus.

Giant-cell tumour or osteoclastoma
Giant-cell tumour or osteoclastoma affects the mature skeleton, in the epiphyseal region close to the joint surface. It has an expanding lytic component, with a definitive zone of transition between tumorous and normal bone (Fig. 7.66). It may act malignantly locally; it is said to metastasize very rarely.

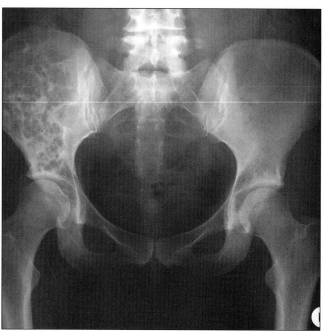

Fig. 7.63 *Fibrous dysplasia affecting the entire right ilium.*

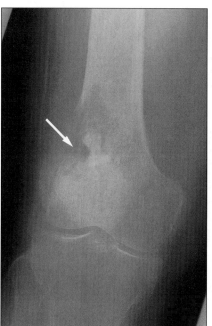

Fig. 7.64 *Destructive lesion in the distal metaphysis of an adult femur (arrow); biopsy revealed malignant fibrohistiocytoma.*

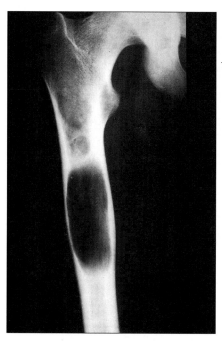

Fig. 7.65 *Simple bone cyst in the upper diaphysis of the right femur. Well-defined cystic lesion in the medulla causing some cortical thinning.*

Haemangioma

The skull and the spine are common sites for the blood vessel tumours known as haemangiomas.

Miscellaneous malignant conditions

Ewing's sarcoma

Ewing's sarcoma is a highly aggressive malignant neoplasm affecting young people. It arises predominately in bone, particularly the long bones, ribs, scapulae, and pelvis. Radiographically, the tumour shows permeated bone destruction, periosteal reaction, and a large soft-tissue mass (**Fig. 7.67**). Extraosseous tumours can also occur.

Lymphoma

Primary bone lymphoma is usually of the histiocytic type, and is relatively rare. Most bony involvement in lymphoma occurs with Hodgkin's lymphoma in the axial skeleton, with the lesions being predominantly lytic or a mixture of lytic and sclerotic (**Fig. 7.68**). Non-Hodgkin's bony disease is exceptionally rare; primary histiocytic lymphoma and lymphoblastic lymphoma are the two predominant types.

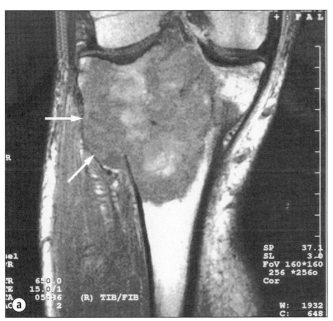

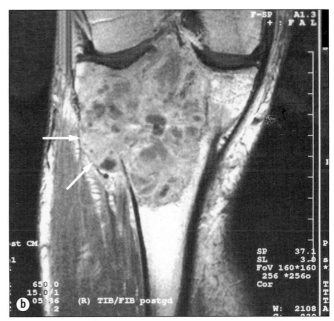

Fig. 7.66 MR (a) pre-gadolinium and (b) post-gadolinium images of a 35-year-old patient with a giant-cell tumour (osteoclastoma) involving the proximal tibia, with some soft-tissue involvement (arrows).

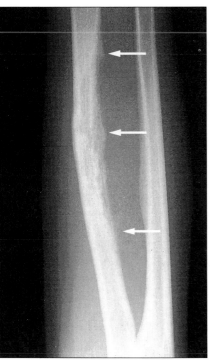

Fig. 7.67 Ewing's sarcoma of the right ulna in an adolescent. Permeated bone destruction with a soft-tissue mass and elevation of the periosteum (arrows).

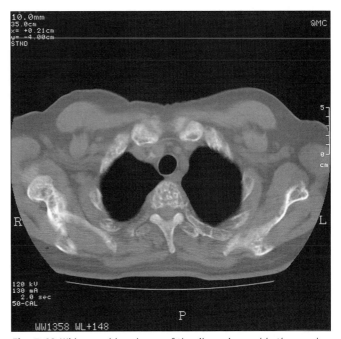

Fig. 7.68 Widespread lymphoma of the ribs, spine and both scapulae in a patient with disseminated disease.

Myeloma

Myeloma is a relatively common primary bone tumour, especially in its multiple form. Characteristically, it produces punched-out lytic deposits throughout the skeleton, with endosteal scalloping (**Figs 7.69a** and **7.69b**). This is the most common primary malignancy of bone. The production of abnormal paraproteins as a result of the plasma-cell dyscrasia leads to renal disease and a high incidence of amyloidosis.

Solitary plasmacytoma

A solitary plasmacytoma is a lytic lesion arising from the medullary cavity, often well-defined and slow growing. It affects the spine, pelvis, and proximal femora and humeri—that is, the red bone marrow areas (**Fig. 7.69c**).

VASCULAR DISORDERS

BONE MARROW DISORDERS
Thalassaemia

Thalassaemia major produces expansion of the marrow, resulting in bone enlargement, thickening of the cortex, and an abnormal trabecular pattern (**Fig. 7.70**). Extramedullary haemopoiesis causes hepatosplenomegaly and paravertebral soft-tissue masses. In thalassaemia minor, there is generalized osteopenia alone.

Sickle-cell disease

There is evidence of bone marrow hyperplasia, bone infarction, and secondary osteomyelitis in sickle-cell disease. Bone infarction produces a characteristic appearance in the hands and in the spine (**Fig. 7.71**).

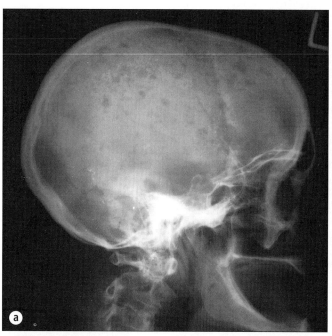

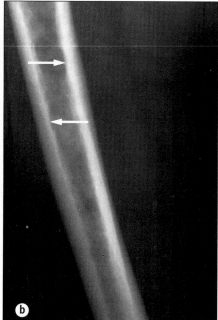

Fig. 7.69 Multiple myloma. (*a*) Multiple defects in the skull vault. (*b*) Coned view of the upper aspect of the right femur showing lytic deposits of myeloma thoughout the marrow cavity causing typical endosteal scalloping found in this condition (arrows). (*c*) A different patient with a large solitary plasmacytoma involving the left ilium (arrows).

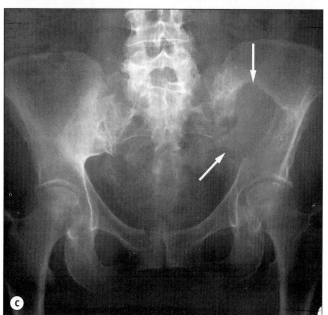

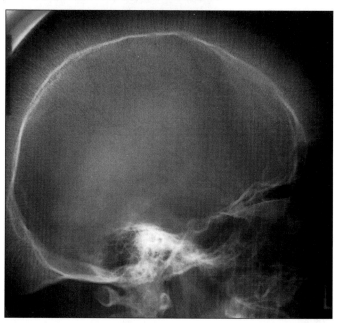

Fig. 7.70 Thalassaemia major. Classical 'hair on end' appearance in a markedly thickened skull vault.

Haemophilia

Bleeding into and around a joint in a patient with haemophilia may produce chronic hyperaemia, leading to abnormal epiphyseal growth, altered trabecular pattern, and premature osteoarthritis, best seen in the knee. Soft-tissue bleeding is common in this condition; if it occurs near a bone, it may produce a pressure erosion defect and a pseudotumour (**Fig. 7.72**).

Leukaemia

In children, leukaemia can cause diffuse or local bony destruction, metaphyseal lucencies, and periosteal reaction (**Fig. 7.73**). In adults, the amount and type of bony involvement are less, and focal areas of bony destruction, identical to metastatic carcinoma, are the most common finding.

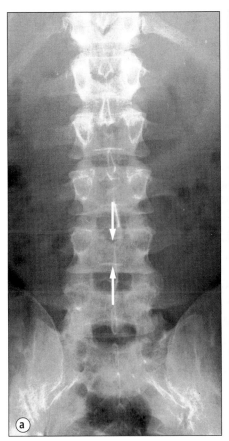

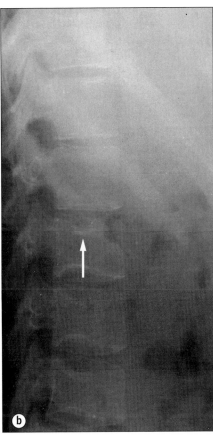

Fig. 7.71 (*a* and *b*) Sickle cell disease, showing characteristic sclerotic areas within the vertebral bodies (arrows).

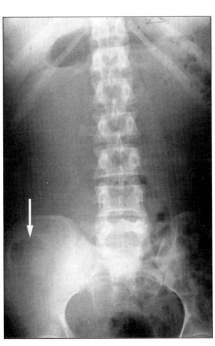

Fig. 7.72 Haemophilic pseudotumour: a large lytic defect in the right ilium (arrow), with a large soft-tissue mass in the right side of the abdomen. The lytic defect is caused by pulsatile pressure from the mass.

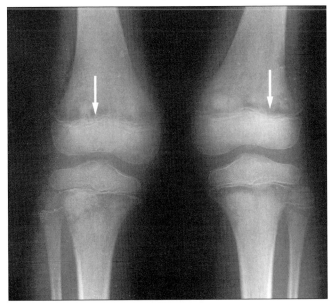

Fig. 7.73 Lucent bands across the metaphyseal areas in a young child with acute leukaemia (arrows).

Myelofibrosis

Widespread replacement of bone marrow by fibrous tissue results in diffuse bone sclerosis in the later stages of myelofibrosis.

Bone infarction

Bone infarcts occur in many conditions, including sickle-cell disease, Gaucher's disease, and polycythaemia; it also occurs in divers and in patients on steroid therapy (**Fig. 7.74**). MR is the most sensitive tool in the investigation of this condition; it offers the additional advantage of its ability to show bone bruises, particularly after trauma around joints.

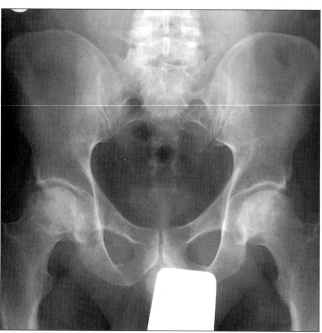

Fig. 7.74 *Osteonecrosis of both femoral heads, with accompanying sclerosis in a patient on long-term steroid treatment.*

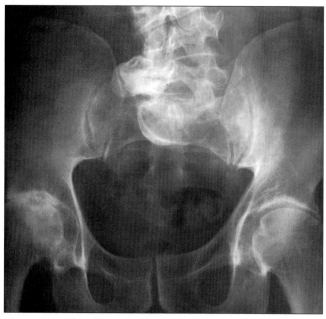

Fig. 7.75 *Pelvic radiography of right hip osteoarthrosis. There is loss of joint space, subchondral sclerosis, and subarticular cysts.*

Gaucher's disease

Gaucher's disease is a hereditary disorder that results in the deposition of glycolipids in the reticuloendothelial cells of the liver, spleen, and bone marrow. Type I, the most common form of the disease, is often found in Ashkenazi Jews. The bony changes in adult life are best seen in the long bones. The abnormalities consist of medullary expansion, with a honeycomb appearance, abnormal metaphyseal modelling, and sclerosis as a result of bone infarction.

DEGENERATIVE CONDITIONS

OSTEOARTHRITIS

The classical primary or idiopathic form of osteoarthritis affects the hand, spine, hip, and knee (**Fig. 7.75**). Secondary osteoarthritis results from any damage to a joint after trauma, osteonecrosis, other forms of arthritides, neuropathic conditions, and many other disorders.

The signs of osteoarthritis are narrowing of the joint space, sclerosis, osteophyte formation, and subchondral cysts. In the hand, these changes are accompanied by Heberden's nodes that involve the terminal interphalangeal joints, or Bouchard's nodes that affect the proximal interphalangeal joints (**Fig. 7.76**).

In the spine, degenerative changes of osteoarthritis involve the synovial joints, the intervertebral discs, and the fibrous articulations and ligaments. A particular form of spinal osteoarthritis is known as diffuse idiopathic skeletal hyperostosis (DISH) or Forestier's disease; it is characterized by extensive ossification of the anterior longitudinal ligament, ligamentous ossification, and osteophyte formation (**Fig. 7.77**).

Excessive and repeated damage to growing bones such as may occur in young gymnasts can result in significant deformity (**Fig. 7.78**).

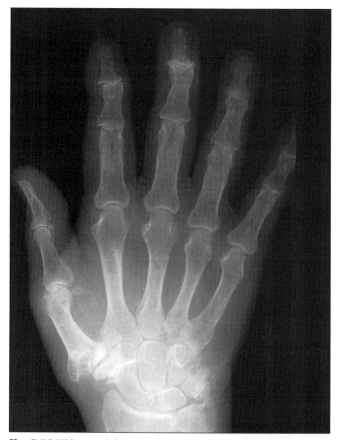

Fig. 7.76 *Widespread degenerative osteoarthritis affecting the base of the thumb and the distal interphalangeal joints with osteophyte formation, sclerosis, and loss of joint space.*

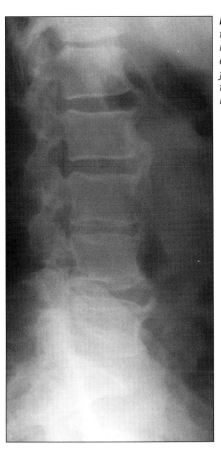

Fig. 7.77 *Diffuse idiopathic skeletal hyperostosis, showing extensive osteophyte formation throughout the lumbar spine, and bony bridging.*

METABOLIC AND ENDOCRINE BONE DISEASE

HYPERPARATHYROIDISM

There are three forms of hyperparathyroidism: primary, secondary, and tertiary. Primary disease is caused by hyperplasia or neoplasia of the parathyroid glands, and is associated with hypercalcaemia. Secondary disease is caused by increased parathormone production as a result of hypocalcaemia, often secondary to renal failure, with hyperphosphataemia. The tertiary form occurs when the parathyroids no longer respond correctly to serum calcium levels and continue to produce parathormone inappropriately; this is usually seen in patients receiving dialysis for chronic renal failure.

Radiological features of primary hyperparathroidism include subperiosteal bone resorption, which is seen particularly in the hands (**Fig. 7.79**), the outer end of the clavicle, and in the loss of the lamina dura around the teeth; the skull shows a typical 'pepper pot' appearance. Cystic changes known as 'Brown tumours' occur in various bones, especially the pelvis, femora, jaw, and shoulder area (**Fig. 7.80**). Soft-tissue, vascular, and cartilage calcification as a result of the hypercalcaemia may occur, but are much more common in the secondary form of the disease. In secondary hyperparathyroidism, the same features are found, but Brown tumours are less common; there is also evidence of areas of increased bone density, particularly in the spine, where the appearances resemble that of a rugger jersey.

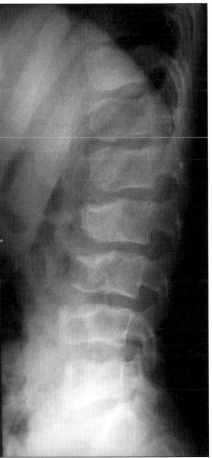

Fig. 7.78 *Osteoarthritic deformity in a 15-year-old gymnast, showing extensive damage to the apophyseal rings of the dorsal and lumbar spine, resulting from chronic flexion and extension injury.*

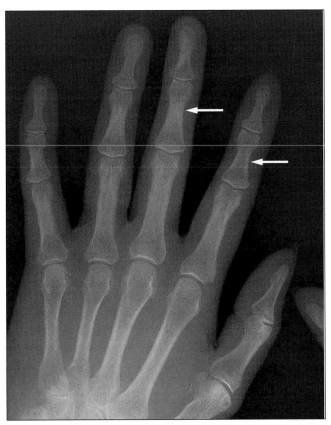

Fig. 7.79 *Hyperparathyroidism, demonstrating the characteristic subperiosteal erosion (arrows), with change in the overall bony matrix.*

OSTEOMALACIA AND RICKETS

Faulty mineralization (calcification) of bone results in rickets in children and in osteomalacia in adults. The causes are dietary (vitamin-D deficiency or reduced absorption from various causes affecting the gastrointestinal tract) or renal (disorders of tubular function and renal osteodystrophy).

Rickets

Changes in rickets are best seen in radiographs of the wrists, where the typical features are flaring of the metaphyses as a result of reduced mineralization of the provisional zone of calcification, widening of the epiphyseal growth plates, localized bone resorption, and bone softening and remodelling (**Fig. 7.81**).

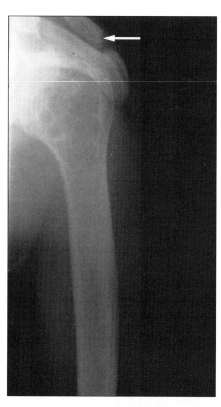

Fig. 7.80 Brown tumour involving the proximal humerus, with erosion of the outer end of the clavicle (arrow), in a patient with primary hyperparathyroidism.

Osteomalacia

In osteomalacia, there is generalized bone loss, accompanied by pseudo-fractures (Looser zones) that are due to stress on the demineralized cortex. These features are seen in the femoral neck, the lateral border of the scapulae, the pelvis, and other long bones (**Fig. 7.82**).

Renal osteodystrophy

In chronic renal disease, there is abnormal vitamin-D metabolism accompanied by hyperphosphataemia and hypocalcaemia, which produces secondary hyperparathyroidism. Thus the radiological features of renal osteodystrophy are a combination of these two conditions.

SCURVY

Vitamin-C deficiency results in a bleeding diathesis causing haemorrhage, and affects the function of osteoblasts, resulting in defective bone formation (osteogenesis). The classic signs are subperiosteal bleeding, with a periosteal reaction and an increase in cortical density of the epiphyses (**Fig. 7.83**).

HYPERPHOSPHATASIA

Hyperphosphatasia is a congenital anomaly of phosphate metabolism; it results in excessive bone turnover, causing a coarse trabecular pattern in all long bones, with bowing deformities (**Fig. 7.84**). This disease is particularly common in Puerto Ricans.

THYROID ACROPACHY

Hyperthyroidism may cause a bubble-like appearance of the periosteum, known as thyroid acropachy. This is best seen in the first metacarpal.

HYPOTHYROIDISM

Childhood hypothyroidism results in delayed skeletal maturation and fragmentation of epiphyses.

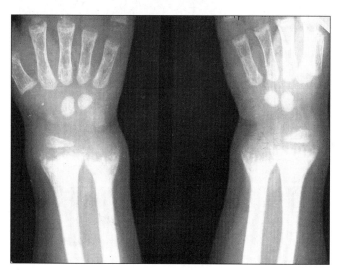

Fig. 7.81 Severe rickets in a young child.

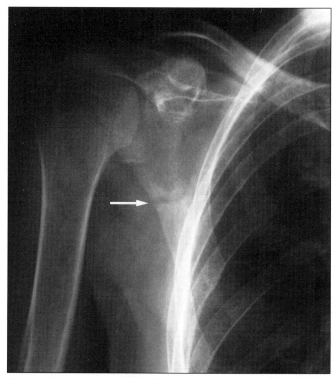

Fig. 7.82 Looser zone (pseudofracture) in the lateral aspect of the scapula (arrow) in a patient with osteomalacia.

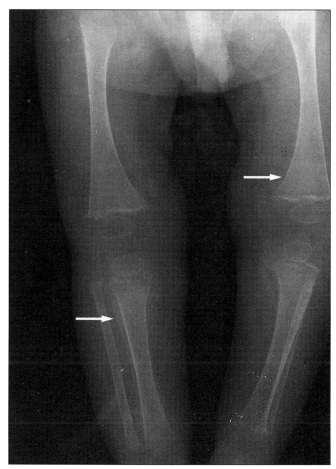

Fig. 7.83 Subperiosteal haematomas (arrows) in a patient with scurvy.

ACROMEGALY/GIGANTISM

Overproduction of growth hormone from the anterior pituitary gland produces, depending on the age of the patient and the stage of epiphyseal fusion, either gigantism or acromegaly.

In acromegaly, the features include the primary pituitary abnormality, with enlargement of the sella turcica in the majority of cases, and the secondary findings of bone overgrowth and soft-tissue enlargement. In the hands, there is generalized soft-tissue enlargement, overgrowth of the tufts of the terminal phalanges, and increased joint spaces. A lateral radiograph of the heel will show marked thickening of the heel pad; in normal individuals this usually measures less than 24 mm, even in obese subjects. The lateral skull radiograph will show, in addition to the pituitary abnormality, increased pharyngeal soft tissue, frontal sinus enlargement, and enlargement and alteration of the angle of the mandible.

TOXIC CONDITIONS

Increased bone density may be the result of chemical poisoning.

Fluorosis

Increased levels of fluorine are endemic in some parts of the world, particularly the Middle East. They can result in the production of dense cortical bone, with ligamentous and tendinous calcification.

Lead poisoning

Lead poisoning is much less common than it used to be, thanks to improvements to public health resulting from the removal of lead water pipes and reduction in the lead content of paints and petrol. Lead poisoning in children results in the production of bands of dense bone at the metaphyseal plates.

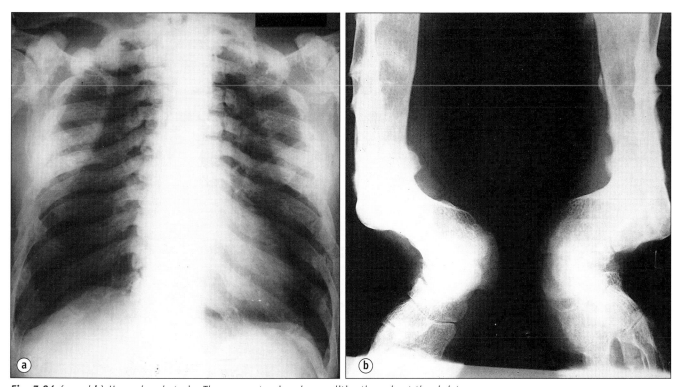

Fig. 7.84 (a and b) Hyperphosphatasia. There are extensive abnormalities throughout the skeleton, including sclerosis, abnormal bony modelling, and bowing deformities.

MISCELLANEOUS CONDITIONS

PAGET'S DISEASE OF BONE

Paget's disease of bone is relatively common, occurs most often after 50 years of age, and has an unknown aetiology. The radiographic appearances reflect the pathological processes of the condition. Initially, there is bone resorption, starting from a bone end and progressing centrally (**Fig. 7.85**). New bone formation follows, with remodelling; the coarse trabeculae produced eventually lead to enlarged, widened bones with a thick cortex (**Fig. 7.86**), accompanied by bowing. The skull shows loss of the diploic space, patchy sclerosis, thickening, and basilar invagination as a result of softening of the bone. Complications include pathological fractures (characteristically, transverse breaks), secondary osteoarthritis of involved joints, heart failure, and the rare development of an associated primary bone tumour, which is usually an osteosarcoma.

SARCOIDOSIS

Bone lesions are present in about 5% of cases of sarcoidosis. They predominantly affect the bones of the hands and feet, and produce lattice-like cystic changes, with some expansion. Very rarely, widespread sclerotic lesions may be found.

INTERVENTIONAL ORTHOPAEDIC PROCEDURES

COMPLICATIONS OF JOINT REPLACEMENT

Dislocation, loosening of the components, and infection are the main complications of total joint replacement. Loosening and infection may result in the appearance of lucent areas around the components. Aspiration, arthrography, and other techniques involving nuclear medicine are required for a full diagnosis (**Fig. 7.87**).

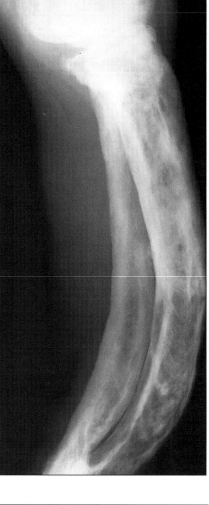

Fig. 7.85 Extensive Paget's disease of the tibia and fibula resulting in bowing.

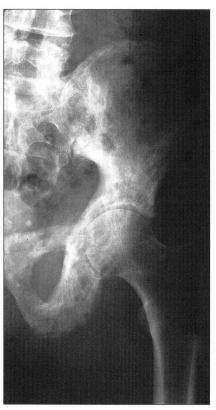

Fig. 7.86 Paget's disease involving the left ilium, showing areas of sclerosis, a coarse trabecular pattern, and bone expansion.

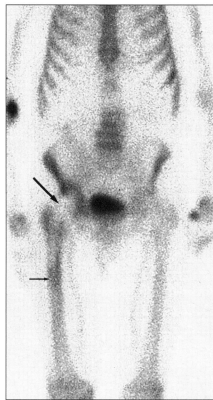

Fig. 7.87 Radionuclide bone scan in a patient with a hip prosthesis on the right, shown by a photon-deficient area (large arrow); the increased area of uptake around the distal femoral component is indicative of loosening (small arrow).

ARTHROGRAPHY

Injection of contrast into a joint cavity to demonstrate the internal anatomy, in conjunction with CT, MR, or plain radiography, can be used in a wide variety of joints. Complications of the technique include soft-tissue damage to neighbouring nerves and vessels, infection, and allergic reactions to contrast media.

BONE BIOPSY

Indications for bone biopsy include possible metastases without a known primary, bone infection, and primary bone tumours. Most biopsies of bone require a core of tissue to be taken for histological purposes. The needles used may be cutting, serrated, or trephine in type; the spring-loaded 'Trucut' cutting needle is best reserved for biopsies of soft tissues.

DISCOGRAPHY

The technique of discography—injecting contrast medium into an intervertebral disc—is used mainly before spinal surgery, to recreate the patient's pain and thereby define the site of the problem (**Fig. 7.88**). Complications include infection, discitis, and soft-tissue damage.

CHEMONUCLEOLYSIS

Chemonucleolysis is a method of injecting a plant substance (chymopapain) into the intervertebral disc, with the intention of reducing disc herniation by means of enzymic effects. Contraindications include allergy to chymopapain, pregnancy, disc herniations at cord level, and non-disc disease.

SOFT-TISSUE TUMOURS

There is an enormous histological variety of both benign and malignant tumours of soft tissue. The advent of CT and MR has made possible significant advances in the diagnosis and staging of these disorders, and hence improvement in their management.

The most common benign tumours, in order of frequency, are lipoma (**Fig. 7.89**), fibrous histiocytoma, fibrous tumours in general, haemangioma, and neural tumours. Malignant tumours, again in order of frequency, include malignant fibrous histiocytoma (*see* Fig. 7.64), liposarcoma, leiomyosarcoma (**Fig. 7.90**), synovial sarcomas, and fibrosarcomas.

Staging of these tumours depends not only on their imaging characteristics, but also on the age of the patient, their history, and the presence of multiple lesions, together with histological typing.

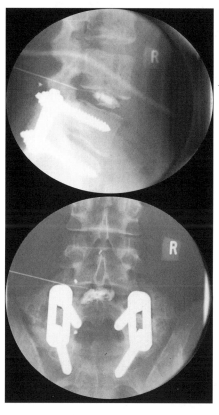

Fig. 7.88 Discography, with injection of contrast into the L4/5 disc. There has been previous Steffi plate fixation of L5 and S1.

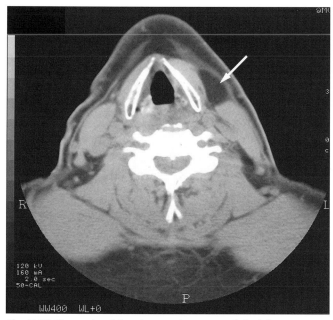

Fig. 7.89 Lipoma involving the anterior aspect of the left sternocleidomastoid muscle (arrow).

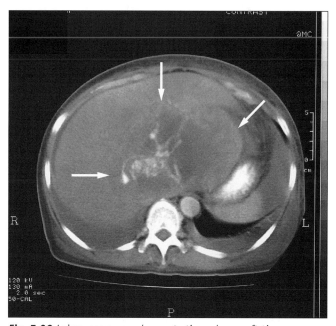

Fig. 7.90 Leiomyosarcoma, demonstrating a large soft-tissue mass, with areas of necrosis and pathological circulation within the lesion (arrows).

chapter 8

Central Nervous System

The modalities used most widely for imaging the central nervous system (CNS) are CT, MR imaging, plain radiography, myelography, and angiography. The neonatal brain is readily imaged with ultrasound, using the anterior fontanelle as an acoustic window. Doppler ultrasound is used to assess the intracranial arteries after subarachnoid haemorrhage, and Duplex ultrasound with colour flow is used in the initial evaluation of the extracranial carotid arteries. Both SPECT and PET are methods that can be used to obtain functional images of the brain: SPECT is most commonly used to show cerebral perfusion, and PET demonstrates metabolism. Fluorine-18, in ^{18}F-deoxyglucose, is the isotope used most frequently in PET imaging of the brain.

There are few indications for imaging the peripheral nervous system, which has been possible only since the advent of MR imaging. Images of the median nerve in the carpal tunnel can now be obtained, and lesions of the brachial plexus are best demonstrated by coronal MR imaging.

CONGENITAL AND NEONATAL ABNORMALITIES

BRAIN ABNORMALITIES

The two most common pathologies diagnosed by ultrasound of the neonatal head are intracranial haemorrhage and hydrocephalus. If more detailed imaging is required in the neonate, or if the anterior fontanelle has closed, MR imaging is the imaging modality of choice, because of its lack of ionizing radiation, excellent tissue contrast, and multiplanar capabilities.

The neonatal brain is incompletely myelinated. Consequently, the normal adult grey/white-matter signal characteristics on MR imaging are reversed at birth, with gradual evolution to the adult pattern by age 2 years.

Neonatal intracranial haemorrhage

Intracranial haemorrhage occurs mainly in preterm infants; four grades are recognized (**Fig. 8.1**). The typical site is the germinal matrix, at the junction of the head of the caudate nucleus and choroid plexus, in the floor of the lateral ventricle (**Fig. 8.2**). Haemorrhage may extend into the ventricular system and the brain; associated complications are hydrocephalus and encephalomalacia.

Subdural haemorrhage is uncommon in neonates, and is more likely to occur in term infants as a result of trauma. In older infants, subdural haematomas, particularly if multiple or containing blood of varying age, are highly suspicious of non-accidental injury.

Hydrocephalus

Neonatal hydrocephalus (**Fig. 8.3**) may be secondary to intracranial haemorrhage or infection such as toxoplasmosis, or may be caused by a congenital abnormality such as aqueduct stenosis or Dandy–Walker malformation (*see* Fig 6.15). It may be diagnosed antenatally.

Classification of neonatal intracranial haemorrhage	
Grade I	Subependymal haemorrhage confined to germinal matrix
Grade II	Intraventricular haemorrhage into normal-sized ventricles
Grade III	Intraventricular haemorrhage with dilated ventricles
Grade IV	Haemorrhage extending into the brain parenchyma

Fig. 8.1 *Classification of neonatal intracranial haemorrhage.*

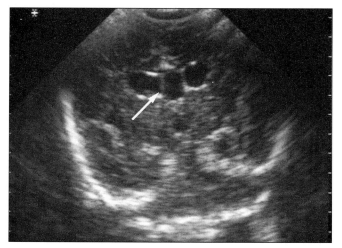

Fig. 8.2 *Ultrasound image of the head of a neonate, showing the site of the germinal matrix (arrow).*

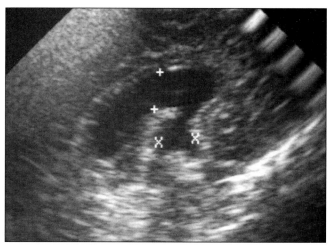

Fig. 8.3 *Ultrasound image of the head of a neonate with hydrocephalus. The lateral and third ventricles are enlarged (crosses).*

Chiari malformations

The group of malformations known as Chiari malformations involve the craniocervical junction, with associated anomalies of other parts of the CNS. Herniation of the cerebellar tonsils through the foramen magnum may obstruct cerebrospinal fluid (CSF) pathways; obstruction of the foramina of the fourth ventricle results in hydrocephalus, and obstruction of the central canal of the cervical cord is implicated in the development of syringomyelia.

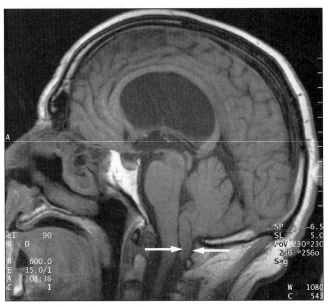

Fig. 8.4 *T1-weighted sagittal MR image of Chiari I malformation, showing herniation of the cerebellar tonsils through the foramen magnum (arrows).*

Chiari I

The cerebellar tonsils herniate more than 6 mm through the foramen magnum in Chiari I (**Fig. 8.4**), the most common type of Chiari malformation. It usually presents in adulthood, and is associated with hydrocephalus and syringomyelia.

Chiari II

With Chiari II malformation, the cerebellar vermis is displaced inferiorly through the foramen magnum, and there is always a myelomeningocele. There are associated anomalies of the tentorium, falx, corpus callosum, and brainstem. Hydrocephalus and syringomyelia are common.

Chiari III

Chiari III is a rare malformation that includes the anomalies of Chiari II, plus a low-occipital/high-cervical encephalocele.

Dandy–Walker malformation

Dandy–Walker malformation is characterized by a cystic structure in the posterior fossa that communicates with the fourth ventricle, with hypoplasia of the cerebellar vermis and, usually, hydrocephalus.

Abnormalities of the corpus callosum

Patients with complete agenesis of the corpus callosum are usually mentally handicapped. The third ventricle is high, and the lateral ventricles abnormally shaped. There may be an associated interhemispheric lipoma. Hypoplasia of the corpus callosum involves the splenium, with or without the body. Lipoma of the corpus callosum can occur without agenesis/hypoplasia, and is then usually an incidental finding (**Fig. 8.5**).

Grey matter heteropias

Grey matter migrates to its normal cortical position. If the migration is incomplete, areas of abnormal grey matter are seen anywhere from

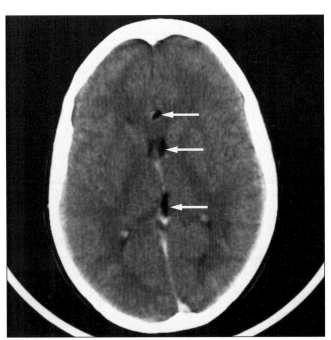

Fig. 8.5 *Lipoma of the corpus callosum. This CT scan shows several small black areas (arrows) in the corpus callosum, that had negative CT numbers on the Hounsfield scale, typical of fat.*

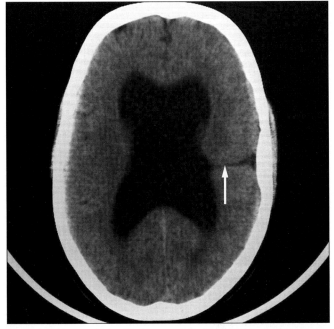

Fig.8.6 *Schizencephaly. CT shows a cleft, lined with grey matter, extending from the lateral ventricle to the brain surface (arrow).*

the ventricular walls to the subcortical area. The abnormal grey matter forms lumps (nodular grey-matter heterotopia) or bands (laminar heterotopia). The clinical presentation is epilepsy.

Rare congenital abnormalities
Lissencephaly
Lissencephaly is characterized by a brain surface that is smooth, without gyri.

Polymicrogyria
The grey matter in polymicrogyria is thickened, with a finely nodular surface that may appear smooth on MR imaging.

Megalencephaly
The term megalencephaly describes a hamartoma that involves the grey and white matter. It can be associated with metabolic disorders.

Schizencephaly
In schizencephaly, there is a cleft extending from the ventricle to the cortex, lined by abnormal grey matter (**Fig. 8.6**).

Holoprosencephaly
Holoprosencephaly is a rare, severe abnormality, with a single, large ventricle.

Septo-optic dysplasia
Absence of the septum pellucidum and hypoplasia of the anterior optic pathways characterize septo-optic dysplasia.

Craniostenosis
Craniostenosis occurs as a result of premature fusion of skull sutures. It is of no clinical significance if only one suture is involved, but if several sutures fuse early, the child will present with an abnormally shaped skull, and may have compression of the underlying brain.

SPINAL ABNORMALITIES
Spinal dysraphism
The term spinal dysraphism refers to a spectrum of abnormalities of the vertebrae, cord, spinal nerve roots, and meninges; those described here frequently coexist. Open spina bifida is seen rarely since the advent of antenatal screening. Lesser degrees of spinal dysraphism are visualized readily with spinal MR imaging. Patients present with varying degrees of spastic paraparesis and bladder dysfunction.

Open spina bifida
In patients with open spina bifida, the neural placode is visible at birth (myelocele) and may be covered with meninges (myelomeningocele). Imaging is indicated for recurrent symptoms after surgical closure, or to look for associated abnormalities such as diastematomyelia or a lipoma.

Closed spina bifida
In closed spina bifida, the midline bony defect is covered by skin that may have a haemangioma, sinus, or hairy patch. MR imaging is indicated to examine the spinal cord, which is usually tethered in an abnormally low position (**Fig. 8.7**).

Intraspinal lipoma
An intraspinal lipoma frequently coexists with closed spina bifida; it consists of intradural fat attached to the cord, cauda equina, or filum terminale (**Fig. 8.7**).

Diastematomyelia
The cord is cleft in two in the sagittal plane by a fibrous or bony band in diastematomyelia (**Fig. 8.8**).

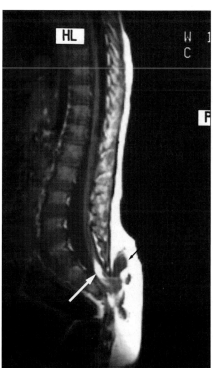

Fig. 8.7 T1-weighted sagittal MR image of lumbosacral spine in a child with a tethered cord, intraspinal lipoma (arrow), and meningocele (small arrow).

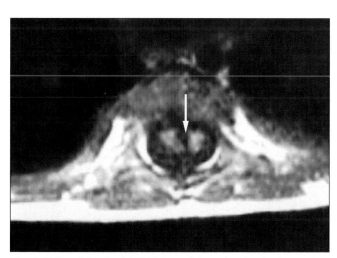

Fig. 8.8 T1-weighted axial MR image of thoracic spine in the same child as in Figure 8.7. There is diastematomyelia, with the thoracic cord cleft in two by a bony septum (arrow).

TRAUMA

HEAD INJURY

Head injury is common; it is a major cause of death and long-term morbidity, particularly in young adult men, and is usually the result of road traffic accidents.

Skull radiographs may show signs of fracture, but can only demonstrate indirect evidence of brain injury (**Fig. 8.9**). Demonstration of a depressed skull fracture (**Fig. 8.10**) is important, as this implies a dural tear; there is commonly intracranial haemorrhage, and epilepsy is a long-term complication. However, if a patient is of reduced conscious level or has focal neurological signs, time should not be wasted in performing skull radiographs. A neurosurgeon's opinion should be sought, and a CT scan performed.

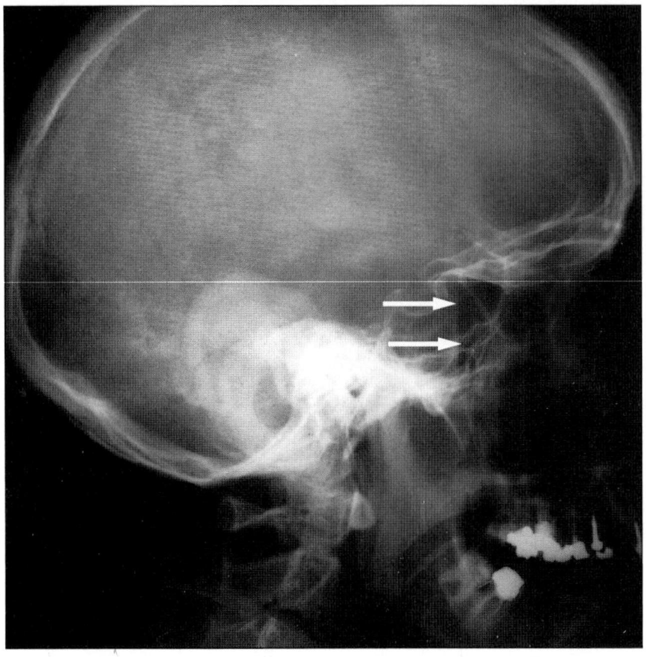

Fig. 8.9 *Lateral skull radiograph taken with a horizontal X-ray beam and the patient supine, showing an air–fluid interface (arrows) in the sphenoid sinus. In a head-injured patient, this is suspicious of a base of skull fracture.*

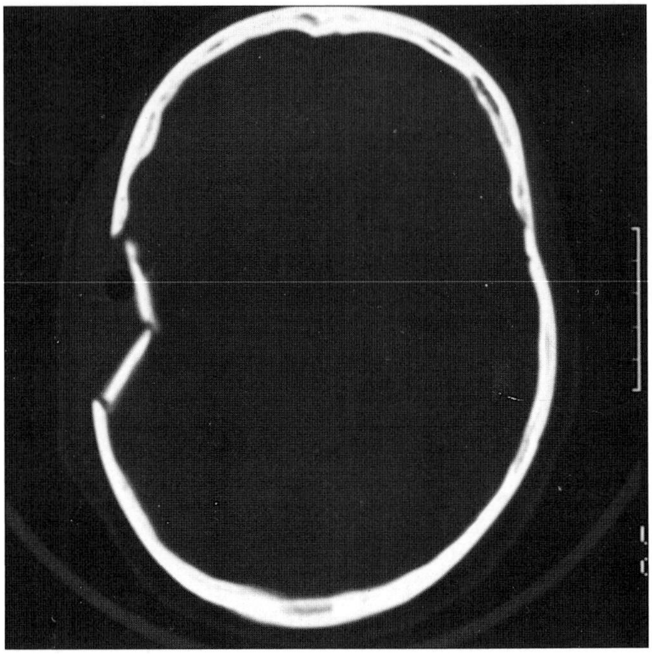

Fig. 8.10 *Depressed skull fracture; this is best seen on CT at bone windows.*

Sites of intracranial haemorrhage	
Extradural	Between inner table and dura
Subdural	Between dura and arachnoid
Subarachnoid	Between arachnoid and brain surface
Intracerebral	Within brain
Intraventricular	Within ventricles

Fig. 8.11 *Sites of intracranial haemorrhage.*

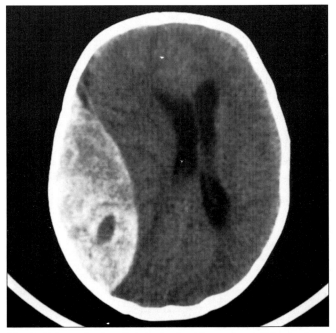

Fig. 8.12 *Large frontopatietal extradural haematoma. Extradural haematomas are recognized by their biconvex shape. There is considerable mass effect, with midline shift.*

CT scanning remains the imaging modality of choice in head-injured patients. It provides rapidly acquired images, with excellent demonstration of brain, fresh blood, bone, and foreign bodies. The design of CT scanners allows free access for patient resuscitation; most current MR scanners provide difficult access to the patient, and necessitate the use of specialized, non-ferromagnetic resuscitation equipment. The development of open MR systems and the increasing availability of non-ferromagnetic equipment are obviating these problems.

Head injury may result in intracranial haemorrhage at five sites, listed in **Figure 8.11**. Blood may be present at more than one site in any individual patient (**Figs 8.12–8.15**). Fresh blood is high density on CT and, at brain windows, appears white. Over time, blood in an intracranial haematoma evolves, with breakdown of haemoglobin. After 2–3 weeks, CT will show a haematoma to be of a density similar to that of brain (**Fig. 8.16**); beyond this time, the haematoma becomes progressively less dense, until it appears the same as CSF (**Fig. 8.17**).

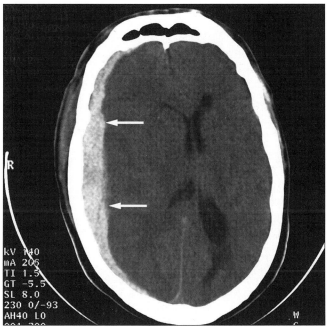

Fig. 8.13 Acute subdural haematoma. This has a typical crescentic shape (arrows). It appears hyperdense compared with brain.

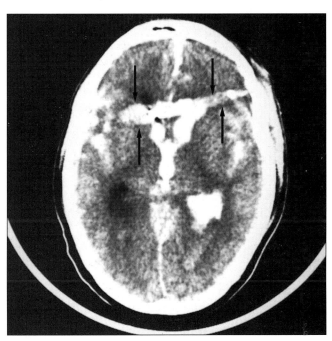

Fig. 8.14 This patient was shot in the head. The missile has left a haemorrhagic track (arrows). There is also subarachnoid haemorrhage, with blood in the sylvian fissures, and intraventicular haemorrhage.

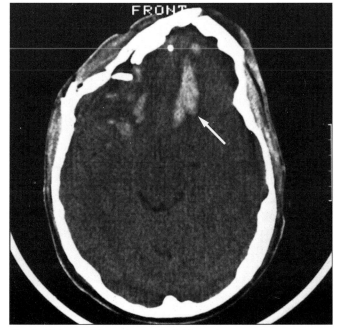

Fig. 8.15 A tree fell on the head of this patient, causing massive frontal injury, with depressed fractures, haemorrhagic contusion, and an intracerebral haematoma (arrow).

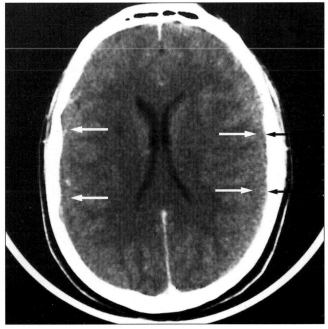

Fig. 8.16 CT of bilateral isodense subdural haematomas (arrows), which are difficult to distinguish from the underlying brain.

Deceleration injury of the brain affects the white matter, and is termed diffuse axonal injury. This is associated with significant long-term disability, but there may be little to see on a CT scan. MR imaging is more sensitive for these subtle white-matter lesions (**Fig. 8.18**), and SPECT scanning may show perfusion deficits.

SPINAL INJURY

Injury to the vertebral column is important, because of the contained spinal cord and nerve roots. The bony component of spinal injury can be seen on plain films, but is best imaged with CT (**Fig. 8.19**), when excellent visualization of vertebral fractures and displaced bony

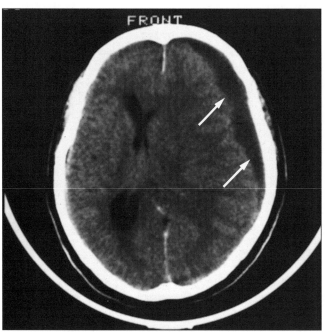

Fig. 8.17 CT of a chronic subdural haematoma (arrows), which is hypodense compared with adjacent brain.

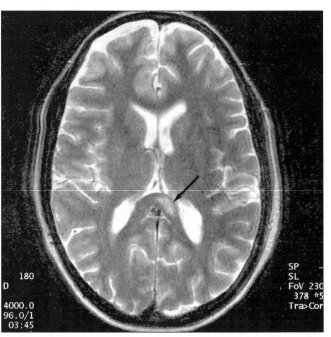

Fig. 8.18 T2-weighted axial MR imaging in head injury, showing high signal in the splenium of the corpus callosum, typical of diffuse axonal injury (arrow).

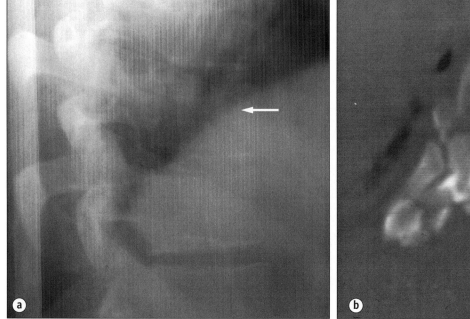

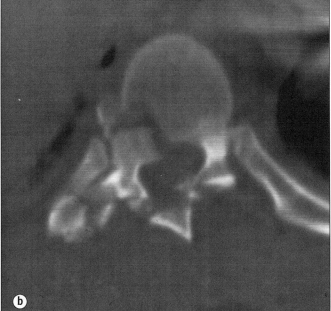

Fig. 8.19 (**a**) Lateral lower thoracic spine radiograph after a road traffic accident. The T10 vertebral body (arrow) shows only minimal abnormality. (**b**) Unstable, comminuted fracture of T10 in the same patient. CT demonstrates fractures through the posterior aspect of the vertebral body, both laminae, and the right transverse process. There is compression of the spinal cord.

fragments can be achieved. However, the extent of bony injury does not correlate with neurological deficit, and CT is extremely limited in its demonstration of cord injury. Compression, haematoma, or oedema of the cord is best seen on MR imaging (Fig. 8.20), and these imaging abnormalities do correlate with the patient's neurological outcome.

MR imaging also provides excellent visualization of complications of spinal cord injury, such as the obstruction of the central canal of the spinal cord after trauma, which results in post-traumatic syringomyelia (Fig. 8.21).

Cervical spine
Fracture, dislocation, or both, of the cervical spine may be fatal, or lead to quadriparesis. Traction injuries to the upper limbs can cause avulsion of cervical nerve roots, which can be shown on MR imaging or cervical myelography.

Thoracic spine
Injury to the thoracic cord can cause paraparesis.

Lumbar spine
Below the level of the conus (L1/L2), lumbar injury may compress the cauda equina, causing lower motor neurone signs in the lower limbs, and urinary retention.

INFECTION

MENINGITIS
The diagnosis of meningitis is based on clinical signs and CSF findings. Imaging is indicated only if there is clinical doubt, to exclude a space-occupying lesion before lumbar puncture.

The majority of patients with meningitis will have a normal CT scan or show meningeal enhancement after intravenous contrast. Chronic meningitis, caused by tuberculosis or fungi, more often shows meningeal enhancement that is most obvious in the basal cisterns.

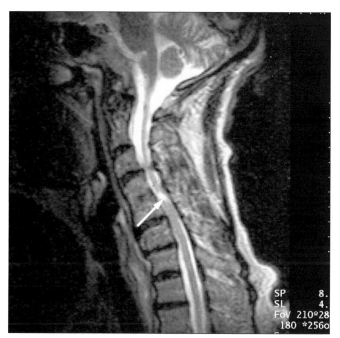

Fig. 8.20 *T2-weighted sagittal MR image of the cervical spine after a road traffic accident. There is high signal in the centre of the cord (arrow), indicating cord injury. The patient was quadriplegic. There is also cervical spondylosis at the C3/4 level.*

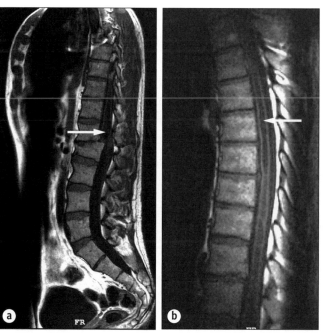

Fig. 8.21 (a) *T1-weighted sagittal MR image of lower thoracic, lumbar, and sacral spine, showing a compression fracture and posterior displacement of L1 causing compression of the conus medullaris. The injury occurred 5 years earlier, and post-traumatic syringomyelia (arrow) has developed. **(b)** T1-weighted sagittal MR image thoracic spine in the same patient, showing extension of the syrinx into the upper thoracic cord (arrow).*

ENCEPHALITIS

Most cases of encephalitis in adults are caused by *Herpes simplex* virus. The temporal lobe is the most common site. Imaging, particularly in the early stages, may be normal, or may show focal swelling with low density on CT (**Fig. 8.22**) and high signal on T2-weighted MR imaging. SPECT scanning can be useful, and reveals a perfusion defect early in the disease process.

CEREBRAL ABSCESS

Cerebral abscess is relatively uncommon and usually results from direct spread from an infection in an adjacent air space in the skull, such as sinusitis, otitis media, or mastoiditis. Haematogenous spread from an infected embolic source such as endocarditis is another cause. CT and MR images show thin-walled cystic lesions, with ring enhancement. Appearances can be similar to those of cerebral metastases, but patients with a cerebral abscess are likely to be pyrexial and more systemically unwell (**Fig. 8.23**).

SUBDURAL EMPYEMA

Subdural empyema can complicate meningitis, or may arise as a result of direct spread from an infected air space. CT and MR imaging reveal a subdural collection of pus, with marked enhancement of the meninges.

SPINAL INFECTION

Spinal infection occurs as a result of spread from adjacent vertebral osteomyelitis (**Fig. 8.24**) or discitis, or by haematogenous spread, resulting in an extradural abscess.

CENTRAL NERVOUS SYSTEM MANIFESTATIONS OF ACQUIRED IMMUNE DEFICIENCY SYNDROME

There are several CNS manifestations of AIDS (**Fig. 8.25**). Many of the lesions are non-specific in appearance and may be caused by various infective agents or neoplasia. Imaging with CT and MR can help to narrow the differential diagnosis but, often, lumbar puncture or brain biopsy is ultimately required.

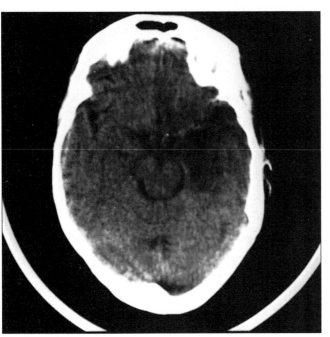

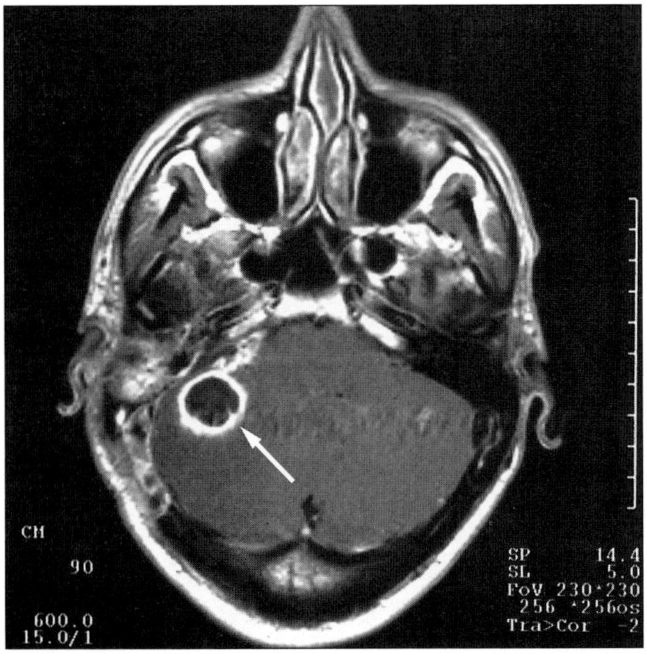

Fig. 8.22 *CT image of herpes simplex virus encephalitis, showing low density in the left temporal lobe.*

Fig. 8.23 *T1-weighted axial MR image post gadolinium showing ring enhancement in the right cerebellar hemisphere (arrow). This is a cerebral abscess due to spread of infection from the right middle ear..*

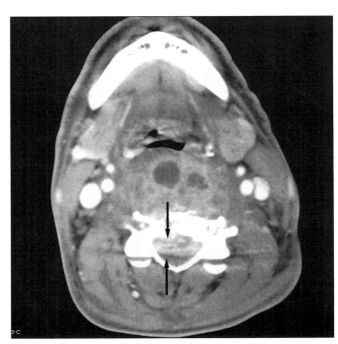

Fig. 8.24 *Cervical vertebral osteomyelitis with extradural abscess (arrows) on CT after contrast. Infection has spread from the soft tissues of the pharynx to the adjacent cervical vertebrae, and then into the spinal extradural space.*

CNS abnormalities in AIDS

AIDS-related disease	CNS abnormality
Human immunodeficiency virus (HIV) encephalopathy	Cerebral atrophy
Progressive multifocal leucoencephalopathy	Multiple non-enhancing white-matter lesions
Toxoplasmosis (most common cause, see Fig. 8.26)	Ring-enhancing mass lesions
Lymphoma Cryptococcosis Cytomegalovirus Mycobacterium tuberculosis (MTB)	Solid-enhancing mass lesions
Cryptococcosis Cytomegalovirus MTB Meningeal spread of lymphoma	Meningitis/meningoencephalitis
HIV Herpes simplex virus Varicella zoster	Myelopathy
Extradural spread of lymphoma Extradural abscess caused by MTB	Cord compression

Fig. 8.25 CNS abnormalities in AIDS.

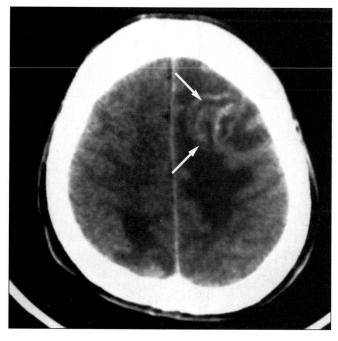

Fig. 8.26 CT in cerebral toxoplasmosis post-contrast. There is an enhancing ring-shaped lesion in the left frontal lobe (arrows) with surrounding oedema.

INFLAMMATORY CONDITIONS

MULTIPLE SCLEROSIS

Multiple sclerosis is the most common inflammatory disease of the CNS. It is probably postviral in aetiology. Pathologically, the lesions are plaques of demyelination in the white matter of the brain and spinal cord. The disease has wide clinical and radiological spectra of severity, which are not necessarily correlated. CT scans of the brain may show no abnormality; demyelination is best seen on proton-density and T2-weighted MR images as multifocal areas of high signal intensity, typically involving the periventricular white matter (**Fig. 8.27**), corpus callosum, visual pathways, brainstem, and cerebellum (**Fig. 8.28**). Spinal plaques are best seen on T2-weighted sagittal (**Fig. 8.29**) and axial MR images of the cord.

ACUTE DEMYELINATING ENCEPHALOMYELITIS

Acute demyelinating encephalomyelitis occurs as a postviral illness and, like multiple sclerosis, results in demyelination. Clinically, the disease has an acute onset and is more severe than multiple sclerosis. Radiologically, the areas of demyelination are more extensive and confluent.

SARCOIDOSIS

CNS involvement with sarcoidosis can give an MR appearance identical to that of multiple sclerosis. Sarcoidosis also has a predilection for involvement of the posterior pituitary, pituitary stalk, hypothalamus, and optic chiasm, and can cause enhancing inflammatory masses that are best seen on T1-weighted MR imaging after gadolinium contrast.

RADIOTHERAPY

Cranial radiotherapy for primary brain tumours or lymphoma can produce areas of inflammatory change and demyelination. It can be impossible to differentiate between changes that occur after radiotherapy and recurrent tumour, even after contrast enhancement on CT and MR imaging; comparison with results from previous examinations is essential. PET scanning with ^{18}F-deoxyglucose can differentiate recurrent tumour (with high glucose metabolism) from scarring (with low glucose metabolism), but is not widely available.

LEUCODYSTROPHIES

Leucodystrophies comprise a rare and heterogeneous group of diseases that result in multiple white-matter lesions. Aetiologies are varied and include inherited, metabolic, and unknown causes. MR imaging shows high signal in the white matter, the distribution of which is characteristic for the different diseases.

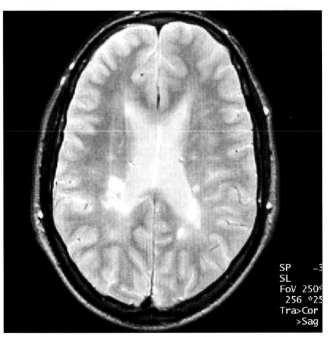

Fig. 8.27 Multiple sclerosis. T2-weighted axial MR image of the cerebrum, showing multiple periventricular high-intensity lesions, which are plaques of demyelination.

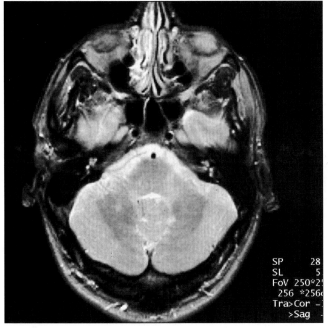

Fig. 8.28 Multiple sclerosis. T2-weighted axial MR image of the posterior fossa. There are several plaques in the pons and cerebellum.

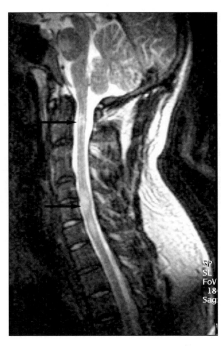

Fig. 8.29 Multiple sclerosis. T2-weighted sagittal MR image of the posterior fossa and cervical cord. There are several plaques (arrows) returning high signal.

VASCULAR DISORDERS

Infarction and haemorrhage are the most common manifestations of cerebrovascular disease. Venous abnormalities and capillary haemangiomas are less common.

INFARCTION

Brain infarction results from sudden occlusion or reduction in perfusion pressure of the carotid or vertebral arteries or their branches (**Fig. 8.30**). If occlusion occurs slowly, sufficient collateral supply may be maintained via the circle of Willis. Imaging is indicated mainly to exclude macroscopic haemorrhage, which will influence secondary preventative treatment such as anticoagulation. At present, there is no overwhelming evidence to support thrombolysis in acute stroke;

should this change in the future, there will be a need to diagnose cerebrovascular occlusion within 6 hours of onset. The modalities likely to be most useful are diffusion and perfusion-weighted MR imaging and SPECT scanning.

On CT, cerebral infarcts are low-density lesions (**Fig. 8.31**) and any haemorrhage into the infarct results in increased density. Large, acute infarcts cause significant mass effect (**Fig. 8.32**); this is most evident with cerebellar infarcts, which can cause loss of consciousness because swelling in the confines of the posterior fossa results in brainstem compression. Old infarcts are areas of gliosis and have reduced volume and density, with dilatation of adjacent CSF spaces.

On MR imaging, infarcts are of low intensity on T1-weighted images and high intensity on T2-weighted images (**Fig. 8.33**).

Causes of cerebral infarction	
Cause of infarction	**Usual site**
Atheroma	Carotid bifurcation
Thromboembolic disease (from cardiac or carotid sites)	Middle cerebral artery
Arteritis (e.g. systemic lupus erythematosus, Takayasu's, radiotherapy, infection)	Smaller peripheral arteries
Dissecting aortic aneurysm	Common carotid, innominate, and subclavian artery origins
Hypotension (e.g. cardiogenic shock)	'Watershed' areas between anterior/middle/posterior cerebral artery territories

Fig. 8.30 *Causes of cerebral infarction.*

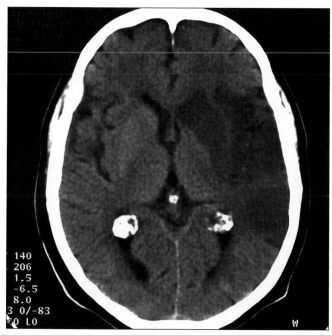

Fig. 8.31 *CT of a recent cerebral infarct. The left middle cerebral territory infarct is of low density compared with adjacent brain.*

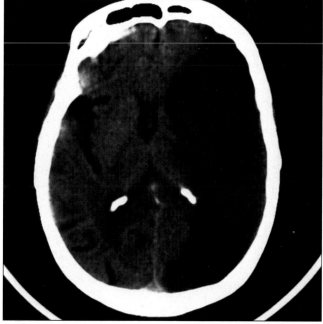

Fig. 8.32 *CT of an extensive left middle cerebral territory infarct. The infarct is swollen and is obliterating the overlying CSF spaces and compressing the left lateral ventricle.*

185

HAEMORRHAGE
Cerebral haemorrhage

Cerebral haemorrhage occurs most commonly as a result of hypertensive vascular change, typically within the distribution of the lenticulostriate arteries. Cerebral haemorrhage may be secondary to an underlying tumour, arteriovenous malformation (AVM) (Fig. 8.34), or aneurysm. CT shows fresh haematoma as a high-density mass.

Subarachnoid haemorrhage

Subarachnoid haemorrhage (SAH) occurs usually as a result of rupture of an intracranial aneurysm (Fig. 8.35), less commonly because of bleeding from an AVM; it can also occur after head injury.

SAH is seen as increased density in the subarachnoid space on CT (Fig. 8.36); if it is extensive, there may also be intraventricular and intracerebral blood. The distribution of blood within the subarachnoid space may indicate the likely site of aneurysmal rupture.

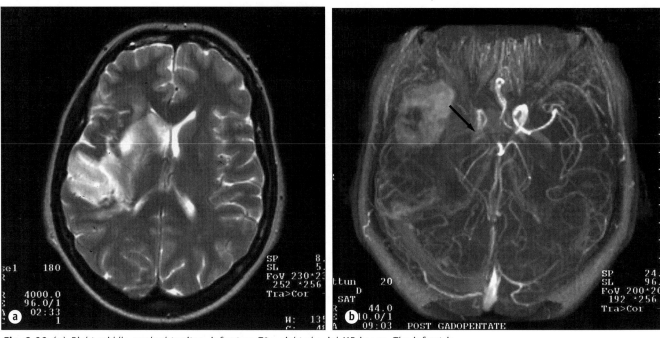

Fig. 8.33 (a) Right middle cerebral territory infarct on T2-weighted axial MR image. The infarct is oedematous and therefore appears bright. *(b)* An MR angiogram in the same patient shows occlusion of the right middle cerebral artery (arrow).

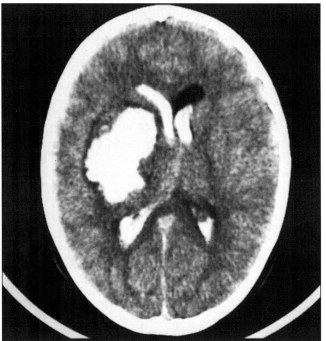

Fig. 8.34 Recent cerebral haemorrhage. CT shows a high-density mass in the right cerebral hemisphere caused by haemorrhage from an AVM. There has also been haemorrhage into the ventricular system.

CT may be negative after a small subarachnoid bleed and lumbar puncture is then required, to look for red cells and xanthochromia.

In proven SAH, cerebral angiography of both carotid and both vertebral arteries is required to demonstrate the underlying vascular abnormality, usually an aneurysm (**Fig. 8.37**). The presence of subarachnoid blood often results in spasm of adjacent arteries, which is obvious at angiography and accounts for much of the morbidity associated with SAH (**Fig. 8.38**). Aneurysms can also be demonstrated

with MR imaging, but as yet the sensitivity for small aneurysms remains inferior to that achieved with conventional angiography.

If an AVM is diagnosed, careful selective angiography is needed to show the feeding arteries and draining veins (**Figs 8.39** and **8.40**).

Frequency of intracranial aneurysms at different sites	
Site	**Frequency**
Anterior communicating artery	30%
Posterior communicating artery	25%
Middle cerebral artery	21%
Terminal carotid artery	13%
Basilar and posterior inferior cerebellar arteries	3%

Fig. 8.35 Frequency of intracranial aneurysms at different sites.

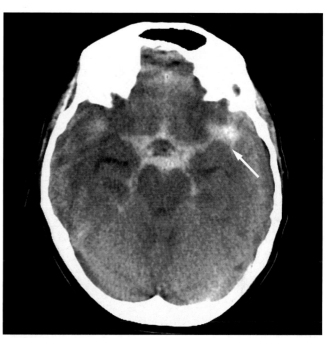

Fig. 8.36 CT after recent subarachnoid haemorrhage. Fresh blood is seen in the suprasellar cistern, ambient cisterns, sylvian fissures, and anterior interhemispheric fissure. Blood is most obvious in the left sylvian fissure (arrow), making rupture of a middle cerebral artery aneurysm the probable cause.

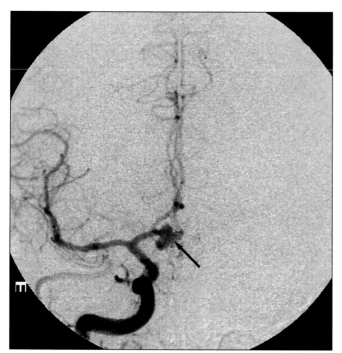

Fig. 8.37 Right common carotid arteriogram. There is a large, lobulated aneurysm of the anterior communicating artery (arrow).

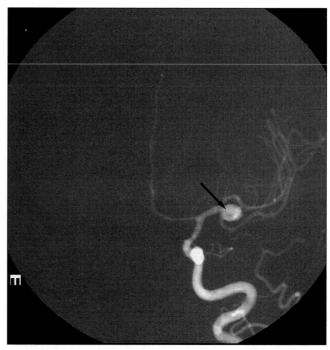

Fig. 8.38 Left common carotid arteriogram. There is an aneurysm of the left middle cerebral artery (arrow), with spasm of the adjacent middle and anterior cerebral branches.

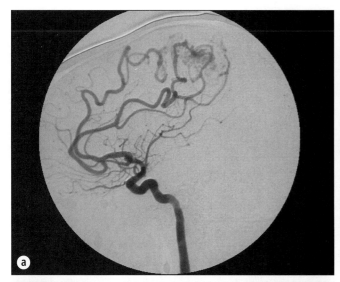

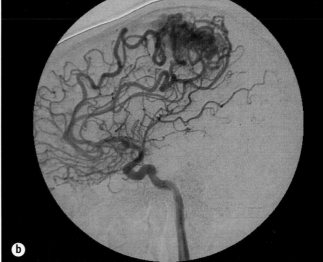

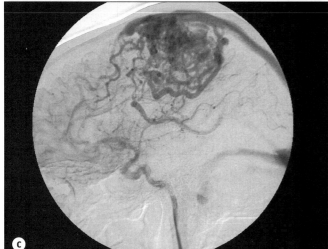

Fig. 8.39 *Left internal carotid arteriograms showing a parietal AVM. (**a**) There are dilated middle cerebral branches supplying the AVM. (**b**) Later arterial phase, with contrast filling the AVM. (**c**) Early venous drainage into the superior sagittal sinus and deep veins.*

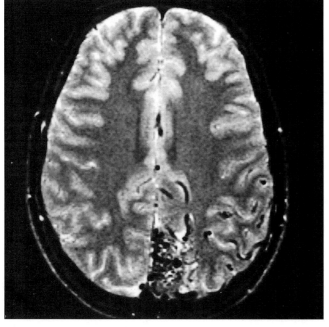

Fig. 8.40 *T2-weighted axial MR image in the same patient as in Figure 8.39. The AVM shows as multiple black flow voids in the left parietal lobe.*

NEOPLASTIC DISEASE

BRAIN

Intracranial neoplasms can be classified as intra-axial and extra-axial. Primary intra-axial tumours are those which arise from the cerebrum, brainstem, or cerebellum; they are further subdivided into those which arise above or below the tentorium. Extra-axial tumours arise from meninges, nerve root sheaths, the pituitary, within the ventricles, and bone. Primary and metastatic tumour may arise in both groups; benign and malignant tumours may occur in both groups. Benign intracranial neoplasms may cause significant neurological deficit because of mass effect; they are often locally recurrent, and may arise at sites to which it is difficult to gain neurosurgical access.

Primary tumours

Intra-axial supratentorial tumours

Gliomas are the most common tumours in the intra-axial, supratentorial group, and range from slow growing, low-grade astrocytomas to the rapidly growing, aggressive glioblastoma multiforme (**Fig. 8.41**), the most common glioma in adults. Generally, the higher the grade of tumour, the more likely it is to show contrast enhancement.

Ependymomas account for about 5% of gliomas. They usually occur in the cerebral hemispheres in young adults, but in the posterior fossa in children. Fifty percent of them calcify.

Oligodendrogliomas account for fewer than 5% of gliomas in adults. They occur typically in the frontal lobes, and commonly calcify (**Fig. 8.42**).

Intra-axial infratentorial tumours

Medulloblastomas are the most common posterior fossa tumours in childhood, and usually present with signs of raised intracranial pressure as a result of hydrocephalus. They occur in the cerebellar vermis in young children, and in the cerebellar hemisphere in young adults. Imaging shows a solid mass, sometimes with cystic areas, without calcification, and showing contrast enhancement (**Fig. 8.43**). Spread is through CSF pathways.

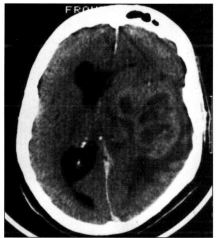

Fig. 8.41 *Glioblastoma multiforme. CT shows a large tumour that is partly solid, partly cystic, and is causing significant mass effect.*

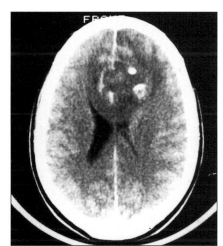

Fig. 8.42 *Frontal oligodendroglioma. CT, shows a midline mass with areas of calcification, and contrast enhancement.*

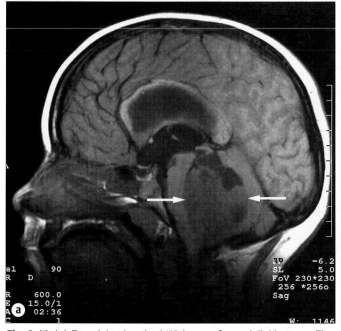

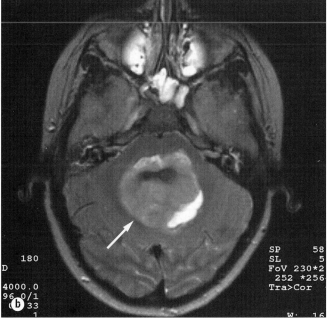

Fig. 8.43 *(a) T1-weighted sagittal MR image of a medulloblastoma. There is a large posterior fossa tumour (arrows) expanding the fourth ventricle and causing hydrocephalus. (b) T2-weighted axial MR image in the same patient.*

Pilocytic astrocytomas are the second most common posterior fossa tumours in childhood, after medulloblastoma. They are usually cystic; with nodules aound the edge that enhance following contrast.

Haemangioblastomas are uncommon tumours that may be cystic, with a mural, enhancing nodule (**Fig. 8.44**), or solid. They occur in the cerebellum and spinal cord, and comprise part of the von Hippel–Lindau syndrome, in which they can be multiple.

Brainstem gliomas account for about 25% of posterior fossa tumours in childhood. They show variable contrast enhancement and must be distinguished from brainstem encephalitis.

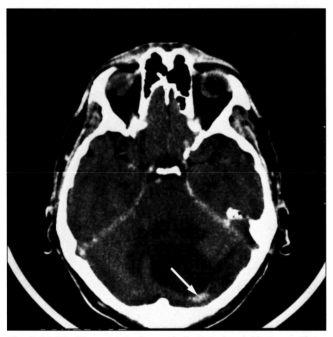

Fig. 8.44 *CT with contrast of a cerebellar haemangioblastoma. There is a cystic mass in the cerebellum, with a small enhancing nodule posteriorly (arrow).*

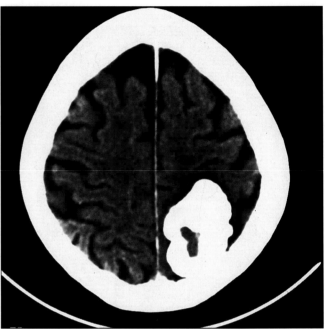

Fig. 8.45 *CT of a heavily calcified meningioma in the left superior parietal region.*

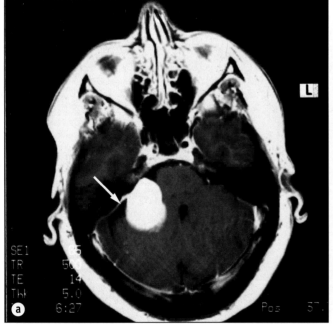

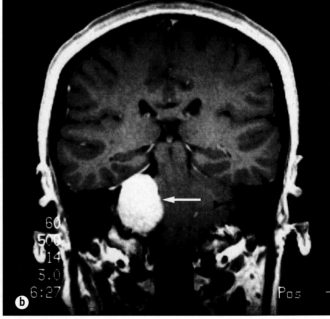

Fig. 8.46 *(a) T1-weighted axial MR image, after gadolinium, of a right cerebellopontine angle meningioma. There is adjacent dural enhancement (arrow), which is non-specific but frequently seen with meningiomas. This lesion presented clinically in the same way as an acoustic neuroma; the imaging features can be similar also.(b) T1-weighted coronal MR image, after gadolinium, of the same lesion (arrow), again showing dural enhancement along the tentorium.*

Extra-axial tumours

Meningiomas are the most common extra-axial tumours in adults, particularly in middle-aged women. They can be multiple in neurofibromatosis type 2 (*see* page 198). These benign tumours almost always have a dural base, can calcify (**Fig. 8.45**), and may be associated with adjacent bony abnormality. Imaging shows a well-defined solid mass, with uniform contrast enhancement (**Fig. 8.46**).

Acoustic neuroma (*see* Chapter 9, pages 210–211).

Pituitary adenoma The most common group of pituitary tumours are microadenomas (<1 cm diameter); they present with endocrine abnormalities (**Fig. 8.47**). Macroadenomas (>1 cm diameter) are usually non-functional and present as a result of compression of adjacent structures—typically, with bitemporal hemianopia caused by compression of the optic chiasm (**Fig. 8.48**).

Craniopharyngioma is a benign tumour that typically has a cystic component containing a variable quantity of protein, with or without fat. The solid component enhances with contrast, and most are revealed as calcified on CT. They usually occur in the suprasellar region (**Fig. 8.49**).

Choroid plexus papillomas are rare tumours; in adults, they usually involve the fourth ventricle, whereas in children they occur in the lateral ventricle.

Although the division of tumours into intra-axial/extra-axial and supratentorial/infratentorial may seem arbitrary, it is important in predicting the type of tumour. For example, a single intra-axial supratentorial lesion in an adult with no known primary malignancy is most likely to be a glioma, whereas a posterior fossa tumour in a child is most likely to be a medulloblastoma.

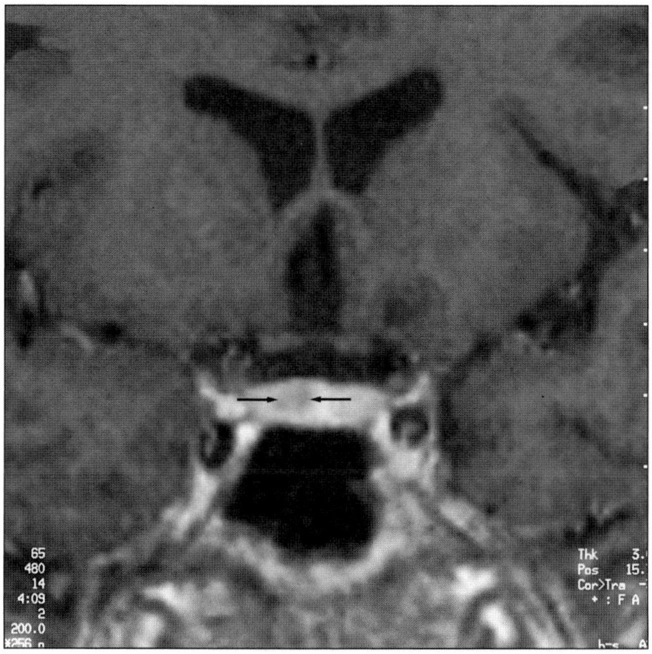

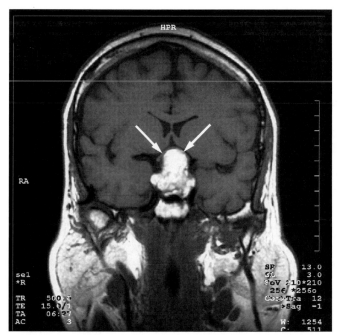

Fig. 8.47 *T1-weighted coronal MR image, after gadolinium, of a pituitary microadenoma. This is the round hypointense area in the right half of the gland (arrows).*

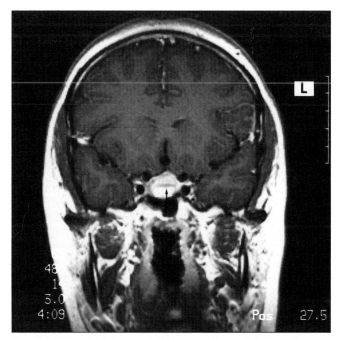

Fig. 8.48 *T1-weighted coronal MR image, after gadolinium, of a pituitary macroadenoma. A large mass expands the pituitary fossa and extends into the suprasellar cistern. It is compressing the optic chiasm (arrows); the patient presented with bitemporal hemianopia.*

Fig. 8.49 *T1-weighted coronal MR image, after gadolinium of a craniopharyngioma. There is a round, predominantly cystic lesion in the suprasellar cistern that contains both fat and fluid, as indicated by the grey band (arrow) caused by MR artefact at the fat–fluid interface.*

Metastases

Intracranial metastases appear on CT as multiple rounded lesions that enhance after contrast and are surrounded by oedema. They can occur anywhere in the cerebral hemispheres and cerebellum (**Figs 8.50** and **8.51**). MR imaging after gadolinium enhancement offers the most sensitive method of demonstrating metastases, but CT is adequate for most purposes.

Metastases can also occur in an extra-axial location and can cause diffuse meningeal involvement (**Fig. 8.52**). This is the method of spread of primary CNS tumours, with tumour seeding along CSF pathways.

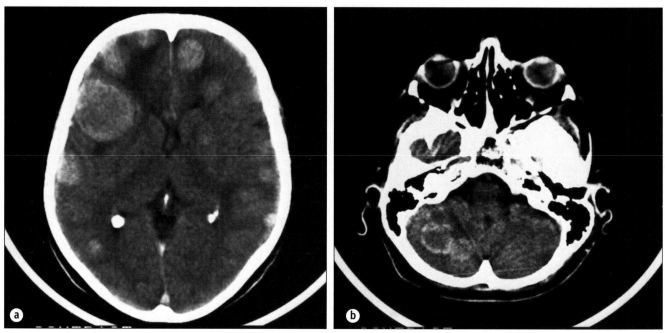

Fig. 8.50 (a) CT after contrast, in a patient with multiple metastases from malignant melanoma. There are multiple, rounded, enhancing soft-tissue masses, some with surrounding oedema, throughout both hemispheres. *(b)* Further metastases are present in the cerebellum of the same patient.

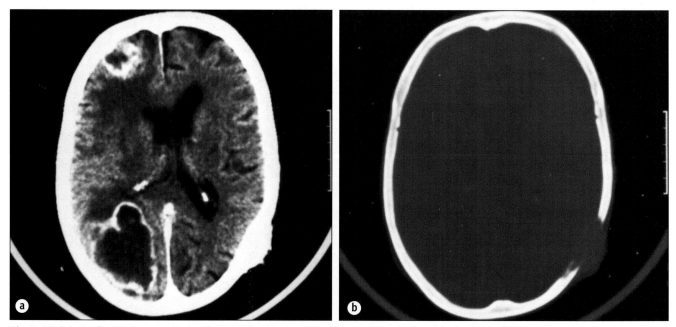

Fig. 8.51 (a) CT after contrast, at brain windows, showing two necrotic metastases in the right frontal and parietal lobes. *(b)* CT after contrast, in the same patient but shown at bony windows, demonstrates a skull vault metastasis also.

SPINE

In common with tumours of the brain, tumours occurring in and around the spinal cord are classified according to their location (**Fig. 8.53**); again, this influences the differential diagnosis. **Figures 8.54–8.58** show examples of imaging of spinal tumours.

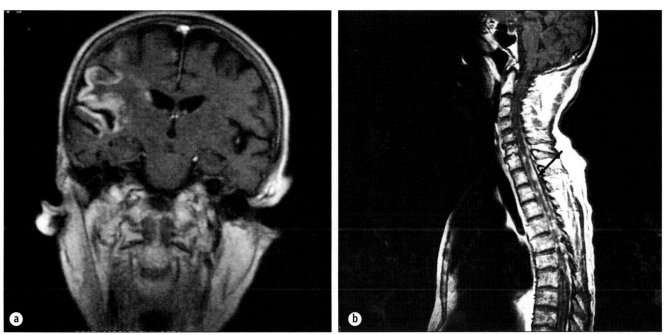

Fig. 8.52 (**a**) T1-weighted coronal MR image, after gadolinium, of a patient with meningeal metastases from a primary, bronchogenic carcinoma. There is enhancement of the meninges in the right sylvian fissure. (**b**) T1-weighted sagittal MR image of cervical and thoracic spine of the same patient, showing nodular enhancement over the surface of the cord (arrow).

Fig. 8.53 Classification of spinal tumours.

Classification of spinal tumours	
Intramedullary	Astrocytoma Ependymoma (*see* **Fig. 8.54**)
Intradural, extramedullary	Meningioma (*see* **Fig. 8.55**) Neurofibroma (*see* **Fig. 8.56**) Neurolemmoma Metastases from primary CNS tumour or with carcinomatosis (*see* **Fig. 8.52b**)
Extradural	Metastases (*see* Fig. 8.57) Primary bone tumours (*see* **Fig. 8.58**) Chordoma

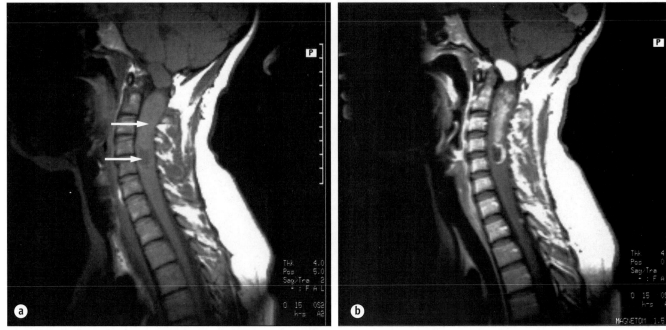

Fig. 8.54 (**a**) *T1-weighted sagittal MR image of the cervical spine, showing expansion and inhomogeneous signal from the upper cervical cord (arrows).* (**b**) *Same patient and sequence but after gadolinium. Note the diffusely enhancing intramedullary ependymoma, and the brightly enhancing meningioma at the craniocervical junction. This patient has neurofibromatosis type 2.*

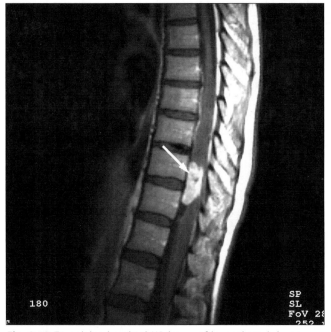

Fig. 8.55 *T1-weighted sagittal MR image of lower thoracic/upper lumbar spine after gadolinium. There is a brightly enhancing intradural, extramedullary meningioma (arrow).*

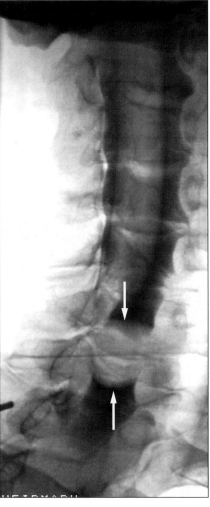

Fig. 8.56 *Cervical myelogram, showing a round mass that is intradural and extramedullary (arrows). This is a neurofibroma.*

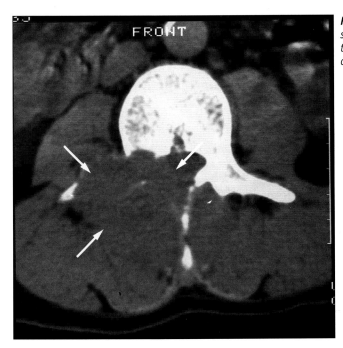

Fig. 8.57 CT showing metastatic tumour destruction in the lumbar spine. Expansile soft tissue (arrows) has destroyed the right pedicle, transverse process, and lamina, and is causing extradural compression of the cauda equina.

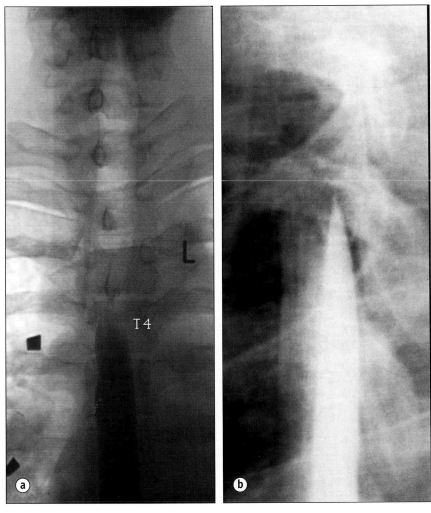

Fig. 8.58 (a) Anteroposterior view of a thoracic myelogram, showing complete block at the T4 level. This was caused by extradural compression from a primary Ewing's sarcoma. The radio-opaque markers are taped to the patient's skin to identify the level of block for neurosurgical decompression. **(b)** Lateral view in the same patient.

DEGENERATIVE CONDITIONS

BRAIN

Atrophy of the brain occurs as part of the ageing process. Focal atrophy is seen in dementias, the most common being temporoparietal atrophy in Altzheimer's disease. This is best demonstrated as reduced temporoparietal perfusion on a SPECT scan (**Fig. 8.59**).

Atrophy is also seen in long-standing multiple sclerosis and in cerebrovascular disease, in which it is associated with multiple small cerebral infarcts. Focal atrophy of the basal ganglia occurs in Huntingdon's chorea; that of the corticospinal tracts is a late finding in motor neurone disease.

Atrophy that disproportionately affects the cerebellum is seen in chronic alcohol abuse, and with long-term treatment with some anti-convulsant drugs, notably phenytoin.

On CT, atrophy is seen as generalized loss of cerebral and cerebellar cortical thickness, with compensatory widening of the sulcal spaces and ventricles (**Fig. 8.60**).

SPINE

Degenerative spondylosis and intervertebral disc disease are common causes of compression of the spinal cord and nerve roots. It is important to appreciate the difference between compression of a nerve root (radiculopathy), which will give lower motor neurone symptoms and signs, and compression of the spinal cord (myelopathy), which will give upper motor neurone symptoms and signs.

Myelopathy

Myelopathy is best investigated with spinal MR imaging (**Fig. 8.61**), the region imaged being determined by the clinical findings. If MR imaging is not available, myelography is the next investigation of choice.

Radioculopathy

At present, although the resolution of cervical roots on MR imaging continues to improve, cervical radiculopathy is best investigated by cervical myelography. Lumbar radiculopathy, however, should be investigated by lumbar CT (**Fig. 8.62**) or MR imaging (**Fig. 8.63**), the latter being preferable because of its lack of ionizing radiation and wider anatomical coverage. If these investigations are contraindicated or equivocal, lumbar myelography should be performed (**Fig. 8.63**).

Compression of the cauda equina as a result of a central lumbar disc prolapse, or by spinal stenosis (**Fig. 8.64**), is best demonstrated by MR imaging or lumbar myelography.

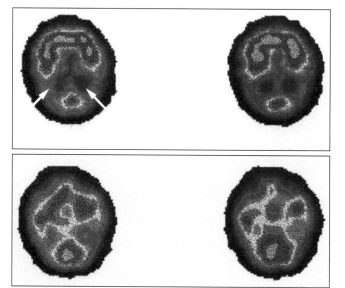

Fig. 8.59 SPECT scan in Altzheimer's disease. There are bilateral perfusion deficits in the temporoparietal regions (arrows).

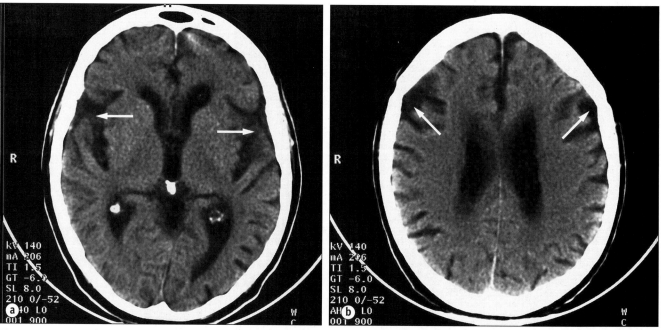

Fig. 8.60 CT in cerebral atrophy, showing (**a**) widening of the sylvian fissures (arrows) and (**b**) prominent sulci (arrows).

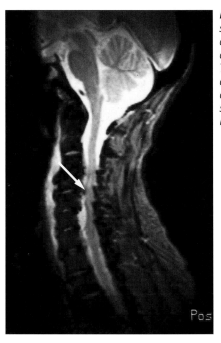

Fig. 8.61 *T2-weighted sagittal MR image of cervical spine in severe cervical spondylosis. There is compression of the mid-cervical cord that is most severe at the C4/5 level (arrow).*

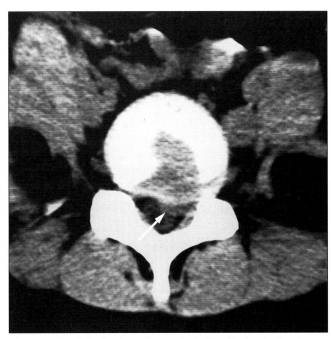

Fig. 8.62 *CT of the lumbar spine at the L5/S1 disc level, showing a left-sided disc prolapse (arrow) compressing the left S1 nerve root.*

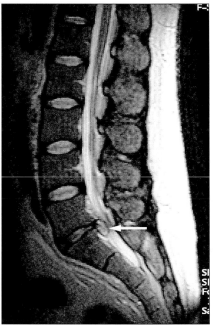

Fig. 8.63 *T2-weighted sagittal MR image of the lumbar spine showing a large L5/S1 disc prolapse (arrow).*

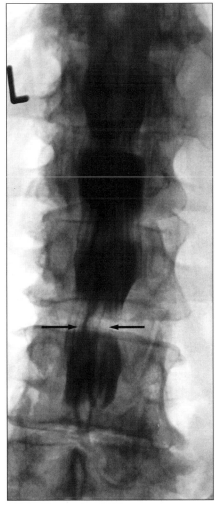

Fig. 8.64 *Lumbar myelogram in spinal stenosis. There is concentric narrowing of the spinal canal at the L4/5 level, causing a complete block. Similar but less severe changes are seen at the level above (arrows).*

METABOLIC AND TOXIC CONDITIONS

Calcification of the basal ganglia

Calcification of the basal ganglia is usually idiopathic. The most common metabolic causes are hypoparathyroidism (**Fig. 8.65**), pseudohypoparathyroidism, and hyperthyroidism.

Wilson's disease

In the disease of copper metabolism known as Wilson's disease, copper is deposited in the basal ganglia, corneas, liver, and bones. MR imaging shows high signal in the basal ganglia on T2-weighted images.

Mucopolysaccharidoses and mucolipidoses

The imaging findings in mucopolysaccharidoses and mucolipidoses include white-matter abnormalities, hydrocephalus, and cerebral atrophy.

Mitochondrial diseases

Mitochondrial diseases are a group of diseases that affect smooth muscle and the CNS. Imaging shows infarcts in the deep grey matter, cerebral cortex, or both.

Central pontine myelinolysis

Patients who are systemically unwell (e.g. with liver disease, malignancies, burns etc.) can develop central pontine myelinolysis, which is possibly related to over-rapid correction of hyponatraemia. T2-weighted MR images show high signal in the pons.

MISCELLANEOUS CONDITIONS

PHAKOMATOSES

Phakomatoses comprise a group of diseases with neuroectodermal abnormalities that have a wide variety of clinical manifestations.

Neurofibromatosis type 1

Neurofibromatosis type 1 (NF1) is 10 times more common than type 2. The neurological abnormalities include optic nerve gliomas (**Fig. 8.66**), plexiform neurofibromas, brain hamartomas, gliomas, and neurofibromas of cranial nerves or spinal roots. Many patients have spinal abnormalities, including kyphoscoliosis and lateral thoracic meningocele. Plain skull radiographs may show a characteristic abnormality called the 'bare orbit', caused by dysplasia of the greater wing of the sphenoid.

Neurofibromatosis type 2

Bilateral acoustic neuromas (**Fig. 8.67**) are classical abnormalities of neurofibromatosis type 2 (NF2). Typical abnormalities of this type are tumours arising from brain and nerve root coverings, that is, meningiomas, schwannomas, and ependymomas. Both NF1 and NF2 are autosomal dominant.

Sturge–Weber syndrome

The diagnostic abnormalities of Sturge–Weber syndrome are a port-wine naevus of the skin, usually in the distribution of the ophthalmic nerve, and leptomeningeal angiodysplasia, usually in the occipitoparietal region of the same side. The intracranial abnormality may calcify, and is often associated with atrophy of the underlying brain.

Von Hippel–Lindau disease

Von Hippel–Lindau disease is autosomal dominant; it is characterized by haemangioblastomas of the posterior fossa or spinal cord that may be multiple. Retinal angiomas also occur.

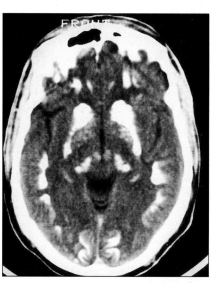

Fig. 8.65 *CT image showing extensive basal ganglia and subcortical calcification caused by hypoparathyroidism.*

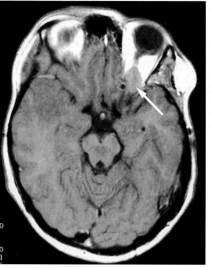

Fig. 8.66 *T1-weighted axial MR image in NF1. There is a glioma of the left optic nerve (arrow). There is also dysplasia of the right greater wing of sphenoid causing asymmetry of the skull base.*

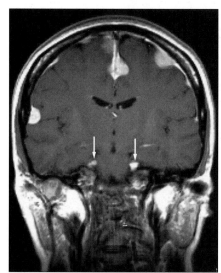

Fig. 8.67 *T1-weighted coronal MR image, after gadolinium, of neurofibromatosis type 2. This patient has bilateral acoustic neuromas (arrows) and multiple meningiomas over the brain convexity and in the interhemispheric fissure.*

Tuberous sclerosis

The clinical features of tuberous sclerosis, an autosomal dominant disease, include facial angiofibromas, epilepsy, and mental handicap. The classical CNS features on imaging are hamartomas, which are usually subependymal or in the white matter; they may calcify.

BENIGN CYSTIC LESIONS
Dermoid

Typically midline in location, dermoids are believed to arise as a result of inclusion of ectodermal tissue during neural tube closure. These lesions contain fat and occur in the spine, suprasella region, floor of the anterior cranial fossa, and posterior fossa (**Fig 8.68**).

Epidermoid

Epidermoids are cystic lesions containing fluid that may be similar to CSF in appearance or contain protein. Typical sites are the cerebellopontine angle, petrous bone (*see* Fig. 9.26), or skull vault.

Arachnoid cyst

Arachnoid cysts have the same imaging appearance as CSF. They usually occur in the sylvian fissure (**Fig. 8.69**), the suprasellar, quadrigeminal or prepontine cisterns, or the cisterna magna.

Colloid cyst

A colloid cysts is a well-defined cyst containing proteinaceous fluid, that occurs at the foramina of Monroe. It results in lateral ventricular hydrocephalus (**Fig. 8.70**).

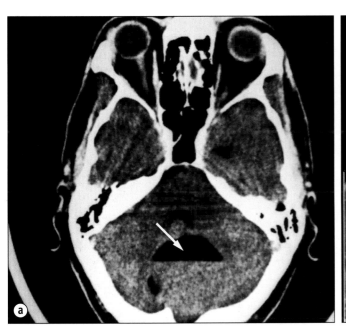
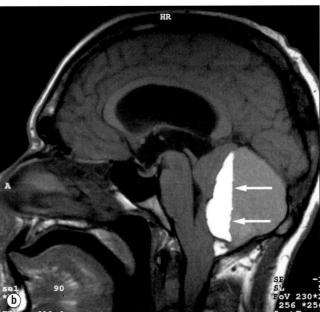

Fig. 8.68 *(a) CT of a posterior fossa dermoid, showing the typical fat contents (arrow). (b) T1-weighted MR image image in the same patient showing a fat–fluid interface (arrows) within the dermoid cyst. The fat appears bright.*

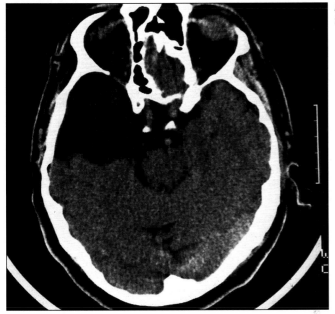

Fig. 8.69 CT of an arachnoid cyst. There is a large CSF space replacing the anterior aspect of the right temporal lobe.

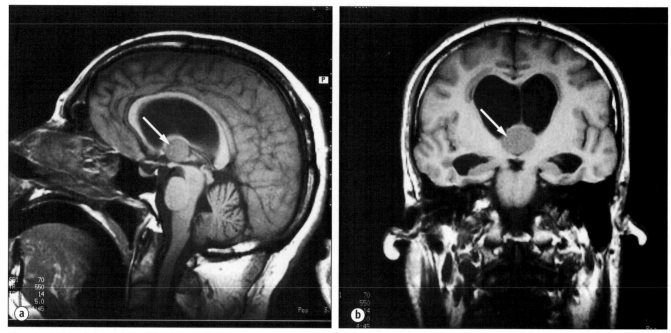

Fig. 8.70 *T1-weighted sagittal MR image (**a**) and T1-weighted coronal MR image (**b**) of a colloid cyst (arrows) that is obstructing the foramina of Monroe and causing lateral ventricular hydrocephalus.*

POSTOPERATIVE APPEARANCES AND INTERVENTIONAL PROCEDURES

Typical imaging appearances after various neurosurgical procedures are illustrated in Figures 8.71–8.75.

Interventional neuroradiology has made possible the treatment of some vascular lesions that were previously either inoperable or associated with considerable operative morbidity. AVMs may be embolized with cyanoacrylate glue (**Fig. 8.76**), and aneurysms may be occluded using detachable metal coils. However, embolization of lesions in the carotid and vertebral territories is a highly skilled procedure, and is not without significant risk. Lesions may not be amenable to embolization because of the arterial or venous anatomy.

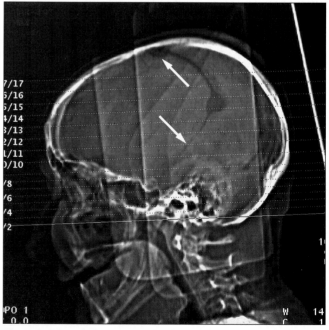

Fig. 8.71 *Lateral CT topogram of the skull showing the appearances of a previous craniotomy (arrows).*

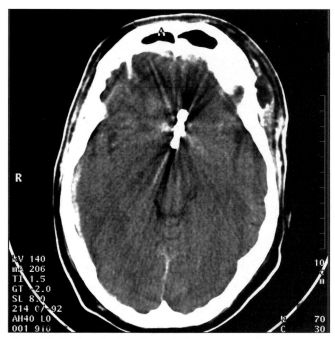

Fig. 8.72 CT after clipping of an anterior communicating aneurysm. The aneurysm clip gives rise to a star artefact.

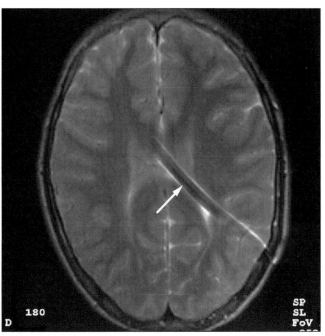

Fig. 8.73 T2-weighted axial MR image showing an intraventricular shunt (arrow) for the treatment of hydrocephalus.

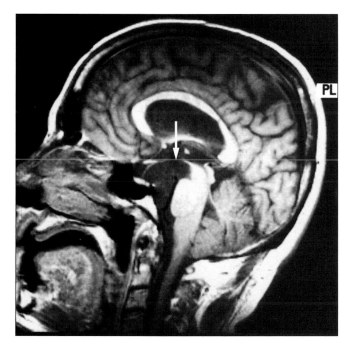

Fig. 8.74 T1-weighted sagittal MR image after third ventriculostomy. A hole is created in the floor of the third ventricle, via an endoscope, for the treatment of hydrocephalus (arrow).

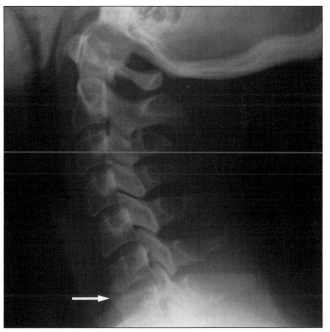

Fig. 8.75 Lateral cervical spine after discectomy and interbody fusion at the C6/7 level (arrow). This procedure is performed for decompression of cervical roots and cord.

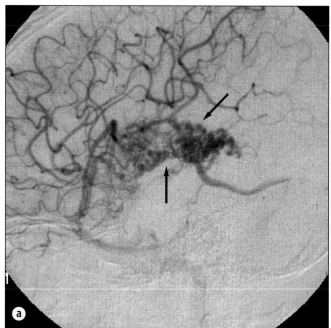

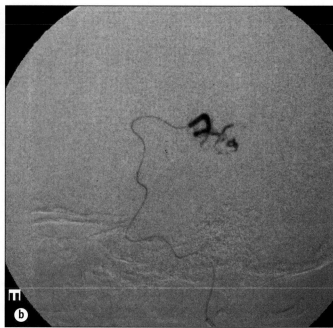

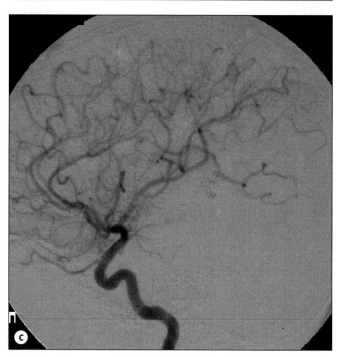

Fig. 8.76 (*a*) *AVM pre-embolization. Right internal carotid angiogram showing a temporoparietal AVM (arrows) filling from branches of the middle cerebral artery with early venous drainage.* (*b*) *Embolization with cyanoacrylate glue; there is a glue cast in the nidus of the AVM.* (*c*) *Post-embolization right internal carotid angiogram showing good obliteration of the AVM.*

chapter 9

Head and Neck

Part 1. Orbits

The imaging modalities used in evaluating orbital pathology are ultrasound, plain films, CT, and MR imaging. Ultrasound is useful for examining the globe, but is limited by cataract and in evaluation of structures posterior to the globe. As in other parts of the body, ultrasound is a dynamic imaging modality that offers better appreciation of pathology during scanning, rather than on isolated images.

CONGENITAL ABNORMALITIES

Absence of the globes (anophthalmia) is rare. Small globes (microphthalmia) are associated with other congenital abnormalities in congenital rubella syndrome, or can occur with persistent hyperplastic primary vitreous or retinopathy of prematurity.

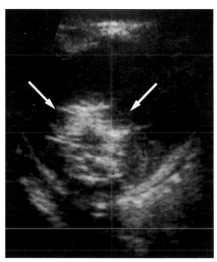

Fig. 9.1 Orbital ultrasound scan of a child with retinoblastoma. There is a mass in the globe that is echogenic, because of calcification (arrows).

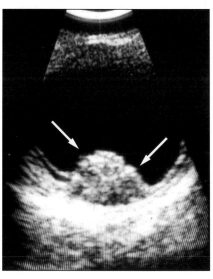

Fig. 9.2 Orbital ultrasound scan of ocular melanoma, showing a mass within the posterior aspect of the globe (arrows).

LESIONS WITHIN THE GLOBE

Retinoblastoma

Retinoblastoma is the most important cause of white pupillary reflex (leucokoria) in a child. These malignant tumours are soft-tissue masses within the globe (**Fig. 9.1**) that may calcify; they are bilateral in 25% of cases. Treatment usually entails enucleation.

Melanoma

The most common ocular tumour in adults is a melanoma (**Fig. 9.2**). Choroidal metastases can have a similar appearance.

Retinal and choroidal detachment

When retinal detachment occurs, fluid accumulates between the sensory retina and the retinal pigment epithelium. Imaging with CT or MRI shows a characteristic V-shaped detachment, with its apex at the optic nerve (**Fig. 9.3**). Subretinal haemorrhage has a similar appearance, but with high-attenuation blood beneath the retina (**Fig. 9.4**). Choroidal detachment occurs after trauma or surgery, or as a result of inflammation. Imaging shows a crescentic lesion in the posterior or lateral aspect of the globe.

Persistent primary hyperplastic vitreous

After retinoblastoma, persistent primary hyperplastic vitreous (PPHV) is the second most common cause of leucokoria. It is caused by persistence of the embryonic hyaloid vascular system. PPHV is associated with microphthalmos, retinal detachment, and vitreous haemorrhage.

Retinopathy of prematurity

Retinopathy of prematurity occurs in premature infants and is believed to be associated with prolonged oxygen therapy. It is associated with PPHV, and the globes may be microphthalmic.

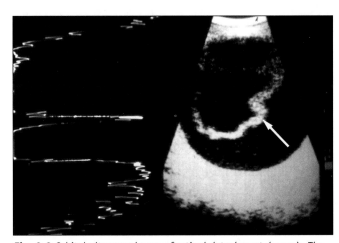

Fig. 9.3 Orbital ultrasound scan of retinal detachment (arrow). The detached retina forms a wavy line, which corresponds to the high-amplitude spike on the A-mode tracing on the left.

Intraocular foreign body

Penetrating injury to the globe occurs particularly among those working with saws and drills, which may project small fragments of wood, metal, or glass into the eye. CT will show most intraocular foreign bodies clearly (**Fig. 9.5**). MR imaging is contraindicated in any patient with a past history of injury that may have left a metal foreign body in the eye, because there is a risk of further ocular injury from movement of such a metal fragment in the magnetic field.

LESIONS OUTSIDE THE GLOBE

Orbital haemangioma

In children, orbital haemangiomas usually occur anterior to the globe,

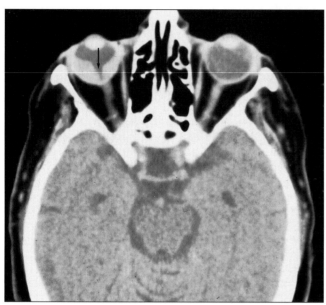

Fig. 9.4 *CT of subretinal haemorrhage. The retina is elevated by high-attenuation blood, forming a V-shape having its apex at the optic disc (small arrow).*

in the superior nasal quadrant, and are capillary haemangiomas. In adults, the most common lesion is the cavernous haemangioma, which occurs posterior to the globe (**Fig. 9.6**) and may calcify. Lymphangiomas and haemangiopericytomas can be indistinguishable on imaging.

Lacrimal gland tumours

Primary tumours of the lacrimal gland are mixed or pleomorphic tumours. The gland can be involved with lymphoma, sarcoidosis, or connective-tissue diseases. In children, dermoid cysts can arise in the lacrimal gland and adjacent orbital wall; they contain fat on CT and may, rarely, have an intracranial extension.

Graves' ophthalmopathy

Graves' ophthalmopathy occurs in patients with Graves' disease of the thyroid, but its activity does not correspond with thyroid status. There is inflammation and oedema of the extraocular muscles, which can lead to optic nerve compression, exophthalmos, and corneal ulceration.

Orbital pseudotumour

The most common cause for an orbital mass in an adult is an orbital pseudotumour, which represents a heterogeneous group of inflammatory disorders. There is a soft-tissue mass, typically involving the retro-orbital fat, extraocular muscles (**Fig. 9.7**), optic nerve, lacrimal gland, or sclera. Lymphoma and Wegener's granulomatosis can have the same appearance on imaging.

Optic nerve lesions

The most common tumours of the optic nerve are meningioma and optic nerve glioma. These may both occur in neurofibromatosis. Other causes of swelling of the optic nerve are optic neuritis (in multiple sclerosis) and sarcoidosis.

Orbital abscess

Orbital abscess occurs as a result of spread of infection from ethmoid sinusitis. Abscess posterior to the globe can be complicated by thrombosis of the ophthalmic vein and cavernous sinus.

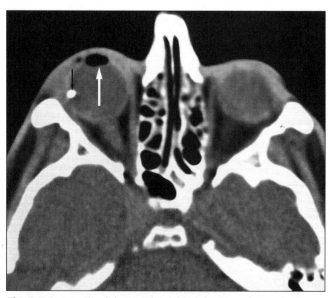

Fig. 9.5 *Penetrating injury to the right globe. There is a metallic foreign body in the lateral aspect of the globe (small arrow), with intraocular gas (large arrow).*

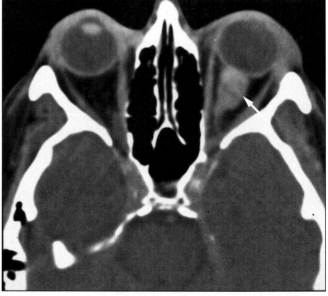

Fig. 9.6 *CT, after contrast, of a cavernous haemangioma posterior to the left globe, demonstrating a well-defined soft-tissue mass (arrow).*

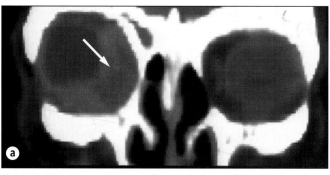
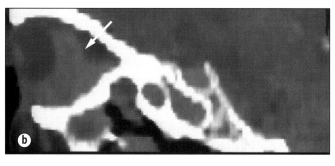

Fig. 9.7 Orbital pseudotumour. Abnormal extraocular soft tissue displacing the right globe superolaterally (arrows) may be seen on both reformatted coronal (*a*) and sagittal (*b*) images.

Part 2. Paranasal sinuses and nose

CONGENITAL ABNORMALITIES

The paranasal sinuses are not pneumatized at birth, and develop gradually during childhood. Hypoplasia is a common normal variant. Abnormalities of the nasal turbinates can predispose to sinus infection.

Choanal atresia

Choanal atresia presents with feeding difficulties in the neonate, caused by obstruction of the posterior nares by a bony septum or membrane. Contrast injected into the nasal cavity confirms the diagnosis.

INFECTION, INFLAMMATORY CONDITIONS, AND ALLERGY

Infection, inflammatory conditions, and allergy constitute the majority of sinus diseases. Most patients with sinusitis never undergo imaging, but if symptoms persist after treatment with antibiotics, decongestants, and topical steroids, imaging is appropriate. Plain film appearances do not correlate with symptoms and are not indicated. CT (**Fig. 9.8**) and MR imaging (**Fig. 9.9**) are the investigations of choice, to document fluid, mucosal thickening, and polyps in the sinuses, to assess the osteomeatal complex (where the maxillary sinus communicates with the nasal cavity), and to exclude other pathology such as tumour.

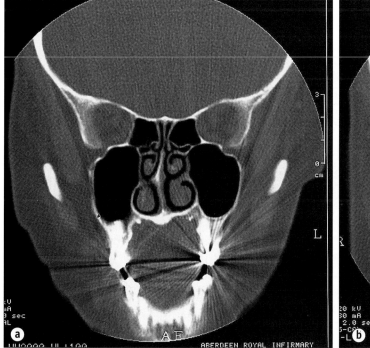
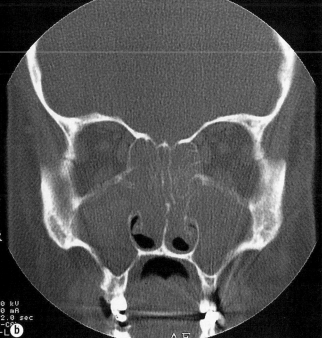

Fig. 9.8 Coronal CT of the paranasal sinuses. (*a*) Normal appearances, with air-filled sinuses.
(*b*) Appearances in pansinusitis, with the frontal, ethmoid, and maxillary sinuses filled with fluid.

Air–fluid interfaces (fluid levels) in the sinuses are seen in acute sinusitis, unless the sinuses are completely fluid-filled, and allergic sinusitis is associated with mucosal polyps; these abnormalities may co-exist in the same patient. Complications of sinusitis include cerebral abscess, subdural empyema, and mucocele, in which secretions accumulate in the sinus, causing bony erosion.

NEOPLASTIC DISEASE

Benign papillomas of the sinuses are rare. It is impossible to differentiate them from malignant tumours on imaging, therefore the two are considered here together.

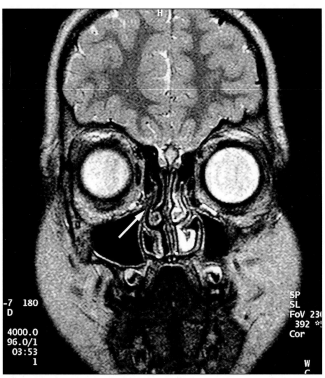

Fig. 9.9 *Coronal T2-weighted MRI of the paranasal sinuses, demonstrating the site of the right osteomeatal complex (arrow).*

Malignant tumours

Epithelial carcinoma is the most common nasal and sinus malignancy. It occurs most often in the maxillary sinus, presenting with pain, epistaxis, and nasal obstruction. CT and MR imaging are the investigations of choice: CT shows bony destruction better (**Fig. 9.10**), whereas MR imaging gives superior demonstration of extension of the tumour into adjacent structures.

Wegener's granulomatosis

The aggressive vasculitic disease known as Wegener's granulomatosis involves the kidneys, lungs, nose, and paranasal sinuses, where it can have a presentation and imaging appearance similar to those of carcinoma.

Cocaine abuse

Abuse of cocaine can result in destruction of the nasal septum.

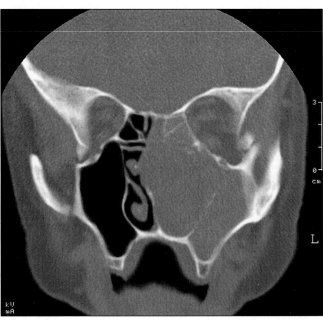

Fig. 9.10 *Coronal CT of a nasal cavity carcinoma. The tumour has arisen in the left side of the nasal cavity, which is filled with soft tissue and expanded. Note the bony destruction and tumour extension into the ethmoid and maxillary sinuses.*

Part 3. Facial skeleton

BONY ABNORMALITIES

Pathology that occurs in other parts of the skeleton, such as metastases, lymphoma (**Fig. 9.11**), and myeloma, may involve the facial bones. Those with a predilection for the facial skeleton are included here.

Osteomas

Osteomas can occur in the walls of the sinuses and are benign, sclerotic lesions (**Fig. 9.12**); they are rarely the cause of obstructive sinusitis.

Fibrous dysplasia

The benign condition of fibrous dysplasia may involve one or more bones in the face, and typically results in an expanded, opaque sinus

that has a 'ground-glass' appearance on plain films or CT (**Fig. 9.13**).

Paget's disease

The maxilla or mandible may be involved in Paget's disease, with expansion and loss of corticomedullary differentiation.

Dental cysts

Dental cysts may occur in the tooth-bearing parts of the maxilla or mandible. They include cysts associated with tooth infection, dentigerous cysts (**Fig. 9.14**), fissurial cysts, and odontogenic keratocysts.

Ameloblastoma

Ameloblastomas are rare, locally invasive tumours that are seen as multiloculated lucencies on plain films (**Fig. 9.15**).

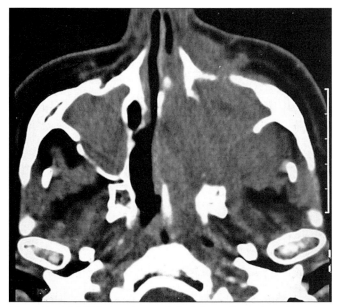

Fig. 9.11 Axial CT in lymphoma of the left maxillary sinus. There is bony destruction, with tumour extending into the soft tissues of the face, nasal cavity, and infratemporal fossa.

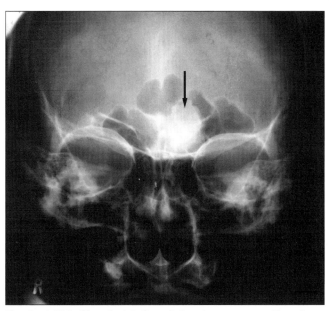

Fig. 9.12 Plain film of a left frontal sinus ivory osteoma. There is a well-defined sclerotic lesion in the left frontal sinus (arrow).

Fig. 9.13 CT of fibrous dysplasia of the right maxilla, which is sclerotic and expanded (arrows).

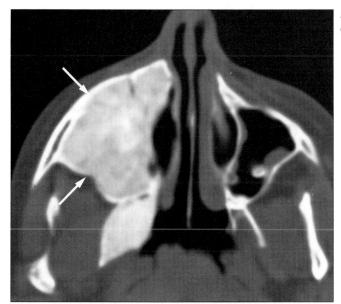

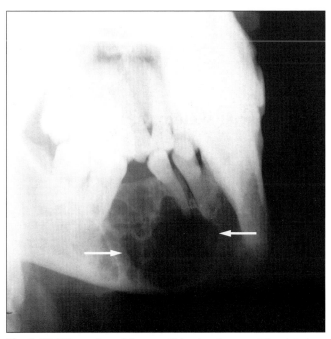

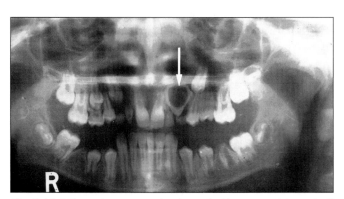

Fig. 9.14 Orthopantomogram, showing a dentigerous cyst (arrow) of the left upper canine.

Fig. 9.15 Oblique view of the mandible, showing a multiloculated lytic lesion caused by an ameloblastoma (arrows).

TRAUMA

Facial trauma is common after road traffic accidents or assault. Injuries to different parts of the face frequently co-exist, and there may be associated brain injury.

Fractures of the facial bones continue to be classified broadly according to the Le Fort system. Le Fort I is a fracture separating the tooth-bearing part of the maxilla from the rest of the maxilla. In Le Fort II, the fracture fragment is pyramidal, with fractures extending through the medial and lateral walls of the maxillary sinuses and through the nasal bones. With a Le Fort III injury, the facial skeleton is completely separated from the rest of the skull, with fractures through the medial and lateral walls of the orbits and through the zygomatic arches. In practice, any patient may have multiple facial fractures, with different types of fracture co-existing (**Fig. 9.16**).

Apart from a fracture, other signs of injury to the facial skeleton are fluid in the maxillary sinuses (**Fig. 9.16**), and gas in the orbital soft tissues, which is called orbital emphysema (**Fig. 9.17**).

Orbital fractures

Fractures involving the orbital walls can distort the orbital contents and cause rupture of the globe, with intraocular haemorrhage (**Fig. 9.18**). Herniation of orbital contents through an orbital floor fracture can cause diplopia; this is most often the result of herniation of orbital fat (**Fig. 9.19**) and fibrosis around the inferior rectus muscle, and rarely caused by herniation of the inferior rectus itself.

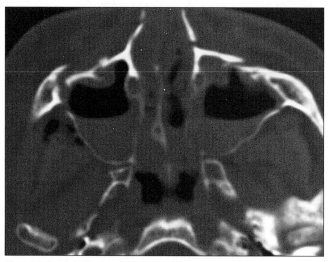

Fig. 9.16 Axial CT of facial trauma. There are multiple fractures of the nasal bones, and of the anterior and lateral walls of both maxillary sinuses, which contain fluid.

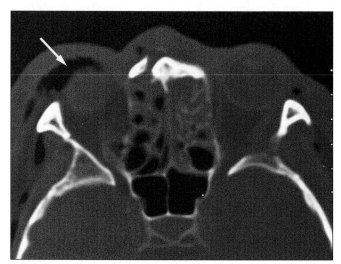

Fig. 9.17 Axial CT after facial trauma, demonstrating right orbital emphysema (arrow).

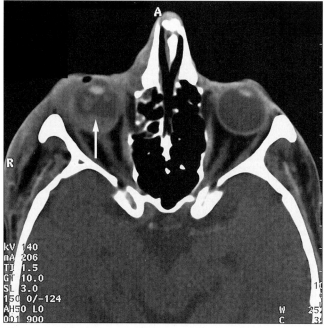

Fig. 9.18 Axial CT after orbital trauma. There has been haemorrhage into the vitreous (arrow) and rupture of the right globe.

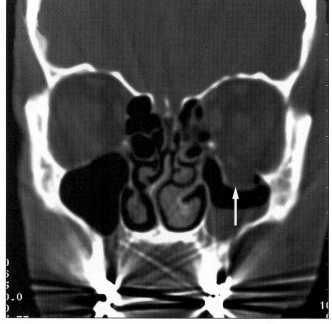

Fig. 9.19 Coronal CT after orbital trauma. There has been a fracture of the floor of the left orbit, with herniation of orbital fat into the left maxilla (arrow); maxillary fluid is also evident.

Zygomatic fractures

The zygoma is analogous to a four-legged table, having processes to the lateral and inferior walls of the orbit, the lateral wall of the maxillary sinus, and the zygomatic arch. A fracture of any one of these is often associated with fractures of the other components (**Fig. 9.20**).

Fractures of the mandible

Fractures of the mandible usually involve the body, the angle or, most commonly, the condylar neck. Those that extend into tooth sockets are compound.

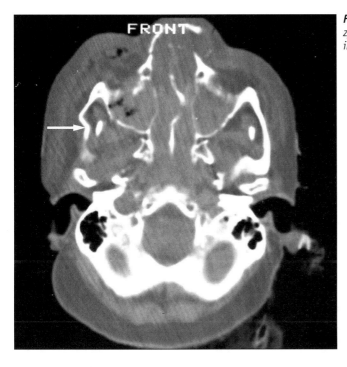

Fig. 9.20 *Multiple facial fractures, including a fracture of the right zygoma that involves the zygomatic arch (arrow) and the lateral and inferior walls of the orbit.*

Part 4. Skull base, petrous temporal bone, and temporomandibular joints

CONGENITAL ABNORMALITIES

Congenital abnormalities of the outer and middle ear may co-exist, and can occur as part of first or second branchial arch dysplasias (**Fig. 9.21**).

Abnormalities of the inner ear comprise a separate group of disorders. High-resolution, fine-section CT of the petrous temporal bones will demonstrate structural abnormalities of the inner ear in 20% of children with congenital sensorineural deafness. The most common imaging abnormality is Mondini's malformation, which is hypoplasia of the cochlea, with absence of the basal turn.

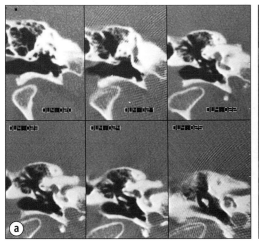
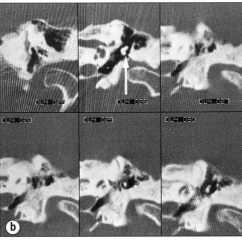

Fig. 9.21 *CT of the petrous bones in congenital aplasia of the left external auditory canal. Coronal reconstructions show no external auditory canal, and hypoplasia of the middle ear cleft and ossicles (arrow) on the left (**b**), compared with the normal right side (**a**).*

TRAUMA

An air–fluid interface in the sphenoid sinus on a lateral skull radiograph, taken with a horizontal X-ray beam and the patient lying supine, should raise the suspicion of a base of skull fracture. The fracture itself is often not seen on plain films; CT is the best investigation.

Most base of skull fractures involve the petrous temporal bone. They are described as longitudinal, which can be associated with conductive deafness (**Fig. 9.22**), or transverse, which can be associated with sensorineural deafness, vertigo, and facial nerve palsy. Clinically, there may be cerebrospinal fluid (CSF) or blood leaking from the external auditory meatus.

INFECTION AND INFLAMMATORY CONDITIONS

Acute otitis media and mastoiditis

Imaging is not indicated in acute otitis media and mastoiditis, unless there is concern of complications such as cerebral abscess or venous sinus thrombosis. Petrous apicitis may complicate acute otitis media if there is pneumatization of the petrous apex. This is best seen on T2-weighted MR imaging (**Fig. 9.23**).

Chronic otitis media and mastoiditis

Chronic inflammatory disease of the petrous bone is the result of Eustachian tube dysfunction. The following complications may arise:

Cholesterol granuloma occurs anywhere from the middle ear cavity to the petrous apex. It contains cholesterol and blood products, and is bright on T1- and T2-weighted MR imaging.

Acquired cholesteatoma occurs as a result of ingrowths of squamous epithelium from the tympanic membrane into the middle ear. A soft-tissue mass forms that erodes either the scutum, epitympanic recess, and into the mastoid antrum, or the ossicles (**Fig. 9.24**).

TUMOURS AND TUMOUR-LIKE LESIONS

Acoustic neuroma

The 8th cranial nerve is the most common site for benign tumours of cranial nerves; after meningioma, these are the second most common extra-axial tumour. If bilateral, they indicate neurofibromatosis type 2. Acoustic neuromas occur anywhere from the

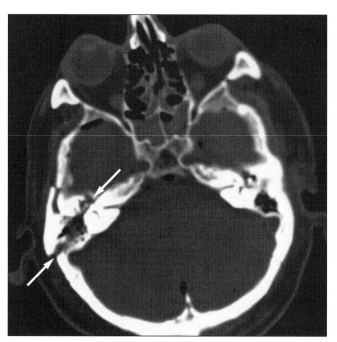

Fig. 9.22 *Axial CT after head injury, showing a longitudinal fracture (arrows) of the right petrous temporal bone.*

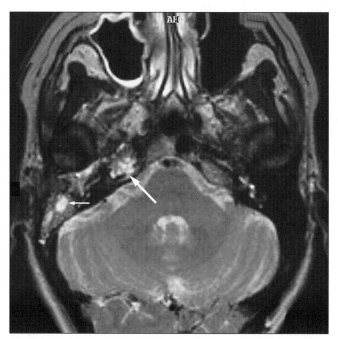

Fig. 9.23 *Axial T2-weighted MR image of the petrous bone in right petrous apicitis. There is high signal in the right petrous apex (large arrow), and right mastoiditis (small arrow).*

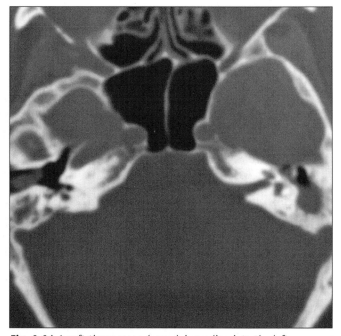

Fig. 9.24 *A soft-tissue mass (arrow) is eroding into the left epitympanic recess; this is an acquired cholesteatoma.*

cerebellopontine angle to the lateral end of the internal acoustic meatus. They are best seen on T1-weighted MR imaging after gadolinium contrast (**Fig. 9.25**). Other lesions that can occur in the cerebellopontine angle are meningiomas (*see* Fig. 8.46), epidermoids, schwannomas of other cranial nerves, and brainstem tumours.

Epidermoid

Epidermoids are also known as congenital cholesteatomas. They are usually of intensity similar to that of CSF, and show no contrast enhancement. They can occur in the cerebellopontine angle (**Fig. 9.26**), or in the petrous bone.

Glomus tumour

Glomus tumours are also termed paragangliomas; they can occur in the jugular bulb (glomus jugulare) or on the cochlear promontory (glomus tympanicum), and are occasionally bilateral (**Fig. 9.27**). They are vascular soft-tissue masses that cause local bony erosion. Their blood supply is from branches of the external carotid artery; thus their embolization before operation can reduce operative blood loss. On MR images, they have a typical 'salt and pepper' appearance, with alternating foci of high and low signal.

Other lesions that can simulate a glomus tympanicum include an anatomically high jugular bulb, congenital variants of the carotid artery, and cholesterol granuloma.

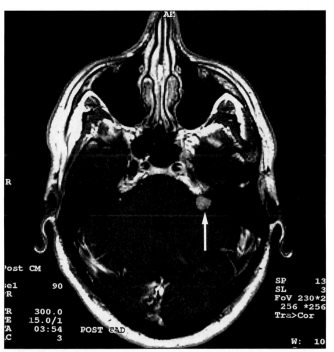

Fig. 9.25 *Axial T1-weighted MR image, after gadolinium, showing a left acoustic neuroma (arrow).*

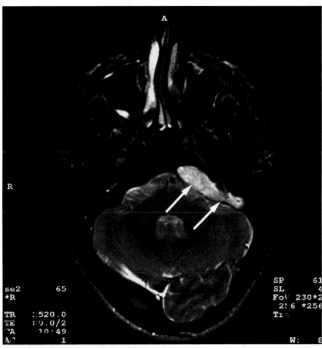

Fig. 9.26 *T2-weighted axial MR image showing a left petrous-bone epidermoid (arrows).*

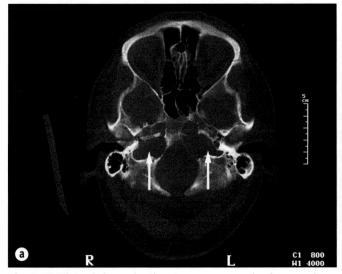

Fig. 9.27 *Bilateral glomus jugulare tumours are causing bony erosion, revealed on CT (**a**; arrows), and show heterogeneous high signal on coronal T1-weighted MR image after gadolinium (**b**; arrows).*

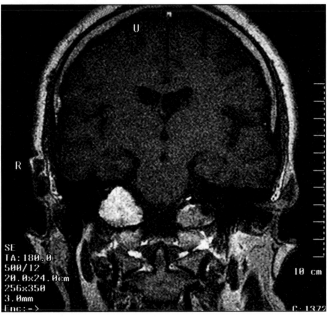

Malignant bone tumours

Metastases are the most common cause of bony destruction of the skull base. Chordoma is a primary malignant tumour of the clivus (that can also occur at the sacrum), which arises from remnants of the notocord (**Fig. 9.28**). Chondrosarcoma is a rare tumour, but has a predilection for the petrous apex.

TEMPOROMANDIBULAR JOINTS

In common with any synovial joint in the body, the temporomandibular joints can be affected by arthropathies such as rheumatoid arthritis. The most common abnormality is termed 'temporomandibular dysfunction' and is caused by displacement of the intra-articular disc during mouth opening. This is best demonstrated on oblique sagittal MR imaging, with the mouth first open and then closed (**Fig. 9.29**).

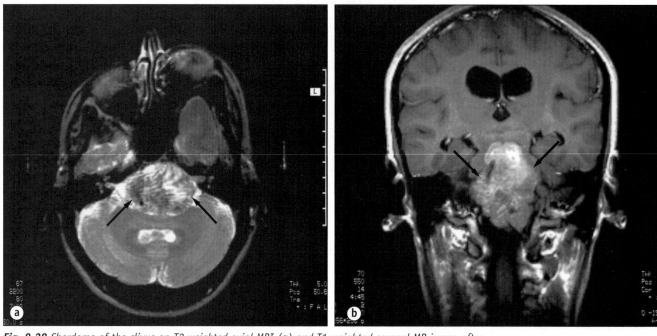

Fig. 9.28 *Chordoma of the clivus on T2-weighted axial MRI (**a**) and T1-weighted coronal MR image after gadolinium (**b**). There is a large extra-axial tumour compressing the pons (arrows).*

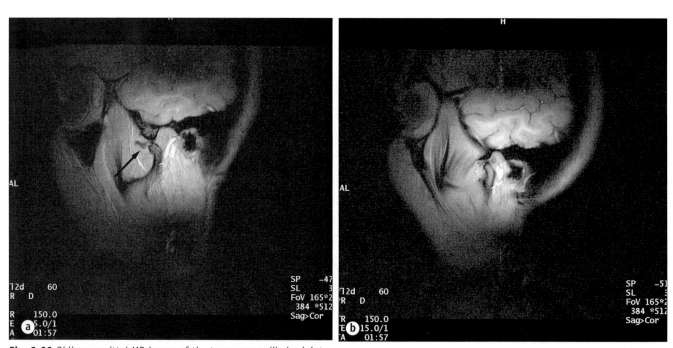

Fig. 9.29 *Oblique sagittal MR image of the temporomandibular joint. (**a**) Mouth open. (**b**) Attempted mouth-closed position. There is anterior displacement of the intra-articular disc (arrow), which prevents normal reduction of the mandibular condyle.*

Part 5. Salivary glands

INFECTION AND INFLAMMATORY CONDITIONS

Any infection of the salivary glands, whether bacterial or viral, may cause stricture formation, which tends to predispose to recurrent infection, calculus formation, and sialectasis (dilatation of the salivary ducts) (**Fig. 9.30**). Patients with human immunodeficiency virus may present with cervical lymphadenopathy and multiple AIDS-related parotid cysts. Mumps is the most common inflammatory disease to affect the glands, particularly the parotid; it may lead to sialectasis.

About 80% of calculi, most of which are radio-opaque, occur in the submandibular duct (**Fig. 9.31**), with the remainder mainly in the parotid duct. Sialography of the parotid or submandibular gland, with cannulation of the duct, is the method of choice for demonstrating duct abnormalities.

Sjögren's syndrome

An autoimmune connective-tissue disorder may result in exocrine failure of the parotid gland, producing a dry mouth. If the disease is limited to the salivary glands, it is termed Sjögren's syndrome. The syndrome also occurs as part of other connective-tissue disorders such as rheumatoid arthritis, Reiter's disease, and scleroderma.

Other inflammatory conditions

The term 'Mikulicz's syndrome' should be reserved to describe salivary and lacrimal gland involvement by sarcoidsosis or, rarely, by tuberculosis or lymphoma.

Heerfordt's syndrome comprises enlarged parotid lymph nodes, facial nerve paralysis, and uveitis; again this condition is caused by sarcoidosis.

A ranula is a retention cyst in the floor of the mouth. It is caused by obstruction of the submandibular gland, and is usually found in children.

NEOPLASTIC DISEASE

Benign tumours

Pleomorphic adenomas account for approximately 70% of all salivary gland tumours, both benign and malignant. On CT or MR imaging (**Fig. 9.32**), the tumour is a well-defined, solid lesion, usually in the periphery of the parotid gland; it may be of considerable size. These slow-growing tumours are common in the 40–60 year age group.

Warthin tumours have the histological appearance of papillary cystadenomas. They occur more commonly in males, may be multiple and bilateral, and are confined essentially to the parotid gland.

Malignant tumours

Mucoepidermoid carcinoma is uncommon in comparison with benign tumours but, despite its slow growth, carries a poor prognosis. It may occur in any of the salivary glands (**Fig. 9.33**), including the minor ones. If it occurs in the parotid gland, it may be associated with facial nerve paralysis.

Adenoid cystic carcinoma is a malignant tumour that is more common in minor salivary glands and the lacrimal gland.

Both primary and secondary lymphoma of the salivary glands are rare but, as the parotid gland contains lymph nodes, systemic lymphoma may produce a lymph-node mass within the gland itself.

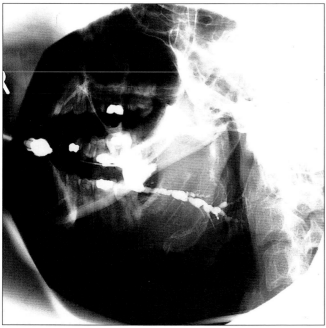

Fig. 9.30 *Parotid sialogram, showing multiple postinflammatory strictures, and sialectasis (dilatation of the salivary ducts).*

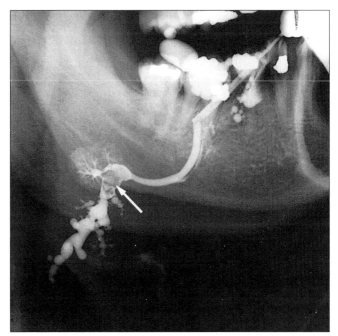

Fig. 9.31 *Submandibular sialogram, showing a large calculus (arrow) obstructing Wharton's duct, with distal sialectasis.*

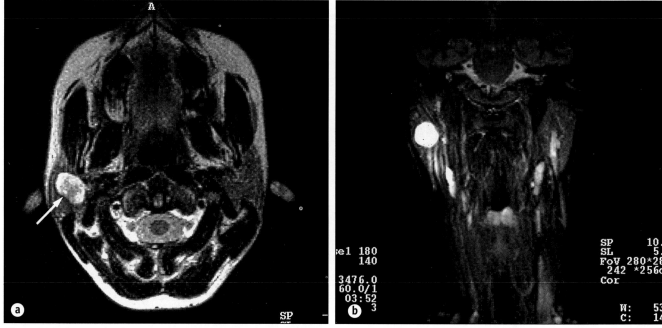

Fig. 9.32 *Right parotid pleomorphic adenoma.* **a:** *T2-weighted axial MR image.* **b:** *STIR coronal MR image. The tumour is well-defined and of high signal intensity (arrow).*

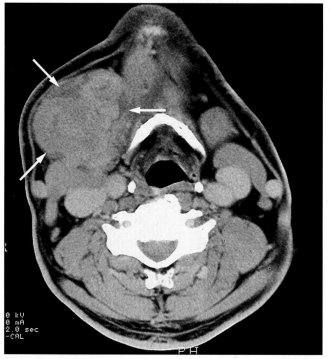

Fig. 9.33 *Axial CT of a large submandibular mucoepidermoid carcinoma (arrows).*

Part 6. Nasopharynx

CONGENITAL ABNORMALITIES

Thornwaldt's cyst is a rare remnant of a pharyngeal bursa; it is seen as a soft-tissue mass in the upper posterior wall of the nasopharynx. Rare midline germ-cell dermoid tumours may present at birth, are more common in females, and may be accompanied by a defect in the skull base.

INFECTION

The pharynx contains lymphoid tissue in the tonsils and adenoids; in children, this tissue is a frequent site of infection, resulting in blockage of the Eustachian tubes and subsequent otitis media.

An abscess in the pharynx usually results from tonsillar infection extending into the parapharyngeal space, or spinal infection into the retropharyngeal space (*see* Fig. 8.24). Penetration by a foreign object such as a fish bone (**Fig. 9.34**) may cause serious soft-tissue infection and a retropharyngeal abscess (**Fig. 9.35**).

NEOPLASTIC DISEASE

Benign tumours

Juvenile nasopharyngeal angiofibroma

Juvenile nasopharyngeal angiofibroma is a rare, highly vascular tumour that principally affects boys aged between 7 and 17 years. It

originates in the superior, posterolateral wall close to the sphenopalatine foramen, and presents as a polypoid nasal mass. Although the lesion is benign, it is locally aggressive and can erode bone (**Fig. 9.36**). As the tumour is highly vascular, external carotid angiography and tumour embolization are often performed before surgery (**Fig. 9.37**). There is recurrence if surgical excision is incomplete.

Malignant tumours

Malignant tumours involving the nasopharynx include metastases, sarcomas, lymphomas, melanomas, plasmacytoma, and adenocarcinoma.

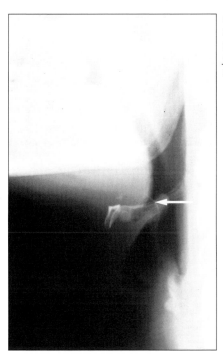

Fig. 9.34 *Lateral soft-tissue radiograph of the neck, showing a fish bone stuck in the epiglottis (arrow).*

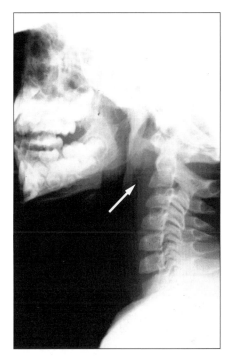

Fig. 9.35 *Retropharyngeal abscess in a child. Note the swelling of the retropharyngeal tissues, which contain gas (arrow).*

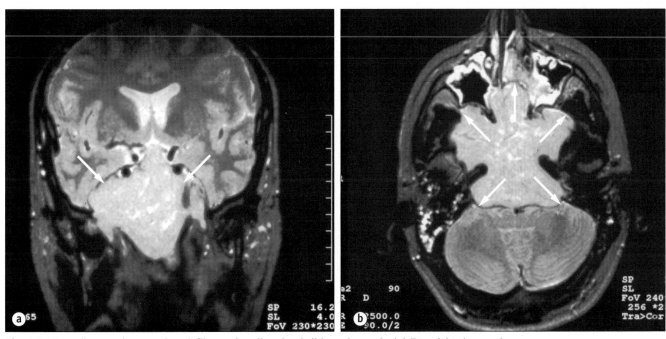

Fig. 9.36 *Juvenile nasopharyngeal angiofibroma invading the skull base (arrows). (**a**) T2-weighted coronal MR image. (**b**) T2-weighted axial MR image.*

Nasopharyngeal carcinoma

Nasopharyngeal carcinomas are common in Chinese patients. The tumours, 80% of which are of squamous cell origin, frequently arise in the lateral pharyngeal recess or fossa of Rosenmuller. CT or MR imaging show the detail of the tumour, its local extent, and any lymphatic spread to the neck through the parapharyngeal space. Bone invasion into the clivus and petrous temporal bones occurs in the late stages of the disease.

Rhabdomyosarcoma

Forty per cent of rhabdomyosarcomas arise in the head and neck, frequently in the orbit and nasopharynx, but also affecting the sinuses, ear, and neck. They originate in the mesenchyme, and can metastasize. This tumour is one of the most common sarcomas in children.

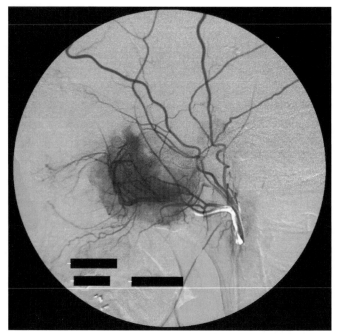

Fig. 9.37 *External carotid digital subtraction angiogram in the same patient as in Figure 9.36. This juvenile nasopharyngeal angiofibroma is a highly vascular tumour, with an intense vascular blush.*

Part 7. Oropharynx

NEOPLASTIC DISEASE

Benign tumours

A dermoid cyst is a midline, embryonic germ-cell tumour that may arise in the submandibular area, the sublingual area, or the floor of the mouth. The patient may not present until their second or third decade of life.

Other tumours include lipomas, which may also develop in the floor of the mouth and—most common of all oropharyngeal masses—the haemangioma/lymphangioma (**Fig. 9.38**).

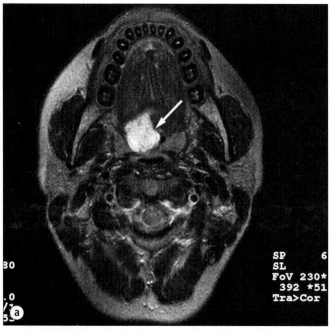

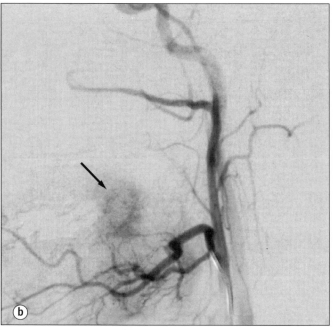

Fig. 9.38 *(a) T2-weighted axial MR image of a haemangioma of the right posterior aspect of the tongue (arrow). (b) Lateral external carotid digital subtraction angiography of the patient shows a vascular blush (arrow), which is supplied by the lingual artery.*

Malignant tumours
Squamous-cell carcinoma
Squamous-cell carcinoma accounts for more than 90% of all oral and oropharyngeal tumours. Men in their 60s and 70s are most affected, and there is an increased risk in heavy smokers and drinkers. Local spread occurs into the tongue, the mandible, and the lateral walls of the oropharynx. There is early lymphatic spread: more than 50% of cases have involved nodes at the time of presentation.

Lymphoma
Deposits of non-Hodgkin's lymphoma can affect the oropharynx, principally in the palatine tonsils.

Part 8. Hypopharynx

CONGENITAL ABNORMALITIES

Thyroglossal cysts
Most thyroglossal duct cysts arise in the midline between the hyoid and the thyroid. They result from the movement of the thyroid from its initial developmental site at the base of the tongue, into the neck during fetal development. A sinus may persist along this line of descent and can be demonstrated by a sinogram (Fig. 9.39).

Cystic hygroma
Cystic hygromas are multiple, dilated cystic lymphatic channels, often found posteriorly in the neck, and sometimes related to other congenital anomalies.

Branchial cleft cysts
Although present at birth, most branchial cysts do not present until adulthood. They are embryonic remnants of the parapharyngeal pouch system; 95% of these cysts relate to the second branchial cleft, and therefore extend from the lower pole of the parotid gland inferiorly to the anterior border of the sternomastoid muscle (Fig. 9.40). First branchial cleft cysts occur between the external auditory meatus and the angle of the mandible. The cysts may become infected and develop a fistulous tract.

NEOPLASTIC DISEASE

Malignant tumours
Squamous cell carcinoma originating in the hypopharynx may be associated with the Paterson–Kelly–Brown (Plummer–Vinson) syndrome, which comprises a postcricoid web, dysphagia, iron-deficiency anaemia, and weight loss. Spread occurs locally into the parapharyngeal space and anteriorly into the larynx, with early lymphatic involvement to the jugulodigastric nodes. This syndrome often affects middle-aged women.

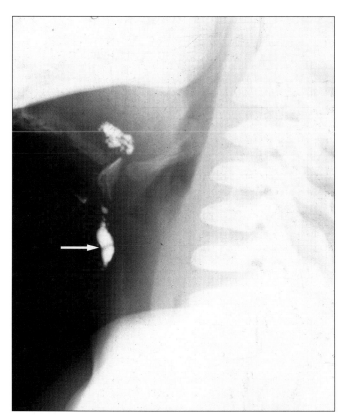

Fig. 9.39 Sinogram of a thyroglossal sinus. Contrast outlines a track from the base of the tongue to the level of the thyroid (arrow).

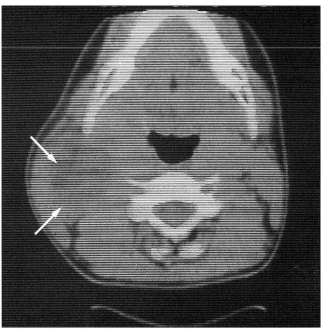

Fig. 9.40 Axial CT of the neck, showing a right branchial cyst arising from the second branchial cleft. The cyst is well defined and lies deep to the right sternomastoid muscle (arrows).

MISCELLANEOUS CONDITIONS

Pharyngeal pouch

A pharyngeal pouch (Zenker's diverticulum) results from weakness of the wall between the fibres of the middle and inferior constrictor muscles, combined with abnormal cricopharyngeus muscle tone. The pressure in the upper aerodigestive tract as a result of spasm of the cricopharyngeus contributes to the production of this diverticulum (**Fig. 9.41**).

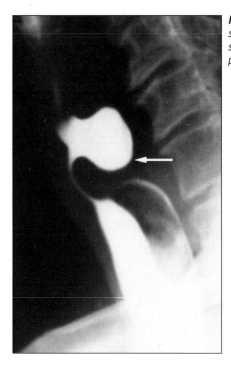

Fig. 9.41 *Barium swallow examination, showing a pharyngeal pouch (arrow).*

Part 9. Thyroid and parathyroid glands

Ultrasound, CT, MR, and radionuclide imaging are all used in evaluating diseases of the thyroid and parathyroid glands. Ultrasound is useful initially, to determine if a lump is solid or cystic, and to guide aspiration and biopsy. Radionuclide imaging is an important source of functional information.

CONGENITAL ABNORMALITIES

Thyroglossal duct cyst is considered on page 217.

Ectopic thyroid

Functionally thyroid tissue can occur from the tongue inferiorly, or can lie lateral to the thyroid gland. Such an ectopic thyroid can present as a lump at the base of the tongue or in the neck. Its nature is best shown with radionuclide imaging.

INFLAMMATORY CONDITIONS

Grave's disease

Grave's disease is an autoimmune disease that results in hyperthyroidism and a diffusely enlarged thyroid, characterized by increased uptake on a radionuclide scan. It is associated with dysthyroid eye disease, although disease activity in the orbits does not always parallel thyroid disease activity.

Hashimoto's thyroiditis

Lymphocytic infiltration in the autoimmune disease, Hashimoto's thyroiditis, causes swelling and tenderness of the thyroid. This condition is a common cause of hypothyroidism, and may co-exist with other autoimmune diseases and with thyroid lymphoma. Radionuclide imaging shows patchy, reduced uptake.

DeQuervain's thyroiditis

The subacute DeQuervain's thyroiditis is associated with upper respiratory tract viral infections. Ultrasound shows a hypoechoic thyroid in acute stages, with patchy uptake on radionuclide imaging.

Riedel's thyroiditis

Riedel's thyroiditis is rare. It results in fibrosis of the thyroid, with fibrous tissue extending into adjacent structures. MR imaging can differentiate this from other forms of thyroiditis.

NEOPLASTIC DISEASE

Benign tumours

Multinodular goitre

Patients with multinodular goitre are usually hypothyroid. Ultrasound shows multiple cystic and solid areas, and radionuclide imaging shows multiple hot and cold areas in an enlarged gland (**Fig. 9.42**).

Thyroid adenoma

Thyroid adenoma may be functioning (giving a hot spot on radionuclide imaging) or non-functioning (giving a cold spot). Thyroid cysts probably represent necrotic adenomas, and may contain solid components (**Fig. 9.43**). Biopsy of non-functioning lesions is required, as they must be distinguished from thyroid cancer.

Malignant tumours

Thyroid carcinoma

The most common thyroid carcinoma is papillary carcinoma, which accounts for 60–80% of all thyroid cancers; follicular and anaplastic carcinomas are less common. Presentation is with a thyroid mass, and radionuclide imaging is the most useful investigation; thyroid cancers are usually 'cold'. However, imaging is not tissue-specific and biopsy is required. CT and MR imaging are important in assessing spread beyond the thyroid, to cervical lymph nodes and distant metastases (*see* Fig. 10.25). Whole-body radionuclide studies with iodine-131 can be used to locate distant metastases.

Medullary carcinoma

Medullary carcinoma arises in the C cells and can occur alone or as part of a multiple endocrine adenopathy syndrome. These tumours may calcify.

Thyroid lymphoma

There is usually a history of previous Hashimoto's thyroiditis in patients with thyroid lymphoma. The tumour is 'cold' on radionuclide imaging with iodine, but 'hot' with gallium.

Parathyroid carcinoma

Parathyroid carcinoma is rare and usually results in hyperparathyroidism; however, only 1–2% of those with hyperparathyroidism have an underlying carcinoma. Imaging is non-specific, and the diagnosis is confirmed only on biopsy or by the presence of invasion into adjacent structures.

HYPERTHYROIDISM

Hyperthyroidism can be caused by Grave's disease, toxic multinodular goitre (**Fig. 9.42**), or a toxic adenoma.

HYPERPARATHYROIDISM

Hyperparathyroidism may be caused by hyperplasia or adenoma of a parathyroid gland, rarely by a carcinoma. Imaging is difficult because of the small size of the glands, and surgical exploration of the neck may be required. Radionuclude imaging using thallium-201 (taken up by thyroid and parathyroid) and iodine-123 (taken up only by thyroid) in a subtraction technique is superior to other imaging modalities (**Fig. 9.44**).

Other manifestations of hyperparathyroidism, such as renal calculi and bony abnormalities, can be seen on plain films.

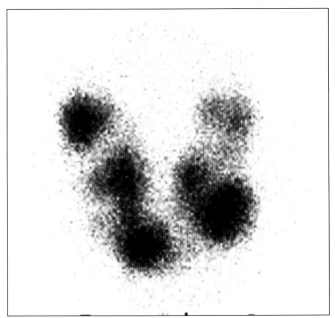

Fig. 9.42 *Radionuclide thyroid scan in a patient with multinodular goitre. The thyroid is enlarged, with patchy increased and decreased uptake.*

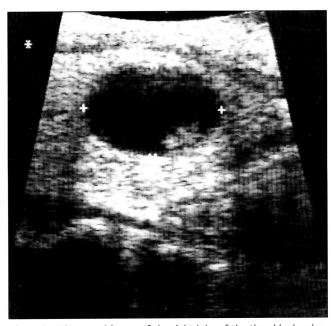

Fig. 9.43 *Ultrasound image of the right lobe of the thyroid, showing a cyst (crosses) that has a small, solid component posteriorly.*

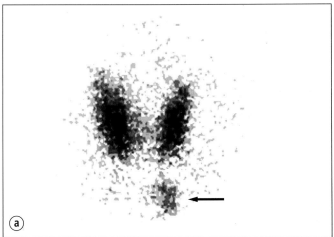

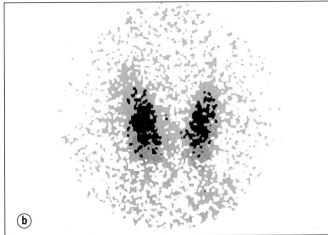

Fig. 9.44 *Radionuclide parathyroid imaging using (**a**) thallium-201 and (**b**) iodine-123 in a subtraction technique. There is a left parathyroid adenoma (arrow), which takes up thallium, but not iodine.*

Part 10. Neck

ANATOMICAL COMPARTMENTS OF THE NECK

A description of the important 'spaces' that occur in the neck is helpful in the understanding of the contents of a particular space and the spread of disease within that space.

Parapharyngeal space

The parapharyngeal space (PPS) extends from the skull base to the great cornu of the hyoid, and is deep to the mandible and parotid glands. It is bordered laterally by the carotid and masticator spaces, posteriorly by the paravertebral muscles, and medially by the tonsillar fossa and the superior constrictor muscle (**Fig. 9.45**).

Infections in the PPS can arise from the teeth, tonsils, nose, paranasal sinuses, external ear, and mastoid. Benign tumours include neurofibromas and the minor salivary gland tumours (*see* page 213). Most malignant tumours in the PPS are metastatic, from oral and oropharyngeal primaries. MR imaging is the best method of showing the lymphatic spread of these tumours in the neck (**Fig. 9.46**).

Carotid space

The carotid space extends from the skull base to the aortic arch. It is bounded by the PPS anteriorly, the parotid space laterally, the pre-vertebral space posteriorly, and the retropharyngeal space medially. Its contents are the carotid artery, internal jugular vein, cranial nerves, sympathetic plexus, and lymphatic vessels and nodes. Benign tumours that affect the carotid space, such as schwannomas and neurofibromas, arise from the neural tissue; paragangliomas, such as the glomus tumour and carotid body tumour, have their origin in the neural crest (**Fig. 9.47**).

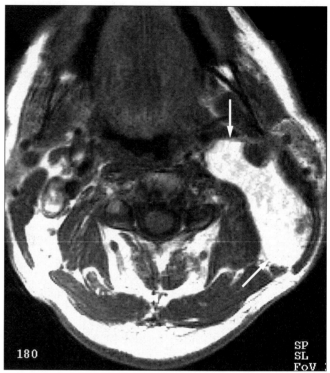

Fig. 9.45 *T1-weighted axial MR image of the neck, showing a left parapharyngeal lipoma. Note the high-signal fatty tissue (arrows) in the left parapharyngeal space.*

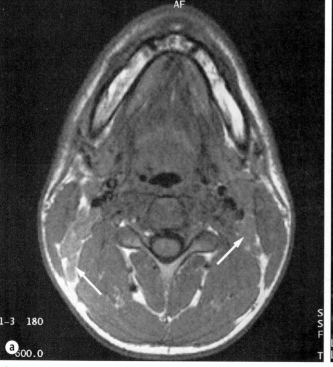
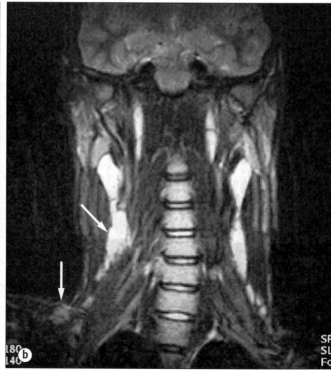

Fig. 9.46 *(a) Axial T1-weighted MR image of the neck, showing lymphadenopathy in the posterior triangles bilaterally (arrows). (b) STIR coronal MR image, on which the lymphadenopathy returns high signal (arrows).*

Masticator space

Attachments to the deep cervical fascia define the boundaries of the masticator space. The superficial suprazygomatic portion was previously known as the temporal fossa, and the deep nasopharyngeal portion as the infratemporal fossa. Infiltration of the masticator space by pharyngeal carcinomas is common.

Prevertebral space

The prevertebral space extends from the neck to the coccyx, and contains the prevertebral and paraspinal muscles. In the neck, it is enclosed by the deep layer of the deep cervical fascia.

Retropharyngeal space

The retropharyngeal space space extends from the skull base to the third thoracic vertebra and contains fat and retropharyngeal nodes only. The visceral fascia lies anterior to this space, and the deep fascia posteriorly.

Posterior cervical space

The posterior cervical space lies behind the carotid space and between the deep layers of the cervical fascia. It contains fat, lymph nodes, vessels, and the brachial plexus.

LYMPHADENOPATHY IN THE NECK

Neck nodes are seen commonly in clinical practice. The major causes include metastatic carcinoma, lymphoma, and inflammatory conditions.

The metastatic carcinomas originate from oral and pharyngeal primary tumours.

Non-Hodgkin's lymphoma is more common in the neck than Hodgkin's disease. It is often bilateral, and tends primarily to affect the middle and lower groups of nodes; lone involvement of the upper groups is rare.

Inflammatory conditions implicated in pathological nodes of the neck include tuberculosis, AIDS-related infection, and sarcoidosis.

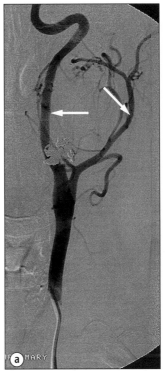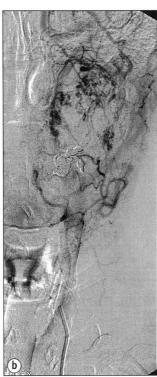

Fig. 9.47 *Left common carotid digital subtraction angiogram in a patient with a carotid body tumour. (**a**) The early arterial phase shows displacement of the proximal internal and external carotid arteries (arrows) because of the tumour. (**b**) Late arterial imaging shows a pathological circulation within this highly vascular tumour. There is artefact from metallic dental fillings.*

Part 11. Larynx

CONGENITAL ABNORMALITIES

Underdevelopment of the larynx or microlarynx may present in infancy, with stridor. Congenital weakness of the laryngeal ventricle may result in the development of an air-filled diverticulum—a laryngocele—which is classified as internal or external, depending on its relationship to the thyroid cartilage (**Fig. 9.48**). Congenital laryngeal polyps also occur.

TRAUMA

Direct injury to the larynx may be penetrating by sharp objects, such as occurs in stabbing, by blunt trauma, as in road traffic accidents, or by strangulation; it often results in haemorrhage that may be fatal. Damage to the larynx and upper trachea, with inflammation, oedema, and fibrosis, may also result from long-term endotracheal intubation. CT is the best method of assessing the anatomy of the larynx and any injury to it (**Fig. 9.49**).

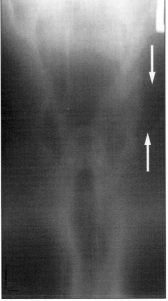

Fig. 9.48 *Coronal laryngeal tomogram, showing a left external laryngocele (arrows).*

NEOPLASTIC DISEASE

Benign tumours

Benign tumours in the larynx are uncommon compared with malignant lesions. Laryngeal papillomas can arise in children as a result of viral infection; those that occur in adults may be a premalignant condition.

Malignant tumours

More than 60% of laryngeal carcinomas arise from the anterior two-thirds of the true vocal cords. Supraglottic carcinomas arise above this level, from the epiglottis, ventricle, false cords, and aryepiglottic folds. Subglottic lesions arise from the undersurface of the true vocal cords, and may extend into the subglottic space of the upper trachea. CT and MR imaging can be used to stage laryngeal tumours, assessing their local invasion and lymph-node spread (**Fig. 9.50**), both of which have important implications for the type of treatment advisable and the prognosis.

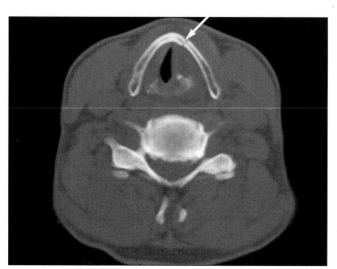

Fig. 9.49 *Axial CT through the larynx of a kick boxer after trauma, showing a fracture of the thyroid cartilage (arrow), with swelling of the left vocal cord.*

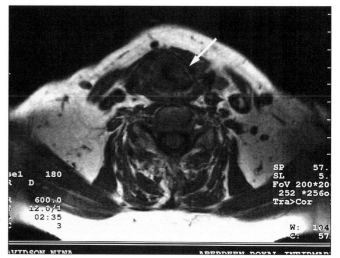

Fig. 9.50 *Axial T1-weighted MR image of the neck in laryngeal carcinoma. There is a soft-tissue mass arising from the left vocal cord, with invasion into the thyroid cartilage (arrow).*

chapter 10

Breast and Endocrine System

Part 1. Breast disease

The variety of acquired pathological conditions affecting the breast is extensive, with a consequently wide, but overlapping, spectrum of appearances on mammography, ultrasound, and MR imaging. The terminology of breast disease also has its own classification. The format here will therefore be to consider congenital abnormalities, but then to base the text on the differentiation of benign from malignant breast disease.

CONGENITAL ABNORMALITIES

Congenital absence of the breast can occur in Poland's syndrome, together with absence of the pectoralis major muscle and varying degrees of shoulder and upper limb abnormalities (**Fig. 10.1**). Supernumerary nipples are also congenital anomalies, as is the presence of breast tissue in the axilla.

BENIGN BREAST DISEASE

TRAUMA

Fat necrosis is believed to be traumatic in origin, but a positive history is found in only about 50% of cases. On mammography, there is a mass, often with calcification, that may be indistinguishable from that found in carcinoma. Traumatic fat necrosis is also seen after breast biopsy, breast surgery, radiation ischaemia, and fibrosis (**Fig. 10.2**).

Haematoma formation may occur after either surgical or accidental trauma. It is usually associated with bruising of the skin.

INFECTION

A patient presenting with a breast abscess is most likely to be a young woman who is lactating. A breast mass, pain, erythema, a retroareolar position, and other clinical features suggest the diagnosis, in which mammography is of little help. Ultrasound (**Fig. 10.3**) shows skin

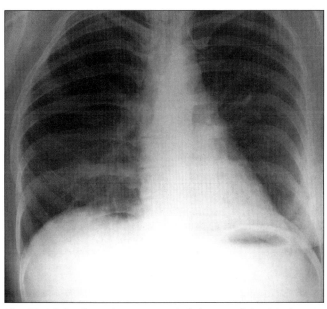

Fig. 10.1 *Poland's syndrome: congenital absence of the right breast and pectoralis major muscle.*

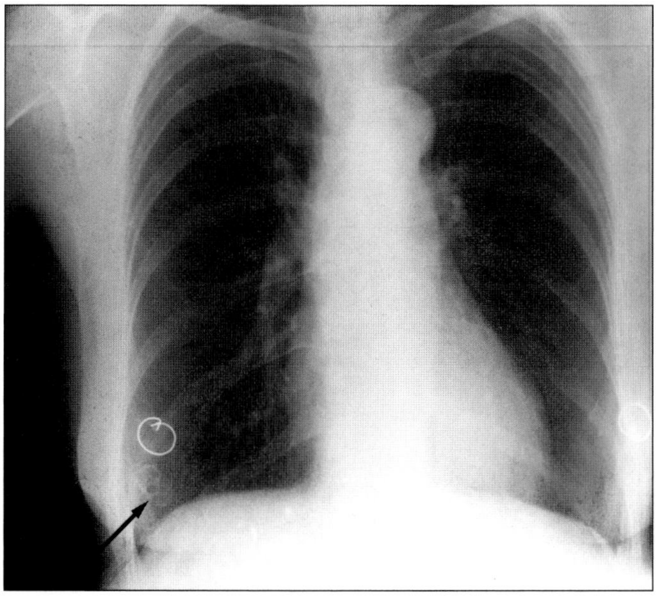

Fig. 10.2 *Chest radiograph showing a calcified lesion in the right breast, caused by fat necrosis (arrow). The radio-opaque circles are nipple markers.*

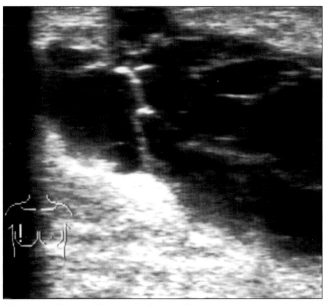

Fig. 10.3 *Ultrasound scan of a breast abscess, showing a multiloculated cavity that contained pus on aspiration.*

thickening, a cavity, and increased blood flow on colour Doppler imaging; it can be used both to determine the site of aspiration and to monitor treatment. *Staphylococcus* is the most common infective organism in these cases.

Other infective conditions may occur in older females, and show clinical evidence of fever, a high white cell count, and signs of local infection. If such infection (or inflammation) is slow to resolve, an underlying neoplasm should be suspected and mammography performed.

INFLAMMATORY CONDITIONS

Inflammatory disorders of the breast include periductal inflammatory disease, which can lead to duct ectasia (**Fig. 10.4**), an inflammatory response, and subsequent fibrosis. Mammography may show the characteristic linear calcifications along the ducts.

FIBROCYSTIC DISEASE

Fibrocystic disease represents a spectrum of benign disease ranging from predominantly fibrotic change to predominantly cystic change; it is a hormone-dependent condition that is most common in the perimenopausal period. Mammography is useful in this condition (**Fig. 10.5**), and ultrasound can be used to characterize the cystic component.

CYSTS

Cysts may also arise from areas of adenosis with duct and acinar dilatation. On mammography, they appear as round or oval, well-defined lesions, occasionally with a rim of calcification. On ultrasound, a confident diagnosis can be made if the cyst shows well-defined margins, a totally echo-free space, and a bright posterior wall—all features indicating a pure liquid-filled cystic lesion (**Fig. 10.6**). Cysts are most common in the perimenopausal period, and are often multiple and bilateral; they recur despite aspiration.

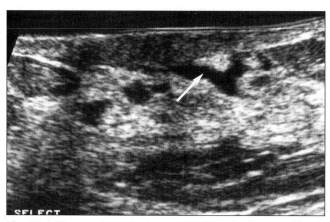

Fig. 10.4 *Ultrasound scan in duct ectasia (arrow). There are dilated hypoechoic channels deep to the nipple.*

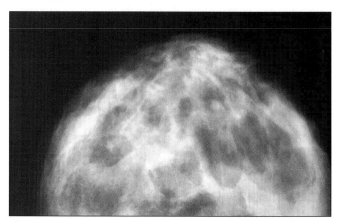

Fig. 10.5 *Craniocaudal mammogram in fibrocystic disease. The breast is of heterogeneous density.*

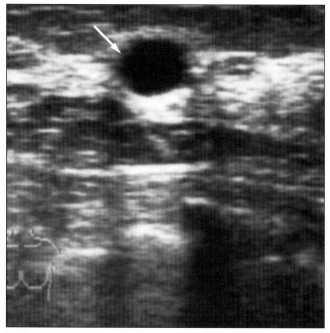

Fig. 10.6 *Ultrasound image of a breast cyst, showing the characteristic features of a round, echo-free lesion (arrow) with a bright posterior wall.*

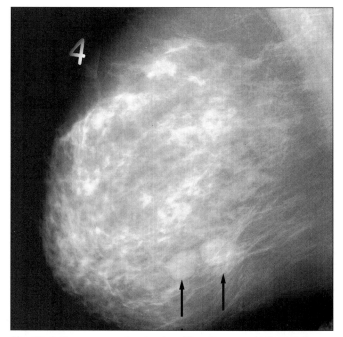

Fig. 10.7 *Mammogram showing two fibroadenomas in the inferior aspect of the breast (arrows).*

THE SPECTRUM OF FIBROADENOMA

Fibroadenomas are the most common benign breast tumours, usually found in the young breast; occasionally they are multiple and bilateral. On mammography, these tumours are often well-defined, round or oval, less than 3 cm in size (**Figs 10.7** and **10.8**), and may contain diagnostic eccentric, coarse calcifications. Because they are glandular in composition, they regress with age.

Cystosarcoma phylloides is a benign tumour, but 20% act locally as malignant; the distinction is made on histological criteria of cellularity. The mass is often large, has characteristics similar to those of fibroadenoma, and derives its name from the leaf-like projections of the tumours into the cystic spaces.

Giant fibroadenoma is another distinct entity in this spectrum of tumours.

PAPILLOMA

If extensive intraductal proliferation occurs in the breast, it causes a retroareolar papilloma. Although this can be shown on ductography, the technique has proved to have little influence on management, and is no longer performed routinely. A papilloma may be indistinguishable from an intraductal papillary carcinoma. Multiple intraductal papillomas can occur, giving rise to the condition of papillomatosis.

RADIAL SCAR

The complex sclerosing lesion known as a radial scar is now believed by some authorities to be a precursor of tubular carcinoma. On mammography, it may be confused with a stellate carcinoma (**Fig. 10.9**).

MALIGNANT BREAST DISEASE

PRIMARY BREAST CARCINOMA
Non-invasive tumours

Ductal carcinoma *in situ* is often associated with calcification, and may be therefore seen on mammography (**Fig. 10.10**). This non-invasive form is believed to progress to invasive intraductal carcinoma in 50–80% of cases.

Lobular carcinoma *in situ* has no specific mammographic appearances and is therefore a pathological diagnosis. The malignant potential of this tumour is less well understood.

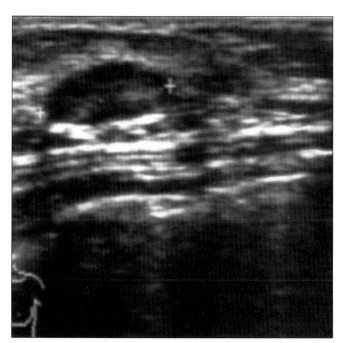

Fig. 10.8 *Ultrasound image of a fibroadenoma (crosses), showing a well-defined soft-tissue mass, with no posterior acoustic shadowing.*

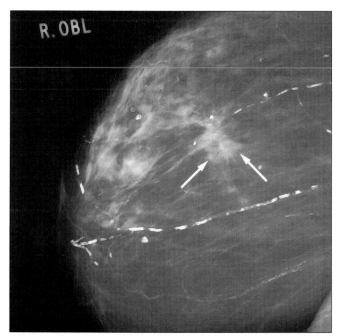

Fig. 10.9 *Mammogram showing a radial scar (arrows). There is a stellate lesion in the centre of the breast. Note also a superficial tumour with skin thickening and extensive benign vascular calcification.*

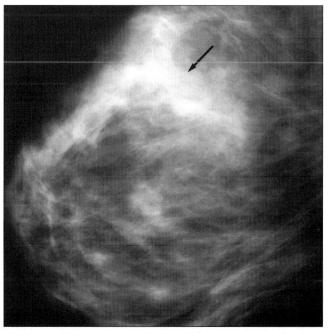

Fig. 10.10 *Mammogram showing a small focus of microcalcification (arrow) caused by ductal carcinoma in situ. This area was subsequently localized and excised.*

Invasive tumours

Invasive carcinomas are ductal, lobular, or special types such as tubular. The most common mammographic abnormality in breast carcinoma is a soft-tissue mass (**Fig. 10.11**), whereas on ultrasound a solid mass with posterior accoustic shadowing typifies the condition (**Fig. 10.12**). MR imaging is becoming increasingly used for certain indications in breast cancer (**Fig. 10.13**).

METASTASES TO THE BREAST

Tumours that metastasize to the breasts include melanoma and disseminated small-cell carcinoma.

MAMMOGRAPHIC APPEARANCES OF BREAST CALCIFICATION

The presence of certain types of microcalcifications is the most sensitive mammographic indicator for carcinoma. The two patterns seen predominantly in malignant tumours are rod-like shapes and a linear arrangement (**Fig. 10.14**); these appearances are attributable to the ductal origin of more than 90% of breast carcinomas. Clusters of calcifications are also seen in these carcinomas; however, they can occur in benign conditions such as fat necrosis, papillomatosis, and adenosis. Benign calcifications include 'eggshell' (**Fig. 10.15**), vascular, secretory, and coarse aggregations.

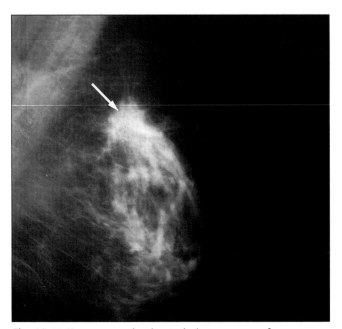

Fig. 10.11 *Mammogram showing typical appearances of a carcinoma. There is a dense spiculated lesion (arrow) in the upper aspect of the breast.*

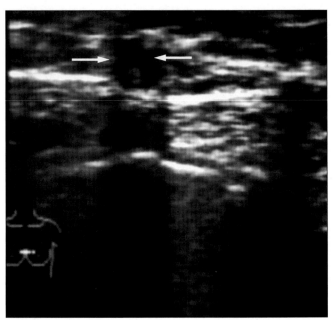

Fig. 10.12 *Ultrasound image of a small breast carcinoma, showing an echo-poor lesion (arrows), and typical posterior acoustic shadowing.*

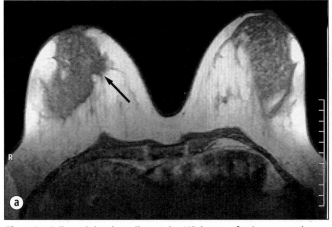
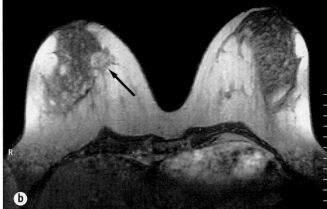

Fig. 10.13 *T1-weighted gradient echo MR image of a breast carcinoma (arrows) before (**a**) and after (**b**) gadolinium, showing typical enhancement.*

PROGNOSTIC INDICATORS FOR SURVIVAL IN PATIENTS WITH BREAST CARCINOMA

- **Tumour size at presentation:** the smaller the tumour, the better the prognosis, hence the importance of accurate measurements on mammography and ultrasound.
- **Tumour grade:** the grading of tumours as 1/2/3 is based on cytological mitotic features, and is therefore a pathological grading.
- **Axillary (locoregional) nodal status:** the role of imaging in assessing the state of axillary node involvement is experimental at this stage; both MR imaging (**Fig. 10.16**) and PET are being used.

BREAST SCREENING

In response to the findings of random controlled trials performed in America and Europe in the 1970s and 1980s, the United Kingdom has established a comprehensive National Breast Screening Programme. This is based on triennial, two-view prevalent and single-view incident screening in women older than 50 years of age.

In the USA, there is no national screening programme, but the recommendations by various National Cancer bodies are followed by many institutions, which run clinics for patients older than 40 years, with repeat cycles averaging 2–3 years.

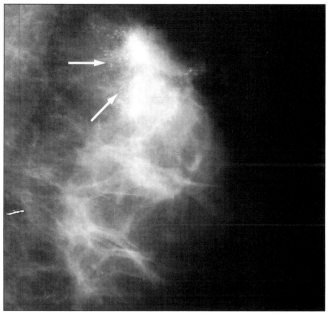

Fig. 10.14 Mammogram showing multiple small rod-like areas of malignant microcalcification associated with a soft-tissue mass. This was an invasive ductal carcinoma (arrows).

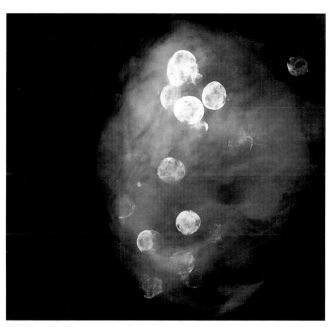

Fig. 10.15 Mammogram showing extensive benign 'eggshell' calcification.

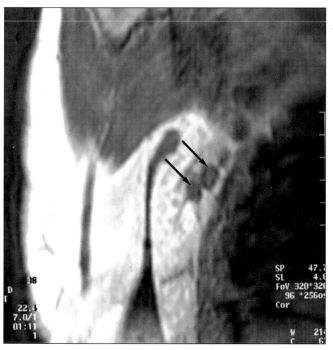

Fig. 10.16 Coronal T1-weighted MR image of the right axilla, showing several enlarged lymph nodes (arrows).

RADIOLOGICAL MANAGEMENT OF FAMILIAL BREAST CARCINOMA

A small proportion (<5%) of breast cancers are known to be familial; to date, two genes linked to breast cancer have been isolated. Medical geneticists are able to calculate relative risk (of developing breast cancer) estimates based on detailed family history; screening for breast cancer in women with a >20% relative risk is now available in some centres. Mammography is the only imaging modality currently used widely (Fig. 10.17); MR mammography may have a role in the future, although this is not yet established.

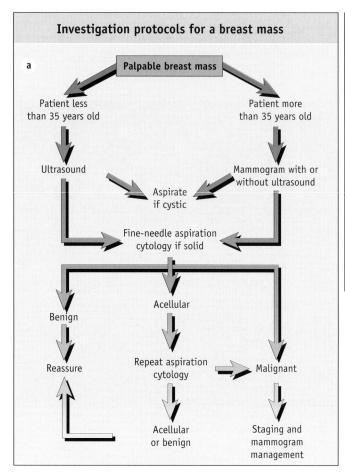

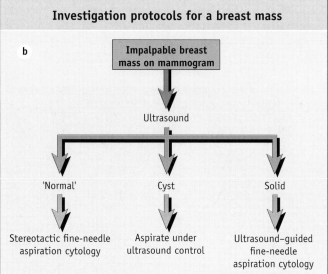

Fig. 10.17 *Investigation protocols for a breast mass.* **(a)** *Palpable breast mass.* **(b)** *Impalpable breast mass on mammography.*

Part 2. Endocrine disorders

PITUITARY GLAND

PROLACTIN

A prolactinoma is the most common actively secreting tumour of the pituitary, causing amenorrhoea and galactorrhoea in females, and impotence and infertility in males. Most prolactinomas are microadenomas, do not cause any enlargement to the pituitary fossa, and are diagnosed by appropriate MR appearances (*see* Fig. 8.47) in conjunction with hyperprolactinaemia.

GROWTH HORMONE

Some of the bony and soft-tissue features of the acromegaly caused by overproduction of growth hormone are described in Chapter 7 (*see* page 171). Other symptoms and signs include hypertension and cardiomegaly, kyphosis, degenerative arthritis, abdominal pain, and hernia formation. There is also an increased risk of associated intracranial aneurysms. The pituitary fossa is enlarged in 80–90% of patients with this tumour (**Fig. 10.18**); as in all forms of pituitary abnormality, gadolinium-enhanced MR offers the best imaging.

ADRENOCORTICOTROPHIC HORMONE

An adenoma of the anterior pituitary gland producing adrenocorticotrophic hormone (ACTH) is one cause of Cushing's syndrome, which comprises hypertension, muscle wasting and weakness, osteoporosis, and abnormal central fat distribution. Ninety per cent of these tumours are microadenomas, often less than 3 mm in size; they can be demonstrated by gadolinium-enhanced MR imaging.

Ectopic production of ACTH is a much more common condition, and is often caused by rapidly growing tumours such as oat-cell lung carcinoma.

NON-FUNCTIONING PITUITARY ADENOMAS

Most non-functioning pituitary adenomas are macroadenomas that present because of compression of adjacent structures, with visual-field defects (typically bitemporal hemianopia), cranial nerve palsies, and increased intracranial pressure (Fig. 10.19). Haemorrhage into or infarction of a pituitary macroadenoma can present as a clinical emergency (pituitary apoplexy), with sudden loss of vision, headache, meningism, and loss of consciousness.

Pituitary adenomas occasionally form part of the multiple endocrine neoplasia syndrome that consists of endocrine pancreatic tumours and parathyroid abnormalities.

ADRENAL CORTEX

GLUCOCORTICOID EXCESS

Cushing's syndrome (hypertension, muscle wasting and weakness, osteoporosis, and abnormal distribution of central fat) may be caused by a pituitary tumour (*see* page 228), or by primary disease of the adrenal cortex, including tumours and hyperplasia, that results in a glucocorticoid excess. Radiological investigation is primarily by CT, which can differentiate hyperplasia from a tumour (Fig. 10.20).

GLUCOCORTICOID DEFICIENCY

Addison's disease results from significant reduction in adrenocortical function. Causes include infection with tuberculosis (Fig. 10.21) and histoplasmosis, haemorrhage, and malignant metastatic tumours, or—the most common cause now encountered—may be idiopathic. Examination of the adrenal glands may reveal the aetiology, but in the idiopathic form there is disappointingly often little to find, with apparently normal-sized glands being present.

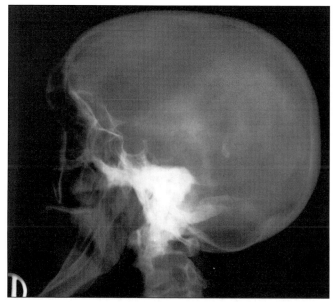

Fig. 10.18 *Lateral skull radiograph in acromegaly. Note the enlargement of the pituitary fossa, the mandible, and the frontal sinuses.*

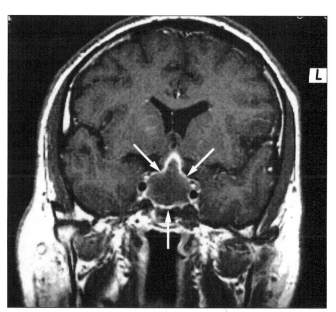

Fig. 10.19 *T1-weighted coronal MR image, after gadolinium, of an infarcted pituitary macroadenoma. There is a large mass expanding the pituitary fossa and extending into the supersellar region, compressing the optic chiasm. The tumour has a dark centre and peripheral enhancement (arrows). This patient presented with pituitary apoplexy.*

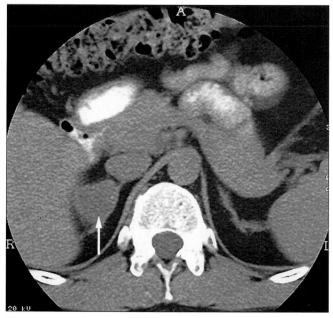

Fig. 10.20 *CT of a right adrenal tumour (arrow).*

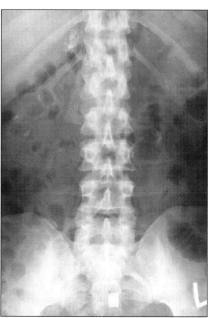

Fig. 10.21 *Plain abdominal radiograph in Addison's disease caused by tuberculosis, showing bilateral adrenal calcification. The patient also has multiple renal calculi.*

MINERALOCORTICOID EXCESS

Conn's syndrome is caused by a unilateral adenoma in the majority of cases, or by bilateral adrenal nodular hyperplasia, either of which results in mineralocorticoid excess. The adenomas are usually small; CT or MR is the imaging investigation of choice (**Fig. 10.22**).

NON-FUNCTIONING ADENOMAS

With the advent of routine CT scanning of the chest and abdomen, the considerable prevalence of adrenal adenomas, familiar in autopsies, has now become readily apparent. Most of these adenomas are small and well defined, and have a low attenuation value because of their tissue constitution. The presence of large lesions (greater than 3 cm) with higher attenuation values suggests either primary or, more commonly, secondary malignancy.

ADRENAL MEDULLA

PHAEOCHROMOCYTOMA

The majority of phaeochromocytomas develop in the adrenal medualla (**Fig. 10.23**), but they may arise outside, in the sympathetic chain. The '10% rule' is useful to remember with these tumours: 10% are bilateral, 10% are ectopic, and 10% are malignant. They are associated with the multiple endocrine neoplasia II syndrome, neurofibromatosis, and von Hippel–Lindau syndrome. The tumour is often several centimetres in size, has soft-tissue attenuation on CT, and is often quite vascular (**Fig. 10.24**).

Metaiodobenzylguanidine (MIBG) is the radiopharmaceutical of choice for demonstrating the sites of phaeochromocytomas in nuclear medicine scanning. These tumours should not be subjected to biopsy, because of the possibility of precipitating a hypertensive crisis.

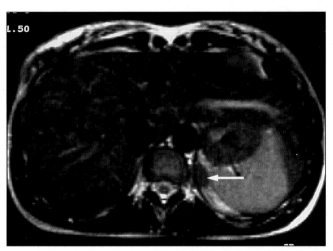

Fig. 10.22 *Axial T2-weighted MR image of the upper abdomen, showing a small left adrenal adenoma (arrow) which was causing Conn's syndrome.*

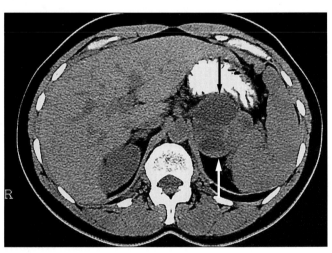

Fig. 10.23 *CT of a phaeochromocytoma of the left adrenal (arrows).*

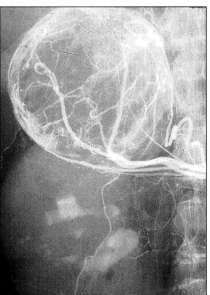

Fig. 10.24 *Right adrenal arteriogram, showing a highly vascular phaeochromocytoma.*

Phaeochromocytomas represent one form of *Amine Precursor Uptake* and *Decarboxylation* (APUD) tumour; other tumours in the group comprise carcinoid tumour, islet-cell carcinoma, neuroblastoma, medullary thyroid carcinoma, chemodectoma, and melanoma. All are highly differentiated neuroendocrine tumours.

THYROID

CARCINOMA

Carcinomas of the thyroid develop either from follicular cells (epithelium) of papillary, follicular, and anaplastic histological type (in order of prevalence), or from parafollicular cells—the medullary carcinoma. In most patients, a mass in the thyroid that is suspected to be malignant should be examined by fine-needle aspiration cytology as the initial investigation. CT and MR imaging can be used for assessment of the primary lesion and for obtaining evidence of local or distant spread (**Fig. 10.25**).

PANCREAS

Endocrine tumours of the pancreas are considered in Chapter 4.

DIABETES MELLITUS

The radiological features of the common disease, diabetes mellitus, reflect its neurological and vascular complications. Atherosclerosis is more extensive and occurs earlier in patients with diabetes mellitus than in non-diabetics; it is often seen as incidental arterial calcification in the hands and feet. The peripheral neuropathy may cause foot ulcers, tarsal fractures, and Charcot's joints (**Fig. 10.26**). Other associations with diabetes mellitus include emphysematous cholecystitis and emphysematous pyelonephritis (*see* Fig. 5.28), in which gas-producing organisms flourish as a result of the abnormal glucose metabolism and the impaired white-cell function.

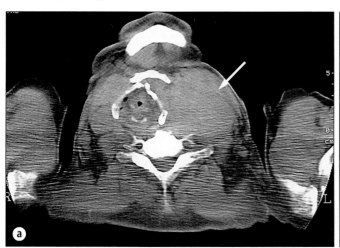
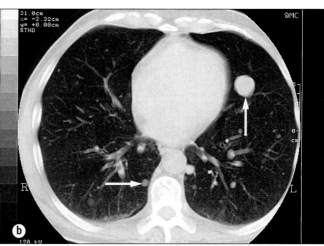

Fig. 10.25 CT in thyroid carcinoma. **(a)** The large mass in the left side of the thyroid gland (arrow) represents the primary tumour. **(b)** Multiple pulmonary metastases (arrows) in the same patient.

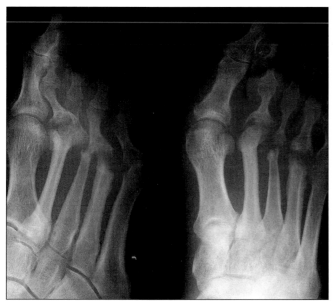

Fig. 10.26 Radiograph of the foot in a patient with diabetic peripheral neuropathy. There are Charcot's joints at the metatarsophalangeal joints, with joint disorganization and destruction of the articular surfaces.

Diabetes mellitus occurs in association with the Prader–Willi syndrome (obesity, mental retardation, and gonadal dysfunction) and is sometimes seen in patients with the Laurence–Moon–Biedl syndrome (polydactyly, retinitis pigmentosa, mental retardation, and genitourinary anomalies).

GONADAL DYSGENESIS

TURNER'S SYNDROME

Turner's syndrome is the name describing the female condition of 45 XO chromosomes. It is characterized by multiple skeletal and connective-tissue anomalies, including craniofacial abnormalities, coarctation of the aorta, abnormal carrying angle of the elbows, short fourth metacarpals and metatarsals (**Fig. 10.27**), and webbing of the neck.

NOONAN'S SYNDROME

Noonan's syndrome is an autosomal dominant abnormality of males and females, who have a webbed neck, short stature, and pulmonary stenosis.

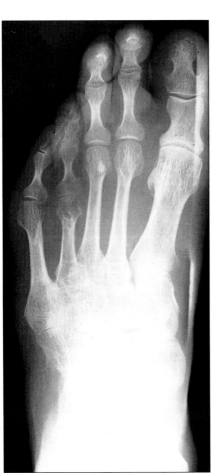

Fig. 10.27 *Radiograph of the foot in Turner's syndrome, showing shortening of the fourth metatarsal.*

GASTROINTESTINAL TRACT

CARCINOID TUMOURS AND THE CARCINOID SYNDROME

Ninety per cent of the neuroendocrine carcinoid tumours arise in the gut, most commonly in the ileocaecal region; the remainder originate in the pancreas or lung. Gut carcinoids may bleed, cause pain, or be sites for obstruction and intussusception. They are locally invasive, but metastatic spread is rare unless the primary origin is the small intestine or the lung, when liver (*see* Chapter 3) and bone are the predominant sites for spread.

The carcinoid syndrome is caused by the production of excess hormones from cell types similar to adrenal medullary cells, resulting in the classical triad of skin flushing, diarrhoea, and right-sided cardiac valve lesions. About 50% of patients with small bowel carcinoid tumours exhibit the syndrome, whereas it is rare when the lung or appendix are the primary sites.

chapter 11

Appendix

PRINCIPLES OF RADIOLOGICAL INVESTIGATION

RADIATION RISKS

In the United Kingdom, the 1988 Ionizing Radiation Regulations dictate good radiological practice and state the statutory aspects of the use of ionizing radiation. It should be remembered that all ionizing radiations, such as X-rays or those from radionuclides, have a potential for harm, even in small doses. The effective dose equivalent of some radiological techniques such as computed tomography (CT) and interventional procedures may be considerable. For example, the dose of radiation from a chest radiograph is low, being the equivalent of 3 days of background radiation; the dose from a CT scan of the chest and abdomen may be as much as 450 times that of a chest radiograph—that is, equivalent to about 4 years of natural background radiation. Thus proposed use of high-dosage radiation procedures should be considered carefully by senior staff, to ensure that the benefit to the patient outweighs the potential risks. Whenever possible, non-ionizing radiation techniques such as ultrasound and MR should be used.

In the United Kingdom, National Guidelines *Making the Best Use of a Department of Clinical Radiology* have been produced by the Royal College of Radiologists, and are of considerable value in advising clinicians on appropriate imaging strategies.

CONSENT

Informed consent is an ever increasing area of concern to patients and their doctors. Many invasive diagnostic and therapeutic procedures potentially have significant complications of which the patient should be aware, so that rational decisions can be made after full discussion. Any investigation that has known complications, and those tests that require local or general anaesthesia, require a consent form to be signed by the patient after the clinician or the radiologist has explained the procedure fully. Depending on the procedure (for example a barium enema in a patient with a prosthetic heart valve), antibiotic prophylaxis may be required, and care must then be taken to ascertain any previous antibiotic allergy.

RADIOLOGICAL TECHNIQUES

PLAIN FILM RADIOGRAPHY

X-rays are man-made ionizing radiation and are produced in an X-ray tube when electrons are accelerated across a vacuum. They are of high frequency and short wavelength, identical to the gamma-radiation that occurs in radionuclide decay. A radiograph is produced when X-rays pass from the X-ray tube through part of a patient onto photographic film. The film emulsion contains silver halide crystals that are blackened by any X-rays reaching the film. Bone absorbs X-rays to a much greater extent than, for example, lung tissue; thus bones appear white on a radiograph, while the lungs are dark because the radiation passes through the lung tissue and blackens the film. Image detectors other than film include image intensifiers and digital detectors, which convey the image to a television monitor.

X-ray mammography is a specific type of plain film radiography that uses low-kilovoltage X-rays and high-resolution film to maximize detection of subtle soft-tissue abnormalities in the breast.

CONTRAST MEDIA

Contrast radiography is a modification of the basic plain radiographic technique. The part of the body of interest is opacified, using a contrast medium. Contrast media contain either barium or iodine, both of which have a high atomic number and, therefore, block X-rays to a greater extent than do soft tissues. Structures containing contrast are thus rendered opaque on the radiograph.

Intravascular contrast agents

The basic constituent of intravascular contrast agents is iodine. Allergic reactions are the most important complications of these agents, and may vary in degree from mild urticaria to acute anaphylaxis. The treatment of complications depends on their severity and includes antihistamines, oxygen, steroids, and adrenaline. There are occasional fatalities when iodinated contrast agents are used, and all procedures using these compounds should be undertaken with full resuscitation equipment available nearby.

Severe anaphylaxis to these agents may present with cardiovascular collapse, bronchospasm, angio-oedema, or pulmonary oedema, or any combination thereof. Treatment comprises 100% oxygen and airway maintenance, 1:10 000 adrenaline intravenously (carefully!), and plasma volume expanders. These measures may be followed by use of antihistamines and intravenous steroids as appropriate.

Barium compounds

Barium suspensions of various consistencies are used in the investigation of gastrointestinal disorders. The compounds are chemically inactive, but complications can arise when barium products enter certain compartments or organs. For example, perforation of the large bowel during a barium enema may cause barium peritonitis, which carries a 50% risk of fatality.

BARIUM STUDIES

Barium examinations of the gastrointestinal tract utilize a double-contrast technique. A small amount of barium is given to coat the mucosa of the relevant viscus, then a second agent, usually a gas, is given to distend the viscus. In the oesophagus, stomach, and duodenum, an oral effervescent agent is given that releases carbon dioxide to provide double contrast. In a small bowel enema, water or methyl cellulose is injected down an orojejunal tube to distend the small bowel. For barium enema examination of the large bowel, air is pumped into the bowel through a rectal catheter, making identification of small mucosal abnormalities easier.

Careful preparation of the patient is essential. For a barium meal examination of the stomach and duodenum, the patient must have fasted for at least 6 hours. A barium enema requires a clean colon, otherwise faecal residue may be confused with polyps or tumour. Standard preparation comprises two sachets of sodium picosulphate (a powerful laxative) on the day before the examination. Both fasting and laxatives are required before a small-bowel enema.

Water-soluble (iodinated) contrast studies have specific indications in the gastrointestinal tract. If there is a risk of perforation, for example in large bowel obstruction, a single-contrast enema using iodinated contrast can identify the site of obstruction. Water-soluble contrast is used in the upper gastrointestinal tract in postoperative patients or, occasionally, to identify the site of a perforation. However, some water-soluble contrast media are hyperosmolar and should not be used in patients in whom there is a risk of aspiration, or in infants in whom there is a risk of dehydration. Non-ionic, iso-osmolar contrast media are available for use in those groups.

INTRAVENOUS UROGRAPHY

Iodinated contrast is excreted by the kidneys and is used commonly to opacify the urinary tract. Clinical indications are frank haematuria and renal colic. No specific preparation of the patient is required.

BILIARY STUDIES

The biliary tree can be opacified in several ways. Oral cholecystography and intravenous cholangiography are techniques that are now seldom performed. Injection of iodinated contrast, via an endoscope or via a transhepatic needle, is used in the investigation of obstructive jaundice. Endoscopic retrograde choledochopancreatography (ERCP) involves cannulating the ampulla of Vater from a side-viewing endoscope and injecting contrast, to outline the biliary and pancreatic ducts; interventions such as sphincterotomy and gall stone extraction are possible. Percutaneous transhepatic cholangiography (PTC) is performed by inserting a long, fine needle through the lateral abdominal wall into the liver until a small bile duct is cannulated. This procedure is indicated when it is not possible to cannulate the bile duct at ERCP, to show dilated bile ducts proximal to an obstructing lesion. A biliary drain or stent can be inserted to relieve obstruction.

ANGIOGRAPHY

Access to the arterial system in order to produce an arteriogram (angiogram) is usually obtained by puncture and catheterization of the common femoral artery under local anaesthesia. Radiographic contrast medium is then injected into the vessel in the area under examination, by manipulating the catheter into the relevant artery. If, for some reason, access via the femoral artery is not possible (e.g. because of iliac occlusive disease or the presence of a graft), alternative sites, such as the brachial or axillary artery, can be used. Angling the radiographic equipment in relation to the patient helps to visualize oblique or tortuous arteries.

All angiographic images are now produced by a digital subtraction technique. Images obtained before any contrast is injected are stored in the computer memory and subsequently subtracted from later images obtained with contrast in the arteries; this leaves an image of the arteries only, with background tissues subtracted. If contrast is injected intra-arterially, the technique is termed 'intra-arterial digital subtraction angiography' (IADSA).

Images of arteries can also be obtained after contrast is injected into a central vein or the right atrium. Such intravenous digital subtraction angiograms (IVDSAs) have poorer contrast than IADSAs, but can be useful in patients with no arterial access.

When the angiographic procedure is finished and the catheter withdrawn from the artery, pressure must be applied for several minutes to ensure haemostasis. All patients should be monitored after femoral artery catheterization. Complications of arterial puncture include bleeding, local haematoma, false aneurysm formation, arterial dissection, and distal embolization. The complication rate is influenced by the size of catheter used, the age of the patient, obesity, and any underlying bleeding tendency. Specialized nursing care in the period immediately after the investigation is important.

VENOGRAPHY

Veins may be visualized in the same way as the arteries, by direct puncture and catheterization. The veins in the upper and lower limbs are imaged by injecting contrast medium via a needle placed in a peripheral vein, such as in the dorsum of the foot or hand, or the antecubital fossa. Alternatively, if imaging from an arterial injection is continued over a prolonged period of time, the arterial, capillary, and venous phases can be recorded and venous anatomy visualized; this is a particularly useful way of visualizing the portal venous system without necessitating direct trans-splenic or transhepatic puncture.

Any patient undergoing an invasive procedure, particularly one involving the use of cutting-needle biopsies for histology or PTC, should have coagulation studies performed to establish if their haemostatic mechanisms are intact. Patients receiving anticoagulation treatment may need to have that treatment withdrawn before undergoing invasive procedures, and special care must be taken in patients who have blood dyscrasias such as leukaemia and thrombocytopenia, who may need fresh frozen plasma or platelet transfusion, as appropriate, before the procedure.

COMPUTED TOMOGRAPHY

The limitation of all plain radiographic techniques is their two-dimensional representation of three-dimensional structures: the linear attenuation coefficients of all of the tissues in the path of the X-ray beam form the image.

Computed tomography (CT) obtains a series of different angular projections of X-rays that are processed by a computer to give a section of specified thickness. The CT image is made up of a regular matrix of small squares termed picture elements (pixels). All the tissues contained within a pixel attenuate the X-ray projections, producing a mean attenuation value for the pixel; this value is compared with the attenuation value of water and is displayed on a scale (the Hounsfield scale) that ranges from −1000 to +1000 Hounsfield units (HU). On the Hounsfield scale, water is arbitrarily assigned an attenuation of 0 HU; air typically has an HU number of −1000, fat is approximately −100 HU, soft tissues are in the range +20 to +70 HU, and bone is greater than +400 HU.

The CT machine consists of a rigid metal frame (the gantry) with an X-ray tube sited opposite a set of detectors. Modern CT machines have a wide detector array and an X-ray fan beam, which encompasses all of the patient's body. The tube and detectors rotate around the patient. Routine acquisition times per slice are 1–4 seconds; newer, spiral scanners have subsecond scan times.

All CT machines, of whatever generation, share similar components. The detectors are gas ionization chambers, scintillation crystals, or ceramic detectors linked to photomultiplier tubes. The signal is digitized by an analog-to-digital converter in the gantry. The digitized signal is transferred to the image processing computer and is subsequently displayed on the operator's console. Images are usually photographed on film (hard copy), using optical or laser cameras. For long-term storage, the data set is transferred to magnetic media (tape or disk), or to optical disk.

No specific preparation of the patient is required for examinations of the brain, spine, musculoskeletal system, and chest. Studies of the abdomen and pelvis almost always require opacification of the gastrointestinal tract, using a solution of dilute contrast medium (either water-soluble or a barium compound). The large bowel may also be opacified using a solution of contrast medium administered rectally, either in a preparation room or when the patient is on the CT table. Examinations of the female pelvis are often performed after the insertion of a vaginal tampon, to facilitate interpretation. Identification of vascular structures may be made on the basis of anatomy alone, but the intravenous injection of water-soluble contrast medium improves visualization of vessels and vascular lesions.

Generally, CT studies are performed with the patient supine, and images are obtained in the transverse (axial) plane. Modern CT machines allow up to 25° of gantry angulation, which is particularly valuable in spinal imaging. Occasionally, coronal images are obtained in the investigation of facial abnormalities.

MAGNETIC RESONANCE IMAGING

Magnetic resonance (MR) imaging combines a strong magnetic field and radiofrequency (RF) energy to study the distribution and behaviour of hydrogen protons in fat and water.

The spinning proton of the hydrogen nucleus can be thought of as a tiny bar magnet, with a north and a south pole. In the absence of an external magnetic field, the magnetic moments of all the protons in the body are randomly arranged. However, when the patient is placed in a strong magnetic field, these magnetic moments align either with or against the field lines of the magnet. A small excess of magnetic moments align with the field, so that a net magnetic vector is established.

RF energy is used to rotate or 'flip' the protons in the static magnetic field. When the RF field is switched off, the protons experience only the effects of the static magnetic field, and flip back to their original position. During this return to equilibrium—a process called 'relaxation'—protons emit a small RF signal. This energy is detected by the antenna in the MRI machine, digitized, amplified and, finally, spatially encoded. The resulting images are displayed on the operator's console and can be recorded on hard copy (for viewing) or transferred to optical disk (for storage).

MR imaging systems are graded according to the strength of the magnetic field they produce. High-field systems are those capable of producing a magnetic field strength of 1–2 Tesla (T), mid-field systems operate at 0.35–0.5 T, and low-field systems produce a field strength of less than 0.2 T. Mid- and high-field systems use superconducting magnets in which the coils of copper wire are kept in a super-conducting state (−269°) by being immersed in a liquid helium bath. Electromagnets are fitted in resistive systems and are limited by heat factors to 0.35 T. Low-field systems use permanently magnetized metal cores, limiting field strength to around 0.2 T.

MR imaging is not associated with any recognized biological hazard. Patients who have any form of pacemaker or implanted electroinductive device must not be examined. Other contra-indications to use of the technique include the presence of ferro-magnetic intracranial aneurysm clips, certain types of cardiac valve prostheses, and intraocular metallic foreign bodies. Generally, it is safe to examine patients who have extracranial vascular clips and orthopaedic prostheses, but these may cause local artefacts. Loose metal items must be excluded from the examination room.

The preparation for an MR examination is simple. Patients wear metal-free clothes and must answer a rigorous safety questionnaire. Antiperistaltic agents (e.g. intravenous hyoscine N-butylbromide or glucagon) are often used in abdominal and pelvic examinations. Software techniques are used to counteract respiratory motion in chest and abdominal imaging. Electrocardiogaphic gating is used in cardiac studies.

MR images may be obtained in any plane. There is a wide range of pulse sequences, each of which provides a different image contrast. An intravenous injection of contrast medium (a gadolinium complex) may be given to enhance the visualization of tumours and inflammatory and vascular abnormalities.

Magnetic resonance angiography

The appearance of blood vessels depends on the pulse sequence used to produce images. With the spin echo technique, the time that elapses between exciting protons and receiving the return signal (the echo time) is such that excited blood has flowed out of the region; this volume of blood is replaced by unexcited blood, which does not produce a signal, resulting in a black vessel in the image (termed a flow void).

Gradient echo sequences use short echo times and more frequent RF excitations, so that protons in stationary tissues do not relax fully, reducing the signal they generate. However, protons entering the slice are fully relaxed and thus produce a high signal (the 'time of flight effect'), so that blood vessels appear as bright structures against a dark background. Images can be displayed as three-dimensional MR angiograms, which can be viewed from any angle.

Another MR angiography technique uses additional magnetic fields to encode the phase of moving protons in blood vessels. A complete assessment of flow requires three acquisitions, each encoded by one of the three orthogonal gradients. These are summed to produce a 'phase contrast' MR angiogram. Phase differences can be quantified to provide estimates of flow velocity.

ULTRASOUND

In contrast with the other imaging modalities referred to in this book, ultrasound does not depend on the use of electromagnetic wave forms. It involves non-ionizing radiation, making it an ideal technique for imaging pregnant women and children.

A sound wave of appropriate frequency (diagnostic range 3.5–10 MHz) is produced by piezoelectric crystals. Both the size and shape of the emitting crystal and its resonant frequency are important factors in determining the course of the sound beam within the tissues to be examined. As the sound beam passes through tissues, two important effects determine image production: attenuation and reflection. Attenuation is caused by the loss of energy from the system, as a result of absorption and reflection, refraction, and beam diver-gence out of the range of the receiver. The greater the attenuation of the sound beam through the tissues, the lower the resultant signal intensity received. Reflection of sound waves within the range of the receiver produces the image, the texture of which is dependent upon differences in acoustic impedance between different tissues. Ultrasound imaging systems are sensitive to the very small changes in acoustic impedance within soft tissue.

Through the application of these basic principles, sophisticated hardware has been developed that converts the pulse echo system, described briefly above, into a real-time two-dimensional sectional image. The addition of the facility to measure blood flow and velocity ultrasonically (using the Doppler principle) has led to the develop-ment of duplex scanners.

The effects of shadowing and enhancement within an ultrasound image are of paramount importance. Systems are designed assuming an average attenuation through a depth of tissue, and are balanced to give an even intensity of signal for deep and superficial tissues. An acoustic shadow occurs when a tissue within the measured depth has a higher than average attenuation; all tissues deep to this will appear with a falsely lower intensity (shadowed). Conversely, a tissue with a lower than average attenuation will cause all tissues deep to it to appear falsely high in intensity (enhanced). Fibrous tissue, calcification, and gas all produce acoustic shadows, whereas fluid-filled structures often cause enhancement.

If a selection of ultrasound transducers with varying frequencies, focusing mechanisms, shapes, and sizes is available, visualization of a wide range of tissues—from neonatal brain to the soft tissues of the hand—becomes possible. Interpretation of the pathology from static ultrasound images is more difficult than that from other imaging modalities, because the technique is highly operator-dependent and provides information on tissue structure and form different from that of other imaging techniques.

Ultrasound of the upper abdomen requires the patient to fast for 6 hours, so that the stomach is empty and the gall bladder full. Pelvic ultrasound is performed with the patient's bladder full, so that gas-containing bowel is displaced and the bladder acts as an acoustic window. Alternatively, in female patients, transvaginal ultrasound gives better resolution of the uterus and ovaries. Transrectal and transoesophageal ultrasound probes are also available for specific indications.

NUCLEAR MEDICINE

Technetium-99m is the radionuclide that is used in the majority of nuclear medicine investigations, because it has certain useful properties. It has a short half-life of 6 hours, emits a gamma-ray at a suitable imaging energy of 140 keV, can be produced simply from a generator, and can be attached to a wide variety of pharmaceutical agents. The radiopharmaceutical agent is usually administered intravenously, and gamma-camera imaging is then performed at appropriate times according to the organ being investigated. Dynamic imaging of the blood flow to the heart, brain, or kidneys is by the rapid acquisition of a series of blood-pool images. In cardiac studies, electrocardiographic gating is used to show changes related to the cardiac cycle. Static imaging allows the particular radiopharmaceutical agent used to accumulate in the organ under investigation, for example bones, thyroid or liver. Images produced in nuclear medicine studies are of lower resolution than most other imaging modalities, but have the advantage of providing functional information that can be quantified, for example to show differential renal function. There are statutory regulations relating to the use, handling, and disposal of radionuclides, and advice on patient care and radionuclide dosages is widely available.

Single photon emission computed tomography imaging

Single Photon Emission Computed Tomography (SPECT) is a technique used to improve resolution, either as sectional images or by three-dimensional reconstruction. Brain imaging and thallium studies of the myocardium are two investigations in which use of SPECT has improved the definition of disease.

Positron emission tomography imaging

Positron Emission Tomography (PET) uses cyclotron-generated, short-lived, positron-emitting radionuclides such as ^{11}C, ^{13}N, and ^{18}F. ^{18}F can be used to label deoxyglucose, forming ^{18}F-deoxyglucose, which has applications in assessment of primary and metastatic tumours.

Index

3